P9-CAO-346

THE PRACTICAL MANAGEMENT OF SPASTICITY IN CHILDREN AND ADULTS

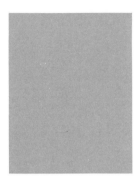

MEL B. GLENN, M.D.

Associate Professor, Department of Rehabilitation Medicine
Tufts University School of Medicine
Boston, Massachusetts

Director, Brain Injury Unit
New England Sinai Hospital
Stoughton, Massachusetts

Director of Rehabilitation Medicine
Greenery Rehabilitation and Skilled Nursing Center
Boston, Massachusetts

JOHN WHYTE, M.D., Ph.D.

Director of Brain Injury Research
Drucker Brain Injury Center
Moss Rehabilitation Hospital
Philadelphia, Pennsylvania

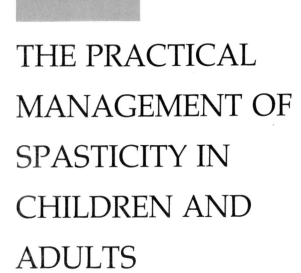

THE PRACTICAL MANAGEMENT OF SPASTICITY IN CHILDREN AND ADULTS

LEA & FEBIGER

1 9 9 0

Philadelphia · London

Lea & Febiger
200 Chester Field Parkway
Malvern, PA 19355
U.S.A.
1-800-444-1785

Lea & Febiger (UK) Ltd.
145a Croydon Road
Beckenham, Kent BR3 3RB
U.K.

Library of Congress Cataloging-in-Publication Data

The Practical management of spasticity in children and adults /
    [edited by] Mel B. Glenn, John Whyte.
        p.   cm.
    ISBN 0-8121-1297-0
    1. Spasticity.   I. Glenn, Mel B.   II. Whyte, John, 1953–
    [DNLM: 1. Muscle Spasticity—rehabilitation.   WE 550 P895]
RC935.S64P73   1990
616.7′44—dc20
DNLM/DLC
for Library of Congress   89-13414
                                                              CIP

Printed in the United States of America

Print Number 5   4   3   2   1

DEDICATION

To our loved ones:
Judith Ashway,
Daniel Glenn,
Hannah Glenn,
and
Tom Wilson Weinberg

PREFACE

Spasticity is one of the most common problems confronting rehabilitation professionals. It is also one of the most challenging. Despite the difficulties it creates and the frequency with which it is encountered, our understanding of this syndrome remains limited. While research continues to bring us closer to a full explanation of this syndrome and our ability to influence it, it is incumbent on those who work in rehabilitation to be aware of the full spectrum of treatments available and the state of the art in each discipline. In this way we may avoid working in isolation from one another, first as team members and also as a field in which one form of treatment may be better developed than another in any given locality.

Thus the title of this book is *The Practical Management of Spasticity in Children and Adults.* Although the neurophysiology of spasticity is addressed, our emphasis is on evaluation and treatment approaches. The final two chapters of the book demonstrate the practical application and integration of interventions through case examples.

The idea for this book grew out of a course of the same title given by the Department of Rehabilitation Medicine at Tufts University School of Medicine and New England Medical Center Hospitals. The interest generated by the course led us to the conclusion that there was a gap between the energy being put into attempts to work with spasticity in rehabilitation patients and the dissemination of information on this subject. This book represents a further attempt to improve communication on this most intriguing phenomenon.

During the writing of this book, we were confronted with the untimely deaths of David Kasdon, M.D. and Kamal Labib, M.D., both of whom have inspired many of us with their teaching on this and other subjects. We are fortunate to have Dr. Kasdon's work among the chapters of this book. Although his direct contribution was not possible, Dr. Labib's influence is represented nonetheless by contributors who worked with him. In particular, one of the editors (M.B.G.) must acknowledge the influence of Dr. Labib's clinical judgment, technical expertise, and teaching skills on the chapter entitled "Nerve Blocks."

The editors wish to thank the contributors for their hard work and perseverance in the face of innumerable other events designed to distract them. In addition, we wish to thank John Groton, Graphic Designer for the Research and Training Center on Rehabilitation and Childhood Trauma, Tufts University School of Medicine and New England Medical Center Hospitals, for the excellent artwork throughout the book.

Boston, Massachusetts   *Mel B. Glenn, M.D.*
Philadelphia, Pennsylvania   *John Whyte, M.D., Ph.D.*

vii

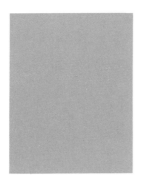

CONTRIBUTORS

JOEL N. ABRAMOVITZ, M.D.
Assistant Professor, Department of
    Neurosurgery, Tufts University School of
    Medicine, Boston, Massachusetts
Chief of Neurosurgery, Veterans
    Administration Medical Center, Boston,
    Massachusetts
Acting Chief of Neurosurgery, St. Elizabeth's
    Hospital, Brighton, Massachusetts

CLIFFORD L. CRAIG, M.D.
Assistant Professor, Department of Orthopaedic
    Surgery, Tufts University School of Medicine,
    Boston, Massachusetts
Chief of Orthopaedic Surgery, Lakeville
    Hospital, Lakeville, Massachusetts

DIDIER CROS, M.D.
Assistant Professor, Department of Neurology,
    Harvard University School of Medicine,
    Boston, Massachusetts
Clinical Neurophysiology Laboratory,
    Massachusetts General Hospital, Boston,
    Massachusetts

PATRICIA A. FELDMAN, O.T.R.
Clinical Instructor, Department of
    Rehabilitation Medicine, Tufts University
    School of Medicine, Boston, Massachusetts
Director of Occupational Therapy, Greenery
    Rehabilitation and Skilled Nursing Center,
    Boston, Massachusetts

BRUCE M. GANS, M.D.
Professor and Chairman, Department of
    Physical Medicine and Rehabilitation, Wayne
    State University, Detroit, Michigan
President and Chief Executive Officer,
    Rehabilitation Institute of Detroit, Detroit
    Medical Center

KAREN B. GIEBLER, P.T., M.B.A.
Clinical Instructor, Department of
    Rehabilitation Medicine, Tufts University
    School of Medicine, Boston, Massachusetts
Director of Physical Therapy, Greenery
    Rehabilitation and Skilled Nursing Center,
    Boston, Massachusetts

MEL B. GLENN, M.D.
Associate Professor, Department of
    Rehabilitation Medicine, Tufts University
    School of Medicine, Boston, Massachusetts
Director, Brain Injury Unit, New England Sinai
    Hospital, Stoughton, Massachusetts
Director of Rehabilitation Medicine, Greenery
    Rehabilitation and Skilled Nursing Center,
    Boston, Massachusetts

DENNIS S. GORDAN, M.D.
Assistant Professor, Department of
    Rehabilitation Medicine, Tufts University
    School of Medicine, Boston, Massachusetts
Medical Director, Weldon Center for
    Rehabilitation at Mercy Hospital, Springfield,
    Massachusetts

STEVEN M. HALEY, Ph.D., P.T.
Assistant Professor, Department of
    Rehabilitation Medicine, Tufts University
    School of Medicine, Boston, Massachusetts
Acting Project Director and Director of
    Research, Research and Training Center on
    Rehabilitation and Childhood Trauma, Tufts
    University School of Medicine and New
    England Medical Center Hospitals, Boston,
    Massachusetts

SUSAN C. HALLENBORG, P.T.
Clinical Instructor, Department of
  Rehabilitation Medicine, Tufts University
  School of Medicine, Boston, Massachusetts
Private Practitioner, Equipment Prescription
  Services, Billerica, Massachusetts

NANCY HYLTON, P.T.
Pediatric Therapist and Consultant, Children's
  Therapy Center, Kent, Washington

CONSTANCE A. INACIO, P.T.
Instructor, Department of Rehabilitation
  Medicine, Tufts University School of
  Medicine, Boston, Massachusetts
Research Assistant, Research and Training
  Center on Rehabilitation and Childhood
  Trauma, New England Medical Center,
  Boston, Massachusetts

DAVID L. KASDON, M.D. (DECEASED)
Former Associate Professor, Department of
  Neurosurgery, Tufts University School of
  Medicine, Boston, Massachusetts
Former Chief, Department of Neurosurgery, St.
  Elizabeth's Hospital, Brighton, Massachusetts

JOAN MORRISSEY, P.T.
Assistant Director of Physical Therapy,
  Greenery Rehabilitation and Skilled Nursing
  Center, Boston, Massachusetts

KEITH M. ROBINSON, M.D.
Assistant Professor, Department of Physical
  Medicine and Rehabilitation, University of
  Pennsylvania School of Medicine,
  Philadelphia, Pennsylvania.

**BHAGWAN T. SHAHANI, M.D., Ph.D.,
D.Phil. (OXON)**
Associate Professor, Department of Neurology,
  Harvard Medical School, Boston,
  Massachusetts
Director, Electromyography and Motor Control
  Unit, Clinical Neurophysiology Laboratory,
  Massachusetts General Hospital, Boston,
  Massachusetts

JAMES A. WHITLOCK, JR., M.D.
Clinical Instructor, Department of
  Rehabilitation Medicine, Tufts University
  School of Medicine, Boston, Massachusetts
Staff Neurologist and Director of Head Injury
  Unit, Northeast Rehabilitation Hospital,
  Salem, New Hampshire

JOHN WHYTE, M.D., Ph.D.
Director of Brain Injury Research, Drucker
  Brain Injury Center, Moss Rehabilitation
  Hospital, Philadelphia, Pennsylvania

SEYMOUR ZIMBLER, M.D.
Professor, Department of Orthopaedic Surgery,
  Tufts University School of Medicine, Boston,
  Massachusetts
Chief of Orthopaedic Surgery, Franciscan
  Children's Hospital, Brighton, Massachusetts

CONTENTS

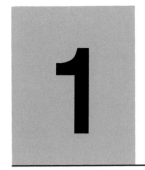

INTRODUCTION

BRUCE M. GANS
MEL B. GLENN

Spasticity is one of the most common features of the motor deficits associated with the upper motor neuron syndrome. It spans a variety of diagnoses and ages, and is one of the most common problems dealt with by physicians and therapists caring for patients with neurologic diseases. This chapter presents an overview of the definitions, bases, and consequences of spasticity, and serves as an orientation and overview of the subject for health professionals.

DEFINITIONS

To discuss the management of spasticity, it is necessary to define tone, spasticity, and a number of other terms. No universal agreement as to the wide acceptance of these terms exists among clinicians or researchers in the field. The definitions presented here do, however, represent the conventions agreed upon by the authors of this book.

WEAKNESS

Weakness (or paresis) describes a lower strength of active muscle contractions than that expected by the examiner with consideration of age, sex, and body habitus. In subtle situations, weakness is tested by contraction against weights or manual resistance by the examiner. In more severe cases, lack of strength is observed when the limb is moved in space against gravity or with gravity eliminated.

PARALYSIS

Complete inability to activate muscle contractions voluntarily is termed paralysis. This term should be reserved for complete absence of contractile ability, while paresis is used more generally for other cases.

FATIGUE

Inability to sustain a work performance level for a voluntary muscle contractile activity at normal levels is described as fatigue. This is typically encountered in clinical circumstances as a diminished capacity to perform an activity for a prolonged period of time.

INCOORDINATION

Incoordination is a decrease in the skilled sequential or contemporaneous control of muscle activation that results in diminished gross or fine motor activity accuracy.

1

TONE

Tone is described as the passive resistance to stretch offered by a muscle group to external manipulation. Two specific abnormal states are noted: decreased (hypotonia) and increased (hypertonia) tone. It is a subjective description of the way a patient's limbs feel when being manipulated by the examiner. More formal and quantitative methods for describing this property of resting limb muscle contractions are discussed in Chapter 5.

REFLEX

A motor reflex is the involuntary motor response of the body or limb segment to a physical agent, such as stretch, touch, vibration, etc. The reflex most significant to the discussion of spasticity is the stretch reflex (e.g., knee jerk). Increased muscle contraction response to a given stimulus is termed hyperreflexia; decreased contraction is termed hyporeflexia.

The terms "phasic" and "tonic" reflexes appear frequently in the literature with inconsistent definitions and usages.[1] "Phasic stretch reflex" is used most commonly to describe the response to rapid stretch seen when deep tendon reflexes or clonus are elicited. The term "tonic reflex" has been used to describe the state of spontaneous and persistent muscle contractions, the resistance of a muscle to being stretched, and the length-dependent excitation that follows a stretch stimulus to a muscle. Because of the confusion and inconsistencies observed, both of these terms are avoided wherever possible in this text.

CLONUS

The sudden application of sustained stretch to a muscle that results in repetitive rhythmic contractions, relaxations, and spontaneous contraction again is termed clonus. It is most commonly elicited at the ankle, but may be observed in almost any muscle group.

SPASTICITY

Spasticity is a syndrome associated with a persistent increase in the involuntary reflex activity of a muscle in response to stretch. Four specific phenomena may be variably observed in the constellation of spasticity: hypertonia (frequently velocity-dependent and demonstrating the "clasp-knife" phenomenon), hyperactive deep tendon reflexes, clonus, and spread of reflex responses beyond the muscle stimulated.[2-5] There is evidence suggesting that spastic hypertonia is associated with a reduction of the threshold angle at which the stretch reflex is elicited.[6]

RIGIDITY[7,8]

Rigidity is an involuntary increase in resistance of muscle to passive stretch that is uniform throughout the range of motion of the muscle(s) being stretched, and which is not velocity-dependent. *Extrapyramidal rigidity* is seen in Parkinson's disease, involving both of an opposing pair of muscle groups about a joint, and may be associated with "cogwheeling." Deep tendon reflexes are not hyperactive. *Decerebrate rigidity* involves extensor muscles of all extremities and *decorticate rigidity* involves extensors in the lower extremities and flexors in the upper extremities. Rigidity is also frequently observed in association with synergies and other primitive motor behaviors.

PRIMITIVE MOTOR REFLEX

Primitive motor reflexes are spontaneous, stereotypical patterns of motor activity, frequently associated with a specific stimulus such as pain, infection, or other noxious stimuli. Head position, contralateral limb position, and body position in space are also stimuli for these primitive motor behaviors. Specific examples include the asymmetric tonic neck reflex, the symmetric tonic neck reflex, and the mass synergies (flexor and extensor) as shown in Figure 1-1.[9]

These patterns of movement are normally present in early development, and

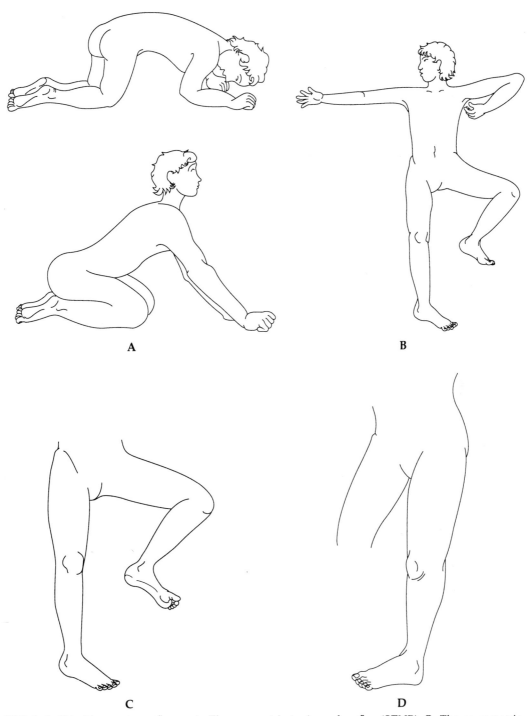

FIG. 1–1. Primitive motor reflexes. A, The symmetric tonic neck reflex (STNR). B, The asymmetric tonic neck reflex (ATNR). C, The flexor synergy in the lower extremity. D, The extensor synergy in the lower extremity. (From Gans, B.M.: Rehabilitation of the pediatric patient. *In* De Lisa et al., eds.: Rehabilitation Medicine: Principles and Practice. Philadelphia, J.B. Lippincott, 1988, p. 396, with permission.)

are commonly seen in normal infants and small children. They become abnormal whenever they are obligate and dominant patterns of movement, or when they persist well past the developmental age when they are normally seen to disappear.

Withdrawal (nociceptive) reflexes are patterns of reflexively mediated movement in response to distal noxious stimuli (typically pain) that appear to be protective in an evolutionary sense. Although they normally persist into adulthood, they are included here as primitive motor reflexes because they otherwise fit this definition. Some authors consider these patterns of movement a component of spasticity; however, they will not be considered so in this book because they are not a manifestation of hyperactive stretch reflexes.

DYSTONIA[8]

Dystonia is an involuntary contraction of muscle that results in a slow, sustained movement and maintenance of joint position in a dystonic posture, in which there is increased resistance to passive stretch in the direction of the resting position. The dystonic movement may be provoked by voluntary motion or may occur spontaneously. Dystonia can be caused by a variety of disorders of the central nervous system.

ATHETOSIS

This term describes one of a number of patterns of movement disorders seen in a variety of neurologic diseases. It consists of slow, writhing movements of the limbs or trunk, usually described as purposeless or adventitious.

In children or adults with cerebral palsy (CP), the term has special meaning as a category of CP (athetoid). In this case, the term includes other phenomena, including dramatic variability of resting tone, and marked persistence of primitive motor reflexes. The typical infant with athetoid CP does not show athetoid movements; rather, hypotonia that becomes rigid hypertonia may be the first motor abnormality seen. Only later (around age 3 to 7) are the writhing patterns of movement typically seen.

UPPER AND LOWER MOTOR NEURON SYNDROMES

Lesions of the motor nervous system are commonly divided into two large categories, upper and lower motor neuron syndromes. These distinctions are both clinically significant and diagnostically important. There are certain disorders (such as amyotrophic lateral sclerosis) where both syndromes may occur simultaneously, but in general they are distinct entities. Sensory disorders may or may not also be present in either syndrome.

UPPER MOTOR NEURON SYNDROME

Lesions of the motor systems occurring in the brain, brainstem, or spinal cord that do not involve the anterior horn cell or peripheral nerve and muscle are described as upper motor neuron lesions. Although some authors include only weakness, spasticity, and extensor plantar responses as the clinical features of this syndrome, this book uses a broader definition that encompasses the following: weakness or full paralysis, spasticity, primitive reflex patterns, athetosis or other hyperkinetic movement disorders, rigidity, dystonia, and preservation of muscle bulk. In general, this syndrome is associated with a number of "positive" signs (Table 1–1) and few negative ones. Typical examples include stroke, cerebral palsy, and traumatic brain injury.

TABLE 1–1. POSITIVE AND NEGATIVE SIGNS IN MOTOR NEURON SYNDROMES

	Upper	Lower
Positive		
Spasticity	+	
Athetosis	+	
Primitive reflexes	+	
Rigidity	+	
Dystonia	+	
Negative		
Weakness	+	+
Paralysis	+	+
Fatigue	+	+
Muscle atrophy		+

LOWER MOTOR NEURON SYNDROME

Disease or damage to the anterior horn cell, peripheral motor nerve, or myoneural junction may be described as yielding the lower motor neuron syndrome. The specific signs include: weakness or paralysis, hyporeflexia, decreased resting tone (hypotonia), and muscle atrophy. Typical examples include diseases such as Guillain-Barré, poliomyelitis, and peripheral nerve injuries.

FUNCTIONAL CONSEQUENCES OF SPASTICITY

A principal consequence of spasticity is diminished capacity of the patient to accomplish useful work with the motor system. This is usually thought of as an exaggerated array of spontaneous motor activity that distorts or precludes useful motor function. For example, the patient with spastic hemiplegia may show a flexor dominance in the hand with a fisted posture. If the flexor activity were less dominant, the residual extensor function under voluntary control could restore more useful hand function. One underlying premise for the management of spasticity is that the reduction in the positive signs allows improved active function if negative signs are not overwhelming.

A second premise is that relief of spasticity may permit better passive function. For example, in the patient with the flexor-dominated hand that is in a fisted posture, even if relief of flexor tone does not improve voluntary extension, the increased ease of passive extension of the fingers may make cleansing of the involved hand easier, faster, and more comfortable. In addition, because the presence of spasticity may lead to soft tissue contractures, treatment of the spasticity may be useful to prevent or manage contractures.

Some of the treatments for spasticity also affect other aspects of the upper motor neuron syndrome. For example, muscle spasms associated with hyperactive nociceptive reflexes may be painful and debilitating. The administration of a medication such as baclofen, which is commonly used for spasticity, might also reduce the painful or disabling spasms. In fact, the treatments for spasticity and the primitive motor behaviors overlap to such an extent that it is not entirely possible to discuss one without the other.

There may be a number of secondary benefits to spasticity in a given patient that need to be considered in clinical decision-making for treatment. For example, the patient may be relying upon the involuntary increased tone during transfers to assist in weight-bearing or limb movement. Further, the preservation of muscle bulk by the reflex activity may protect the skin against pressure and be cosmetically pleasing to the patient. The metabolic work performed by spastic muscles may help to consume calories and avoid weight gain by the patient. Finally, spastic activity may have the beneficial effect of retarding the development of osteoporosis.

DECIDING WHETHER TO TREAT SPASTICITY

The choice of whether or not to intervene in the spastic state must be made based on the establishment of specific goals of treatment to identify expected benefits. The most obvious criterion is that spasticity treatment should result in improvement of the patient's active or passive function, or comfort. A special case is reserved for the determination of the etiology of the spasticity, particularly when a change in the degree of spasticity is noted and thought to be clinically significant.

While the basic cause for the presence of spastic patterns may be well known (a spinal cord injury, for example), the specific stimulus producing a patient's pattern and degree of spasticity may need specific elucidation. Spasticity may increase in response to any noxious stimulus in the body, and in fact may be thought of clinically as a physical manifestation of pain. This is particularly important in the patient who is unable to experience pain (e.g., complete spinal cord injury) or unable to communicate (e.g., severe brain injury). Thus, when a patient shows a sudden change in spasticity, a search for a causative agent (perhaps unrelated to the nervous system disorder) should be undertaken. Common causes for increases in spasticity include bladder and bowel problems; occult fractures below the level of the neurologic lesion; skin irritations such as sunburn, pressure sores, and ingrown toenails; occult abdominal problems, and many other agents. When a specific cause is identified, treatment may well secondarily reduce the exaggerated spasticity.

DECIDING HOW TO TREAT SPASTICITY

Once the decision has been made to treat, and goals have been defined, the choice of specific methods must be made. This book describes a host of interventions: physical agents and modalities, drugs, peripheral ablative procedures, and central ablative and stimulating methods. The treatment should be targeted to the scope and severity of the problem. In broad terms, as limited an intervention as possible should be chosen. When the problem is topographically limited to a particular muscle or nerve group, local intervention should be considered. When it is widespread, systemic or generalized agents should be considered.

The cost-benefit and risk-benefit ratios of any intervention should be considered. Thus, for example, high-risk neurosurgical interventions should be limited to extreme situations. True costs should be considered. While a "dose" of physical therapy may be less expensive than a surgical procedure, if the total amount of therapy needed is priced out, the surgical intervention could prove to be the more cost-effective choice.

The practicality of the treatment should also be considered. It may be more realistic to accept the one-time costs and risks of a nerve block, for example, than to expect a patient to keep up with a four-times-daily medication schedule for months or years.

The side effects or other consequences of

treatments should also be considered. Drugs, for example, may cause other problems including fatigue, gastrointestinal distress, or addiction. Physical agents may consume great amounts of time and limit lifestyles. Devices may cause skin problems. Surgery may cause pain, scars, and the risk of infection. The risk of side effects must enter into the decision-making process.

Finally, therapeutic interventions should be considered in combination more than in isolation. Daily or twice-daily range-of-motion exercises should remain as constant treatments regardless of whether other interventions are used as well. Drugs too, may be used in combination (although compliance may become more problematic) or with other interventions (such as casts or braces).

In the end, all treating clinicians must recognize that the treatment of a patient's spasticity is not typically sufficient to resolve completely all of the signs and symptoms of the disorder. There is not, unfortunately, a neurologically normal person hiding below the surface of a spastic exterior in most patients. Therefore, the goals of treatment must be consistent with the entire neurologic, physical, medical, and psychologic status of the patient. As a corollary, there are times when spasticity is best left untreated, either because it may be providing the patient with some benefits, or because its treatment is not likely to result in functional gains.

CONCLUSION

With a proper understanding of the nature of spasticity, its causes, and functional problems it causes, intelligent decisions may be made to effect treatment and management. While not curative, the various options described in this book allow effective betterment of the patient's condition.

REFERENCES

1. Little, J.W., and Merritt, J.L.: Spasticity and associated abnormalities of muscle tone. *In* Rehabilitation Medicine: Principles and Practice. Ed. J.A. DeLisa et al. Philadelphia, J. B. Lippincott, 1988.
2. Bishop, B.: Spasticity: Its physiology and

management, Part I: Neurophysiology of spasticity—classical concepts. Phys. Ther. 57:371–376, 1977.

3. Bishop, B.: Spasticity: Its physiology and management, Part II: Neurophysiology of spasticity—current concepts. Phys. Ther. 57:377–384, 1977.

4. Bishop, B.: Spasticity: Its physiology and management, Part III: Identifying and assessing the mechanisms underlying spasticity. Phys. Ther. 57:385–395, 1977.

5. Bishop, B.: Spasticity: Its physiology and management, Part IV: Current and projected treatment procedures for spasticity. Phys. Ther. 57:396–401, 1977.

6. Lee, W.A., Boughton, A., and Rymer, W.Z.: Absence of stretch reflex gain enhancement in voluntarily activated spastic muscle. Exp. Neurol. 98:317–335, 1987.

7. DeJong, R.N.: Case taking and the neurologic examination. *In* Baker, A.B., and Baker, L.H.: Clinical Neurology. Vol. 1. Ed. R.J. Joynt. Philadelphia, J.B. Lippincott, 1988.

8. McDowell, F.H., and Cedarbaum, J.M.: The extrapyramidal system and disorders of movement. *In* Baker, A.B., and Baker, L.H.: Clinical Neurology, Vol 3. Ed. R.J. Joynt. Philadelphia, J.B. Lippincott, 1988.

9. Gans, B.M.: Rehabilitation of the pediatric patient. *In* Rehabilitation Medicine: Principles and Practice. Ed. J.A. De Lisa et al. Philadelphia, J. B. Lippincott, 1988.

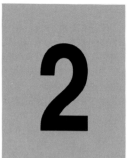

2 NEUROPHYSIOLOGY OF SPASTICITY

JAMES A. WHITLOCK, JR.

"The essence of knowledge is, having it, to apply it;
not having it, to confess your ignorance."
—Confucius

SENSORIMOTOR SYSTEMS REGULATING REFLEX, TONE, AND MOVEMENT

Knowledge about the functional organization of motor systems offers the possibility of application in attempts to design solutions to clinical problems resulting from neuropathology. Advances in neurophysiology have changed views on spasticity greatly over the past 10 years. Although no major new therapeutic interventions have resulted directly from new knowledge, the type and methodology of therapeutic techniques are changing as the physiologic basis of various spastic states is clarified.

The alterations in resting muscle tone, reflexes, and motor control that define spasticity can best be understood within a review that considers the basic functional organization underlying normal tone, reflex, and motor control.

THE MOTOR UNIT

The active changes in muscle associated with spasticity are representative of the state of their associated motor neurons. The motor unit, Sherrington's "final common path,"[1] consists of a single alpha motor neuron (α MN) and each of the muscle fibers innervated by its axon branches. Differences in motor unit size and organization correlate with different functional roles. The most numerous small α MNs innervate aerobically-metabolizing, very slowly fatiguing, small, "red" (histologic type 1) muscle fibers. These units have relatively few muscle fibers per neuron. Large α MNs, fewer in number, drive many large, rapidly fatiguing, anaerobically metabolizing "white" (histologic type 2) fibers. Between the two extremes are many intermediate-sized units that span a functional and anatomic spectrum.[2]

The α MNs of ubiquitous small motor units have a low firing threshold and are largely responsible for the active component of normal motor "tone." Frequent asynchronous discharging of small motor neurons within a "motor pool" innervating a muscle or group of muscles influences their state of active tension. These small motor units can be thought of as tonic units.

Large motor units have high-threshold α MNs that are normally called into play only when a motor act requires more speed or power than smaller units together can provide. They are phasic power units.

Most muscular activity reflects an economy of effort based on a recruitment order first described by Henneman.[3] Small motor units are activated before progressively larger units. Recruitment order is mirrored by a corresponding derecruitment order whereby the largest active units cease firing first as net motor output declines. This recruitment order is rarely, if ever, violated and applies to both reflex and voluntary motor output.

When considering pathologic changes that can occur in motor disorders, the above described match between α MN and muscle fiber types becomes especially important (and will be discussed in more depth later). Muscle fiber type appears to be under the direct influence of specific neuronal innervation by means of the discharge frequency of that neuron. If innervation to a specific muscle fiber changes (as in reinnervation of denervated units or in various experimental preparations), the muscle fiber adapts to the new input even if it means changing from a large, pale, fast fiber to a small, red, slow one.[4]

A new and important class of motor neurons has been described.[5] Beta motor neurons (β MNs) are small neurons that are unique in that each innervates both main muscle fibers and intrafusal (spindle) fibers. β MNs may have an important role in regulating reflex activity and postural tone.

THE AFFERENT LIMB OF THE STRETCH REFLEX ARC

Within skeletal muscle are self-tuning length transducers consisting of specialized sensory receptors or "spindles." Afferent endings of cell bodies located in dorsal root ganglia are attached in unique fashion to small, specialized motor fibers. The entire assembly, each containing several "intrafusal" motor fibers, is encapsulated and attached to the connective tissue within the muscle belly. The density of spindles in a given muscle generally correlates with its functional versatility, with distal upper extremity musculature being especially spindle rich, while proximal limb musculature is relatively sparsely populated.[6]

Afferent volleys from spindles encoding information on length of muscle and change in length are transmitted through rapidly conducting, large-diameter group Ia afferents. Smaller group II afferents are sensitive only to static length. The principle of spindle operation depends upon the facts that: (1) they are within the muscle body and thus are in parallel with the forces deforming muscle longitudinally (stretch or contraction); (2) the intrafusal fibers to which the afferents attach have to adjust their own length actively for spindles to remain sensitive to extrafusal muscle length. The latter is accomplished through the gamma (fusimotor) system (Fig. 2–1).

When extrafusal muscle contracts, muscle spindles within its body are passively shortened. The length-sensitive spindle would be unable to provide the CNS with feedback at shortened muscle lengths were it not for some compensatory mechanism which allows them to retain their sensitivity over an assortment of muscle lengths. The γ MN provides this compensation by means of innervating small intrafusal muscle fibers which, paradoxically, put the spindle on stretch when they are stimulated to contract. Thus, Ia afferents may be activated as readily in a shortened as in a lengthened position.

Small gamma motor neurons (γ MNs) are mixed with corresponding α and β MNs of the spinal motor neuron pool supplying a muscle. Activation of gamma motor discharge is closely linked with activation of α MNs, although descending and intraspinal influences on the two systems are different. The principle of coactivation of associated α and γ MNs helps to ensure the accurate reflection of change in muscle length within its most functional range during real-time activities.[7]

Both Ia and II afferents are key components in the regulation of motor performance at the segmental level. They also constitute the afferent limb of monosynaptic (chiefly Ia) and polysynaptic (II) reflexes. Although their input is not required for motor output (as long as some other sensory pathway is intact), they provide essential feedback to higher levels of the neural hierarchy during the learning of new skilled motor tasks. These are the afferents that transmit the most important proprioceptive

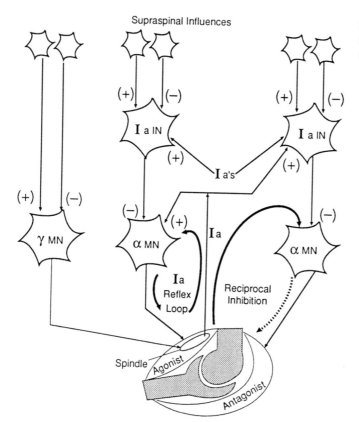

FIG. 2–1. The gamma fusimotor system, stretch reflex loop, and reciprocal inhibition.

information relating to the difference between an intended and an accomplished movement. The central connections of these afferents and the influences exerted upon them by local and remote control loops are discussed further in later sections. (See "Stretch Reflexes and Motor Organization," "Factors Influencing Motor Unit Discharge," and "Hyperreflexia and Hypertonia as Velocity-Sensitive Responses" below.)

GOLGI TENDON ORGANS AND TENSION TRANSDUCTION

The mechanics of muscle action are described by length, tension, and dynamic relationship. Effective neural control requires feedback regarding both. Spindles provide the length information. Tension feedback is mediated by highly sensitive receptors located within muscle tendons. These Golgi tendon organs (GTOs) are connected to rapidly conducting Ib afferents. Like Ia afferents, their cell bodies lie within the dorsal root ganglia. Unlike Ias, which have some direct feedback connections to α MNs, with Ibs information is processed through interneurons which, in turn, influence agonist/synergist-antagonist pairs (Fig. 2–2).[8]

In general, the Ib tension-feedback system helps to define an upper limit to an overly stressed system by exerting a net inhibitory influence on agonists while facilitating antagonists. Thus, an agonist exerting "too much" tension will be inhibited. At the same time, decline in muscle tension associated with fatigue leads to decreased Ib transmission and a corresponding decrease in Ib-mediated agonist inhibition. This helps to compensate for loss of power. Ib interneurons are facilitated by low-threshold cutaneous (touch) and joint receptors. This allows their probable role in buffering against undue, potentially injuri-

Supraspinal and Propriospinal Influences

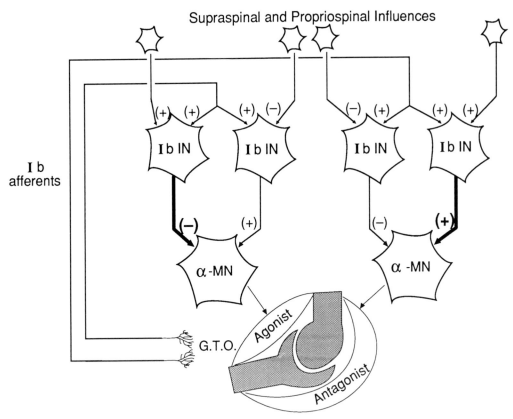

FIG. 2-2. Pathways whereby Ib-afferent information from an agonist exerts influence upon activity in agonist-antagonist pair. (The Golgi tendon organ: A review and update, by Moore, J.C. Am. J. Occup. Ther. *38*:232, 1984. Copyright (1984) by the American Occupational Therapy Association, Inc. Reprinted with permission.)

ous increase in tension associated with the unexpected obstruction of a moving limb.[9]

STRETCH REFLEXES AND MOTOR ORGANIZATION

Without the ability to perform certain fast, functionally useful motor acts independent of volition or deliberation, we would be forever at the mercy of perturbations to positional stability in a world where gravity reigns. One of the beauties of hierarchical CNS organization is the existence of intraspinal mechanisms for making rapid and advantageous motor corrections without requiring the processing abilities of higher centers.

Reflex responses to muscular stretch (Sherrington's "myotatic reflex") reflect measurable behaviors to physical variables.

Most such physical variables can be well controlled in experimental settings. Much of what has been learned about motor system organization has been derived from study of mechanical and electrophysiologic correlates of stretch reflex activity in animals and man. Through stimulation or ablation of various higher centers, descending influences on such reflex activity have been elucidated.

Two basic physical changes happen when a muscle is passively stretched. Its length changes during the stretch and it assumes a new length when the stretch is complete. The monosynaptic reflex loop generates a phasic change in length that is mediated by Ia afferents. The unbridled response to diffuse Ia afferent input from a stretched muscle would be increased α MN activity. If, at the moment stretch occurs, there is substantial activity in antagonist

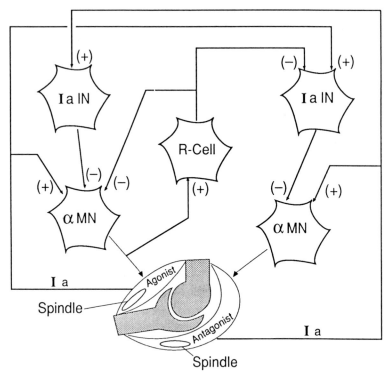

FIG. 2–3. Renshaw circuit.

muscle groups, the discharge of stretched units can be rendered ineffectual as agonist and antagonist fight against each other.

Reciprocal inhibition of antagonists, mediated by Ia interneurons (Ia INs) belonging to the agonist pool, acts to prevent such motor discord (Figure 2–1). Spindle output of the agonist would be increased by passive muscle stretch. This spindle activity not only facilitates agonist motor neuron discharge by way of the segmental reflex loop, it also tends to inhibit discharge of the antagonist α MN by way of an associated Ia IN.

This mechanism almost certainly has a bearing on the effectiveness of *active* contractions as well. If the antagonists were also to contract in response to spindle stretch and Ia excitation during an active movement, undesired stiffening or oscillation might result without inhibition of the Ia afferent volleys from the antagonist. This tendency is reduced or at least buffered through reciprocal inhibition by means of agonist Ia afferents, triggered by γ MNs

which are activated in concert with α MNs (coactivation). This circuit is thus viewed as an important mediator of balanced contractions of agonist-antagonist pairs and is a central control point for descending supraspinal signals.[10]

Ia INs may be viewed as promoting high gain in the reflex arc by decreasing the forces acting against members of its motor pool. Variable control of the gain is provided in the form of Renshaw (R) cell-mediated recurrent inhibition (Fig. 2–3). In the Renshaw circuit, α MN discharge excites neighboring R-cells by means of an axon collateral. R-cell discharge then sends inhibitory signals back to the discharging α MN ("recurrent inhibition"). R cells act as a neural brake on both α and γ MNs of their pool and synergists.[11] They tend to promote the active firing of only those MNs within their domain that are being driven hard enough to overcome their own recurrent inhibition. They highlight the activity of the most active members of a synergy group while inhibiting the rest. In addition, R-cell discharge sends inhibitory signals to Ia INs associated with the α MN of the antagonist. The negative influence on the Ia IN of the antagonist helps to allow the antagonist α MN to react to stretch by means of its Ia afferent circuit. Although the descending controls on R cells are unclear, studies of R-cell-mediated inhibition in spastic subjects by Katz and Pierrot-Deseilligny suggest that removal of their control may indeed give rise to difficulty in grading the strength of attempted contraction and in voluntary control of movements that require regulation of reciprocal Ia inhibition (in which R-cells participate (Fig. 2–3)).[12]

In the normal, healthy resting state, the stretch reflex is of low amplitude and probably of little functional importance. In the course of active motor behavior, stretch reflex elements become more useful under the moderating control of many descending tracts. In pathologic states, abolition or exaggeration of segmental reflexes provides valuable clues to the nature and progression of clinical motor system dysfunction.

FLEXOR REFLEX AFFERENTS

In general (excluding the Ib tension feedback system discussed above in "Golgi Tendon Organs and Tension Transduction"), nonspindle afferents mediate flexor associated movements that have tissue-protective value. Such "flexor reflexes" have a physiologically slower time course than stretch reflexes, a function of the fact that they are mediated through interneurons (polysynaptic reflexes) and transmitted over generally smaller-diameter, more slowly conducting group II and III axons.[13] Unlike segmental reflexes, they often represent coordinated discharge of motor pools spanning many segments, sometimes bilaterally.

Receptors in joints, skin, connective tissue and extrafusal muscle whose afferents are involved in polysynaptic flexor reflexes have been termed "flexor reflex afferents" (FRAs). With certain exceptions, FRA-mediated reflexes demonstrate stimulus and location specificity. Evoked motor responses are focused on the withdrawal from or reaction to the area from which the

stimulus came in a manner which varies with the strength and type of stimulus.[14] Thus a gentle superficial stimulus may evoke reflexive scratching while a stronger stimulus evokes focal withdrawal and an even stronger (painful) stimulus to the same site results in a flexion withdrawal and contralateral extension (the crossed-extensor reflex).

FRA pathways are extremely complex and may involve any spinal interneuron between the FRA itself and the MN that becomes the actor in an evoked reflex. This includes long and short propriospinal interneurons (whose neuronal processes travel within gray and white matter of the spinal cord, spanning one or many segments) and Ib interneurons of the tension-feedback loop. FRAs have been attributed a gating function in modulating descending influences on MNs.[15] They may also mediate transmission of corollary discharges or "efference copies" to higher levels of the neuraxis, providing ongoing feedback about activity within spinal reflex networks that forms the basis for updated commands dependent on cerebellar processing (Fig. 2–4.[16,17] FRAs are also one local source for GABA-mediated presynaptic inhibition of Ia afferents.[18]

FACTORS INFLUENCING MOTOR UNIT DISCHARGE

The neural complexity of segmental and intersegmental networks engaged by primary afferents and motor neurons reminds one of how abstract some of the simple schematics of reflex and control pathways are. Still, clinical and physiologic schemas have predicted the existence of anatomic substrates that were subsequently found and described (e.g., Renshaw cells, crossed-spinal connections at the segmental level, long propriospinal pathways). Anatomic and physiologic work continue to feed each other, allowing the grand scheme of neural organization to become ever more complex and thereby reflective of the true state of things.

Physiologic studies beginning with Sherrington's at the turn of the century demonstrated the behavioral richness of the spinal cat and dog, whose hindlimbs could be re-

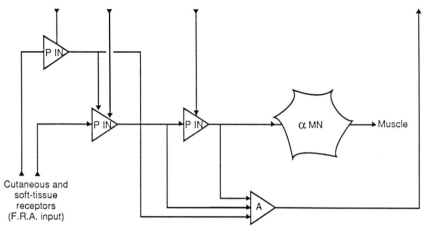

FIG. 2-4. Flexor reflex afferent pathways.

flexively engaged in alternating movements akin to walking.[19] Brown was soon to prove that these walking movements in spinal animals could be obtained briefly even after the dorsal roots had been sectioned.[20] This finding nourished the idea that complex spinal networks were capable of autonomously generating meaningful patterns of movement.

Renshaw cells, Ia INs, and Ib INs are a few types of spinal interneurons whose functions are becoming understood. There are many more interneurons whose functions remain clouded in ambiguity. The wealth of intersegmental connections mediated by long and short propriospinal interneurons (P INs) are well known to anatomists who have observed the thick skirt of their funiculus from around the ventral horn to the dorsolateral cord.[21] In monkeys, up to 50% of Lissauer's tract fibers may be propriospinal as well.[22]

Relatively few of the classic highly arborized, compact Golgi II type interneurons are found in the spinal cord. Instead, most propriospinal interneurons (P INs) have relatively long axonal processes, which may span short distances between one to several segments or across the midline (short propriospinals) or can link cervical to lumbar segments (long propriospinals). Propriospinal axons typically give off many collateral branches in their ascent or descent.

Relatively little is known about the phys-

iology of most P INs and their active behavior in networks. Long P INs can mediate either excitatory or inhibitory effects on MNs directly or through an additional interneuron. The existence of such elements and what *is* known about them reinforces conceptual models of spinal networks subserving motor subroutines (such as those of Loeb).[23] The tapestry of propriospinal connections makes it possible to conceive of a relatively small number of descending control signals from a higher program resulting in a very complex motor output. The P IN mediated interconnections between both efferent and afferent components of motor output stages are also thought to allow monitoring of complex patterns of spinal activity by higher centers which receive signals that reflect the state of INs (whose state, in turn, reflects the activity of a larger neural network). This function may be mediated through spinocerebellar pathways.[24]

There are many possible ways to conceptually lump or split the pathways exerting descending influence on spinal motor systems. Each is artificial and oversimplifying in one way or another. Many of the pathways studied in animals are thus far extremely difficult to study in humans. Major interspecies differences in their function have sometimes appeared. Descending systems are herein grouped according to extensor versus flexor facilitation (Table 2–1). The following summary is based largely

TABLE 2–1. SUPRASPINAL INFLUENCES
ON SPINAL MOTOR CIRCUITS

Lateral vestibulospinal tract, medial (pontine) reticulospinal tract:	Corticospinal tract, corticorubrospinal tract, corticoreticulospinal tract:
Phylogenetically older	Phylogenetically younger
Widespread spinal connections	Focused, discrete connections
Extensor-oriented	Flexor-oriented
Postural maintenance	Fractionated/isolated movement

upon Brodal's synopsis[21] with an attempt to integrate additional information contained in Brooks[25] and others.

The brainstem reticular formation appears to give rise to two functionally different reticulospinal systems in animals—one originating in the pons and the other in the medulla. The pontine system, first described by Rhines and Magoun,[26] facilitates extensor α and γ MNs. It may be less influenced than its medullary counterpart by cortex, but does appear to receive some input from the sensorimotor cortex and possibly the supplementary motor area. Additional facilitory afferents come from the cord. Fibers of this so-called medial reticulospinal tract tend to remain ipsilateral during their descent in the ventral funiculus, with some crossing near their segmental terminae. This system is fairly diffuse and not subject to somatotopic organization. The anatomy of analogous pathways assumed to exist in man is unclear.

The lateral vestibulospinal tract is another source of descending extensor facilitation. Large and small cells in the lateral vestibular nucleus of Deiter's descend in the ventromedial cord throughout its length. There is somatotopic organization to this nucleus and tract whose fibers terminate adjacent to the motor neuron pools of the ventral horn. Bilateral effects of each nucleus are presumed to be exerted through spinal interneurons. Stimulation of Deiter's cells results in direct EPSPs on extensor α and γ MNs. Vestibulospinal stimulation also gives rise to inhibition of physiologic flexors. This system is under cerebellar control by means of afferents from anterior and flocculonodular lobes as well as the fastigial nucleus. Fastigial input is excitatory, whereas cerebellar cortical influence on both fastigial and vestibular nuclei is inhibitory.

The pontine reticular formation and the lateral vestibular nucleus together have a positive extensor facilitory role that can be dramatically unmasked in animal lesion experiments wherein lesions interrupt the extensor inhibitory (or flexor-facilitory) influences with which they are normally in balance.

The medullary reticular formation of the cat has been described as the seat of an extensor inhibitory effect that contrasts with its pontine counterpart.[27] Referred to as the lateral reticulospinal system, its fibers descend ipsi- and contralaterally in the lateral funiculus to form inhibitory synapses upon extensor MNs and Ia INs. Influence is exerted on both α and γ MNs. Excitatory afferents to medial reticular formation come from cortex. A dorsolateral component to this system is thought to exert its inhibitory effects on segmental FRA and Ib networks, thereby decreasing the background activity impinging upon α MNs and increasing their receptivity to other descending signals.

A review of some of the phenomena discovered during lesion stimulation studies in the decerebrate cat provides insight regarding the interplay of the foregoing systems. The extreme extensor rigidity of a midbrain-sectioned cat promoted by release of the cortically-facilitated medullary reticulospinal extensor inhibition areas leaves the extensor facilitory pontine reticulospinal and lateral vestibulospinal systems free to exert unfettered dominance. Facilitory influences ascending from the cord to pontine reticulospinal neurons are intact in such a preparation. But even amidst this forced collaboration between reticulospinal and vestibulospinal systems, there is a domineering force from the lateral vestibular nucleus, inhibition of which markedly reduces extensor rigidity. The rigidity can be abolished at once in a limb by section of its dorsal roots, suggesting that the fusimotor system was mediating much of the extensor tone. In the decerebrate cat, γ MN activity is markedly increased. For a long time this finding (among others) helped fuel the search for fusimotor disinhibition as an explanation of human spasticity for which decerebrate preparations were considered models. Granit believed that because of the γ MNs' small size, a given amount of descending α-γ facilitation from pathways like the reticulospinal would have a proportionally greater effect on γ MNs, and the concept of gamma rigidity was born.[28] Well before Granit, it had been shown that ablation of the anterior lobe of the cerebellum of decerebrate cats gave rise to an extensor rigidity that could not be abolished by dorsal root section.[29] This so-called "alpha-rigidity" was assumed to be due to marked and overriding vestibulospinal facilitation from a Dieter's nucleus removed from direct and indirect (by means of fastigial nucleus) cerebellar inhibition. This phenomenon was important in showing that hypertonia could exist even after dorsal root section (and removal of Ia afferent feedback), fueling the notion that the fusimotor system influence might not be as important as was thought. The concept of alpha-rigidity may also have a bearing on explanations of failure in permanent relief of spastic hypertonia after dorsal rhizotomy in humans.

The medullary extensor inhibitory center may be viewed as part of a larger cortico-reticulospinal flexor biasing system. The corticorubrospinal and corticospinal systems also have a flexor orientation and are organized differently from all other systems.

Rubrospinal fibers come from small and large cells of the red nucleus in the midbrain. Somatotopic organization is apparent in cats. In man, the rubrospinal tract travels adjacent to the lateral corticospinal tract after crossing in the brainstem. It probably extends to the sacral cord. Claims that this system is rudimentary in man are unfounded.[30]

Primate studies have shown abundant cortical input from precentral and adjacent cortex and supplementary motor areas to somatotopically oriented red nucleus cells. Even though little is known about such connections in man, a precentral corticorubral projection has been identified. The terminae of axons in the rubrospinal tract of primates are in the same area of cord as the terminations of corticospinal neurons. Many rubral cells seem to receive direct, noncollateral corticorubral fibers, suggesting a high degree of focused control by cortical motor centers. Rubral cell axons have a tendency to split, with one process descending to spinal cord while the other goes to cerebellum. The heavy cerebellar input to the red nucleus raises some interesting possibilities of possible integration or comparator function in these cells which mediate both corticorubrospinal traffic and a cerebellorubrocerebellar side loop. That is, the pattern of rubral cell activity may represent the sum or difference in the activities of these separate motor system components.

The corticorubrospinal system exerts an indirect excitatory influence upon contralateral flexor α and γ MNs and an inhibitory effect on corresponding extensor MNs. All identified effects on MNs are mediated through interneurons, most of which receive Ia and/or FRA afferents. In animals, as the somatotopic organization implies, this flexor-facilitory system is much more focused and represents a higher degree of organization under cortical influence than bulbopontine extensor facilitation.

The principal protagonist of fractionated volitional movement in man is the corticospinal system. Cells principally from layer 5 of Brodman's areas 3 (a and b), 1, 2 ("primary sensory cortex"), 4 ("primary motor cortex"), 6 (including the supplementary motor area), and 5 are contributors to this pathway. Only a minority of the 2 million pyramidal fibers come from the large Betz cells of primary motor cortex.[31] Somatotopically arranged corticospinal, corticobulbar, and corticorubral fibers from sensorimotor cortex coalesce into a thick ribbon which twists about a half turn as it descends in the posterior part of the internal capsule. After passing through the middle portion of the cerebral peduncle, the ribbon splits into clusters of fibers, some of which pass through the basis pontis while others synapse with neurons of the pontine nuclei through which the clusters are passing. Final assemblage to form the medullary pyramid precedes the crossing of most corticospinal fibers at the decussation of the lower medulla. The crossed fibers give rise to the large, grossly cylindrical lateral corticospinal tract—a variable minority of fibers remaining uncrossed as the ventral corticospinal tract. Some uncrossed fibers remain in the lateral corticospinal tract (inspiring clinicians to wonder what potential role they might have—or be coaxed into—in recovery of motor function after hemispheric lesion).

In primates, most of the corticospinal impact upon spinal motor neurons is indirect, but there are monosynaptic contacts with MNs in monkeys, and there is no reason to doubt that a similar condition prevails in man. In monkeys, these direct connections arise from cells in cortical areas 3a and 4 and are found in segments innervating distal extremity musculature. Net corticospinal effect tends to be flexor-facilitory and disynaptically extensor-inhibitory (largely by way of Ia INs) with similar effects exerted on α and γ components of the spinal motor pool.

Two major feature of this system deserve special mention within the context of a consideration of suprasegmental influences on motor unit discharge. The first feature involves the rich collateralization of descending upper motor neuron fibers. The second relates to a gross functional division between relatively "fast" and "slow" fiber components.

Animal studies have shown that cortical cells of the motor system which are ultimately destined to reach the cord give off many collaterals to structures at all levels of the motor heirarchy. Collateralization of corticospinal fibers even takes place at the level of the cord.[32] At the same time, direct noncollateral contacts between sensorimotor cortex and motor nuclei occur, at least in basal ganglia and brainstem. This implies that the discharge of one cortical motor neuron *may* result in an EPSP on a striatal neuron, whereas discharge of a cortical neighbor might (for example) result in EPSPs occurring with an anatomically-ordained temporal order on cells in thalamus, red nucleus, reticular formation, cervical and lumbar cord. Little is known about exactly what patterns of focused or coinnervation exist in man, but the possibilities suggested by animal studies are awesome (Fig. 2–5). The questions raised are correspondingly legion. Of the numerous possibilities, what collateral-mediated connections actually occur in the human nervous system? With what statistically proportional frequency? With what proportional degree of synaptic influence on a given nucleus or motor pool relative to other inputs? What is the cortical distribution of cells having similar collateral distribution and what physiologic/metabolic features do

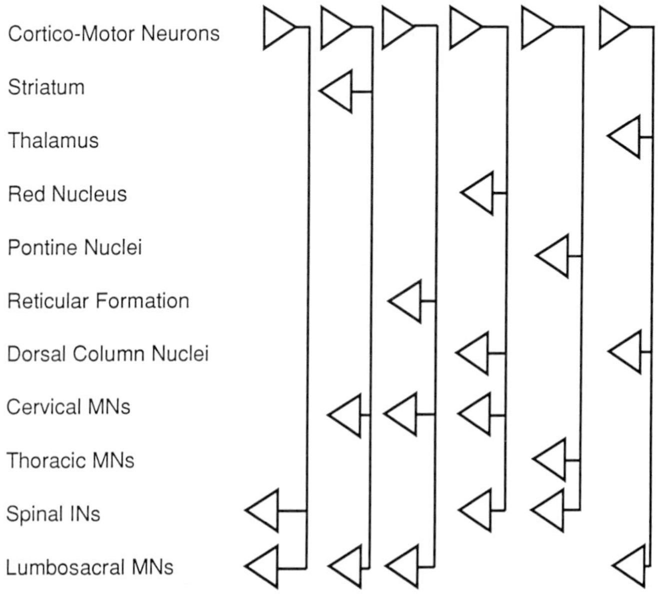

FIG. 2–5. Conceptual diagram of multilevel corticospinomotor innervation via collateralization.

Cortico-Motor Neurons

Striatum

Thalamus

Red Nucleus

Pontine Nuclei

Reticular Formation

Dorsal Column Nuclei

Cervical MNs

Thoracic MNs

Spinal INs

Lumbosacral MNs

they share? Presumably, richly collateralized motor neurons whose processes span large distances with the CNS impose a greater metabolic demand for their maintenance. Are they, in fact, "selectively vulnerable" to conditions that affect metabolic processes? If they are, is reversible injury to such cells manifest by preservation of proximal synaptic communication after sacrifice of more distal axonal segments and their contacts? Does the pattern of collateralization predict the nature and distribution of clinically observable motor deficit (or vice versa) following anoxic or other metabolic insult? When incomplete volitional influence exists over motor units after central nervous system injury, what are the implications of collateralization for motor retraining? Is there any possibility of separately facilitating more direct corticospinal pathways in some instances? Likewise, is there any way to influence collateral pathways through training or physically induced inhibition or facilitation so that a desirable result is obtained (i.e., if effects of neuronal discharge on a damaged pathway affect a certain spinal level preferentially, can intact pathways with collaterals to the affected area be restructured by therapy to allow improved cortical control over the denervated structure)?

With respect to the gross physiologic division possible between fast and slow corticospinal neurons, animal studies (mammalian and primate) have shown that there are two conduction velocity peaks within the corticospinal conduction spectrum, one at approximately 14 m/sec and the other at 42 m/sec.[33] In general, the fast fiber system seems to supply ventral cord regions while slow fibers end more dorsally. In primates, this division corresponds to an anatomic division between fibers arising from areas 3a and 4 (more classically "primary motor"), which end in more ventral areas of spinal grey matter and pyramidal fibers from "sensory" cortex, which end dorsally. This has raised the specter of a primary role for fast fibers in more direct spinal motor control, whereas slower pathways may modulate sensory (e.g., FRA) and interneuronal pathways involved in segmental motor discharge patterns.

The raphe-spinal pathways are thought to be a component of the endogenous analgesia system. Most of what is known about this system comes from studies in the cat. Serotonergic neurons projecting to spinal cord come from nuclei in the pons and medulla. Their myelinated and unmyelinated processes descend in mainly dorsolateral cord and terminate preferentially in the dorsal horn, intermediolateral cell column, and ventral horn, and around the central canal.

Raphe-spinal fibers exert a tonic inhibitory influence over the flexion reflex pathways of decerebrate animals, probably mediated mainly by effects on dorsal horn interneurons. Somatic α and γ MNs are influenced by this system as well, although the nature of their potentially facilitory or inhibitory influence is unclear. Serotonin appears to enhance the excitatory effects acting on motor neurons in the cord. Raphe-spinal fibers may influence by means of indirect modulatory chemical action rather than direct synapse. That is, they may act through exerting a widespread release of their transmitter that affects the firing threshold of entire neuronal subsystems in the cord. The role of the raphe-spinal system in humans is unknown.[34]

The dorsolateral pontine tegmentum is the conspicuous home of the locus coeruleus (the "blue place"). Nearby is the nucleus subcoeruleus. These centers of norepinephrine-mediated neural transmisson in the CNS send and receive fibers throughout. Locus coeruleus neurons (LCNs) collateralize to supply cortical and cerebellar cortices as well as spinal cord. In the cat, every LCN appears to send a collateral to cord and this is thought to be the major source of spinal catecholamine. The system in the cat appears to be fairly diffuse and most terminals occur in cervical and lumbar intumescenses, suggesting a primary role in limb rather than axial innervation. Some direct motor neuron connections seem to exist, although it appears that the analgesic effect of locus coeruleus stimulation is mediated by inhibitory contacts on dorsal horn interneurons. Descending coerulospinal volleys are thought to facilitate IN-mediated presynaptic inhibition of FRAs. The catecholaminergic facilitation of monosynaptic reflexes in cats is due either to activation of excitatory MN input or (more likely) inhibition of tonically active inhibitory pathways.[35]*

The cerebellum as a potential modulator for spasticity and/or rigidity has been of special interest ever since it was found that ablation of the anterior lobe of decerebrate cats led to a rigidity that did not respond to deafferentation (i.e., alpha rigidity).

Recent studies have examined the role of the cerebellum in modifying stretch reflex responses. Glaser and Higgins found that, in decerebrate cats, the anterior lobe tended to have a dynamic regulatory effect on stretch reflexes with net stabilization of such reflexes, diminishing tendencies toward oscillation. Overall function tended to ensure stability of position control and voluntary movement at initiation. Mechanisms for compensation that occurred after cerebellectomy were assigned to brainstem vestibulocephalic reflex systems.[36]

Ebner and associates studied the effects of paravermal cerebellar cortical stimulation in partially decorticate monkeys. In their carefully controlled experiments, they found that a tendency toward normalization of reflex response to passive limb movement was sensitive to stimulus quality and location. Application of certain stimuli to the same location actually exaggerated some abnormal responses.[37]

Hopes of favorably modifying spasticity have led to neurosurgical attempts to ameliorate human spasticity (see Chapter 12). Penn reviews such efforts and points out that, while a mounting body of uncontrolled evidence suggests that cerebellar stimulation in cerebral palsy can at times ameliorate deficits and improve function, controlled studies fail to demonstrate consistently favorable results. The reader is referred to his comprehensive review of the subject.[38]

---

*Author's note: Although I have expected and looked for alterations in tone and reflexes in closed head-injured patients with complex motor deficits after they were placed on noradrenergic agonists to increase general arousal, I have yet to discover any noteworthy clinical alteration in spastic phenomena in these patients. More rigorous laboratory conditions might well detect salient (and therapeutically meaningful) changes that escape gross clinical detection.

PATHOPHYSIOLOGY OF SPASTIC PHENOMENA: CLINICOPATHOLOGIC CONSIDERATIONS

In general, a clinical and pathophysiologic division exists between the epiphenomena of spasticity caused by isolation of the cord and that caused by cerebral lesions that leave brainstem influences intact (although they are indirectly affected themselves). Table 2–2 outlines some of these differences.

The boundaries of pathology rarely respect those of neuroanatomic systems. Still, clinically complete spinal lesions do remove most, if not all, descending brainstem and cortical input to motor neuron pools, interrupting some afferent pathways involved in reflex and motor behavior as well. Depending on the level of the lesion, one might expect varying degrees of effect on long propriospinal circuits. In cortical, capsular, or peduncular hemiplegia, brainstem effects on cord continue to exist (though probably always in modified form), whereas variable amounts of corticospinal input to α, γ and β MNs, spinal interneurons, and dorsal horn afferents are removed. Reticulospinal and rubrospinal activity is presumably disrupted to a greater direct extent than that of other brainstem sensorimotor systems in view of the significant flow of cortically-originating information they receive. As a result, there is a

TABLE 2–2. SPASTICITY-ASSOCIATED CLINICAL PHENOMENA

Spinal	Cerebral
Flexor pattern in lower extremities	Tone predominant in antigravity muscles
Flexor spasms common (early)	Flexor spasms rare
Clasp-knife phenomenon common	Less clasp-knife phenomenon
Clonus prominent "Paraplegia in flexion"	Clonus less prominent "Hemiplegic pattern"
Spinal shock 1–16 weeks	Cerebral shock, 2–3 weeks
Exaggerated exteroceptive reflexes	Superficial abdominal and cremasterics gone
Autonomic dysreflexia	Autonomic phenomena absent

net loss of their flexor-oriented direct and indirect facilitation. Brainstem lesions can be expected to exhibit a plethora of clinical and physiologic effects, depending on the location and extent of involvement. The ability to derive thorough analogies of animal studies of experimental brainstem lesions and human conditions will probably always be prevented by the fact that all common brainstem pathologies (vascular, traumatic, demyelinative) tend to be anatomically irregular and unique from individual to individual.[39]

HYPERREFLEXIA AND HYPERTONIA AS
VELOCITY-SENSITIVE RESPONSES

A clinically oriented approach to the explanation of spasticity in humans tends to artificially separate elements which are rarely, if ever, found in isolation. Yet the different clinical features of spasticity underscore different sources of physiologic discord that together comprise the basis of spastic motor dyscontrol.

Perhaps the weakest distinction on a physiologic level lies in any attempt to divorce hyperreflexia from velocity-dependent, unidirectional increases in resistance to passive muscle stretch (spastic hypertonia). Although exaggerated tendon reflexes are in themselves unlikely to be of any functional consequence, their association with spastic states and their amenability to study have fostered a vast literature. Because of the velocity-dependent nature shared by spastic hyperreflexia and hypertonia, it has been expected that elucidation of mechanisms of one would shed light on the other.

Attempts to explain hyperactive tendon jerks focused for a long time on the classical myotatic reflex arc. Within this model it appeared that reflex changes attending isolation of spinal segments from descending influences had to rest in increased α MN excitability, increased Ia-mediated facilitation of motor discharge, or a combination of the two. As details regarding the fusimotor-spindle system emerged, it appeared that increased fusimotor excitability with secondary hypersensitization of velocity-sensitive spindles could be the source of reflex perversion in spasticity. Descending influences upon γ neurons were viewed as primarily inhibitory in nature and their interruption logically suggested that γ MNs would become unnaturally sensitive to local or brainstem facilitory influences. For many years this "gamma release" hypothesis was regarded as the primary factor behind spasticity. A review of some of the work that changed the view of spastic pathophysiology over the past 30 years follows.

In the early sixties, most researchers viewed the decerebrate cat as a good model of human spasticity. Rushworth, one of these researchers, considered his ability to abolish hyperactive reflexes in the cat model as well as in human hemiplegic spasticity using dilute procaine to achieve selective neural blockade of small nerve fibers (demonstrated electrophysiologically) as strong evidence for gamma-based pathophysiology. Clinical conditions featuring hypertonia resistant to procaine block were thought to be caused by alpha-rigidity[40] (see previous section entitled "Factors Influencing Motor Unit Discharge").

During the same epoch, Granit echoed the physiologic zeitgeist of his time and pointed out that the coactivation of α and γ neurons probably helped to ensure the exaggerated muscular responses to γ-mediated increases in spindle sensitivity. But he also issued a subtle warning that knowledge of the relationship of experimental findings to the human condition was incomplete. He suggested complicated interactions among system components that were just beginning to be understood.[41]

The early 1970s were major transition years for thinking on the subject. Dietrichson reported a disproportionately large evoked muscle response from calibrated tendon tap as opposed to electrically elicited (H) reflexes in spastic subjects as further evidence for primary mechanoreceptor hyperactivity. He also inferred that increased α excitability underlay the increased ratio of maximal electrically elicited H response to direct evoked muscle (M) response which he observed in his subjects (see Chapter 3). Anecdotally adding observations that chemical neurolysis abolished resistance to quick passive movements in each of the subjects in which it was used, he seemed comfortable that the gamma release hypothesis was secure.[42]

But in the 1960s it had been discovered that vibration could *inhibit* monosynaptic reflexes in normal man (see Chapter 3). It also appeared that this vibratory reflex inhibition (VRI) was rather specifically mediated by primary afferents.[43] This notion contradicted the classical view of the afferent limb of the reflex arc as always committed to a facilitory role. Furthermore, vibration of muscle or tendon had been found to have a second effect whereby motor neurons were activated with the latent emergence of a contraction of muscles in the vibrated group—the tonic vibration reflex (TVR).[44]

While vibratory paraphenomena added tremendous puzzlement to the picture of motor physiology, vibration added significantly to the limited armamentarium available for studying the functioning human motor system. It joined quantitative mechanical stretch and electrophysiologic measures (especially H reflex). The utility of vibratory techniques combined with these other measures was soon proven.

Delwaide's work was important in advancing an alternative to the gamma-release hypothesis of human spasticity. He showed that VRI was absent on the affected side and normal on the unaffected side of hemiplegics. He also noted that quantitative assessment of VRI was normal in Parkinson's disease patients and in non-neurologically diseased persons with overtly exaggerated reflexes. Surmising that there was loss of a segmentally active inhibitory mechanism in "pyramidal hyperreflexia," he had to prove that the source of afferent input to this mechanism was truly mediated by Ia fibers from homonymous muscles. He demonstrated that short, passive, relatively slow sinusoidal mechanical movement of the ankle produced H-reflex inhibition without stimulating antagonist spindles (as happens during application of a vibratory stimulus). This inhibition could not be increased by the addition of a vibratory stimulus to the Achilles tendon but *was* in-creased by cutaneous stimulation. This, in turn, suggested that large afferents (rather than cutaneous afferents) mediated vibratory as well as sinusoidal movement-derived inhibition (i.e., vibration had no effect because afferent pathways were already busy with mechanically induced neural traffic). He then proceeded to deliver quantitative phasic stretches to the Achilles tendon of immobilized joints while measuring the H-reflex during different points in the stretch. He discovered that H-reflex responses were inhibited by even slight stretching of the mechanically-isolated triceps surae. This mechano-electrophysiologic analog to VRI was further proof of an Ia mediated inhibition of the reflex arc. The inhibition occurred even though the overall excitability of motor neuron pools was not depressed. It thus seemed to be a presynaptic inhibition. Delwaide hypothesized that Ia INs were the prime sources of inhibitory synapses on the terminal arborizations of neighboring Ia afferents. In spasticity, removal of descending facilitory influences acting on these interneurons was conceived of as the basis for a decrease in their local presynaptic inhibitory action (Fig. 2–6).[45]

Observations of others complicated the emerging "presynaptic inhibition" hypothesis. Disparate bits of information had to be reconciled. Ashby and Verrier described potentiation of VRI during spinal shock that outlasted the period of shock only to fade with chronicity.[46] They also found VRI enhancement in early hemiplegic spasticity which yielded to marked attenuation in the chronic state. They attempted to explain the dissociation between Achilles tendon evoked muscle responses and H reflex responses observed in chronic lesions[42] as still best explained by increased fusimotor drive. They thought that this increased gamma motor excitability was perhaps applicable only to the chronic state. Hypertonia, on the other hand, they attributed to an emerging decline in spinal inhibitory mechanisms as dorsal root afferents sent new sprouts to fill synaptic vacancies left by degenerating supraspinal fibers. The sprouts would be devoid of the presynaptic inhibitory influence of their unaffected Ia associ-

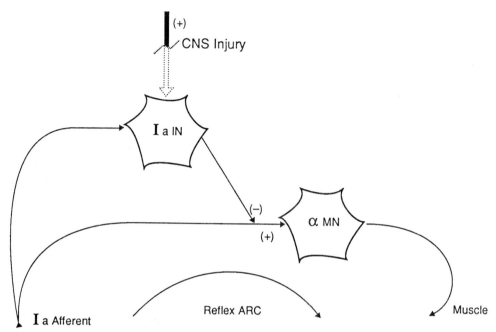

FIG. 2-6. Loss of descending facilitation of Ia Interneuron (Ia IN) mediating presynaptic inhibition results in exaggerated stretch reflex.

ates. Temporal changes in Ia-mediated reflexes and tone were thereby viewed as tied to the temporal requirements of degenerative and regenerative central nervous system processes.[47,48]

Axonal sprouting in animal (cat) spinal cord after rostral lesions had been demonstrated by McCouch and colleagues in 1958 and was offered by them at the time as an anatomic substrate for temporal changes in physiologic behavior underlying spastic motor phenomena.[49] Chambers, Liu and McCouch subsequently reviewed a substantial body of evidence accruing thereafter which gave credence to consideration of axonal sprouting as a real and salient factor in neural re-organization of cord after higher lesions. They acknowledged much less (though some) contribution from "denervation hypersensitivity" of the type described in the classical work of Canon and his associates.[50,51]

Sprouting has continued to be thought of as a primary element behind some of the temporal changes in reflexes and tone occurring as sequelae of certain CNS injuries. Other mechanisms are thought to be involved in the immediate course of such injuries (the consideration of which is beyond the scope of this chapter).

As the 1970s came to an end, it appeared that the "gamma-release" hypothesis of human spasticity was on its way out. Burke reviewed accrued information of fusimotor activity in normal humans and found no evidence for its involvement in regulating reflex arc gain, mediating enhancement maneuvers (such as Jendrassik's) upon tendon reflexes, or affecting resting spindle activity.[52] In normal subjects, it looked as though gamma motor functions could be linked only to voluntary activity. Similar reviews of fusimotor function in human spasticity (with the patient at rest) had failed to demonstrate any fusimotor hyperactivity. In an excellent, comprehensive later review of fusimotor involvement in abnormal reflex and tone states, Burke concluded that there was no evidence to support fusimotor regulation of proprioceptive (stretch) reflex gain, spastic hypertonia or cerebellar "hypotonia" in humans.[53]

The study of human responses to musculotendinous vibration in health and disease led to some seemingly contradictory phenomena. Vibration of normal skeletal muscle can at once facilitate motor neurons leading to tonic muscle contraction (TVR) and inhibit the phasic (tendon jerk) reflex of the same motor pool. Furthermore, expression of a masseteric reflex in normal humans is facilitated by chin vibration, unlike the inhibitory effect noted in limb musculature. Desmedt attempted to explain these phenomena within a hypothetic framework supported by his work with Godaux and findings of his predecessors.[54] They viewed the fixed recruitment order of MNs within a motor pool as determinants of the response to vibratory spindle afferent input. But just as Ia afferents mediate growing recruitment of neurons of increasing size and threshold, they are also exerting an amount of presynaptic inhibition on adjacent Ia afferents. This inhibition hampers further recruitment of MNs and, as a side effect, dampens response of lower threshold components of the MN pool to phasic reflex recruitment. The recruitment order determines that lower threshold units fire first. But in vibrated limb muscles, strong homonomous presynaptic inhibition of afferents mediating phasic stretch responses effectively raise the threshold of the motor pool and impede responses of MNs not yet actively engaged in mediating the TVR contraction (Fig. 2–7). A "pure" facilitory effect in jaw closure musculature (for both tonic

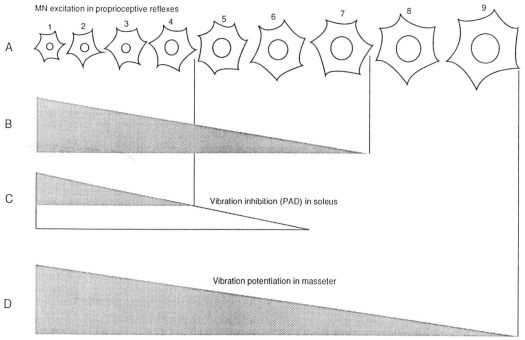

FIG. 2–7. MN recruitment by steady vibration. A, MNs are recruited in a fixed order from left to right in proprioceptive phasic or tonic reflexes, and also in voluntary contractions (Henneman's size principle). The actual amount of resulting synaptic activation (indicated by vertical width of black triangles in B to D) is larger for MNs first recruited, decreasing from left to right. B, Synaptic activation by a standard proprioceptive volley recruits MNs 1 to 7. C, In the presence of steady vibration of soleus, presynaptic inhibition of spindle afferents reduces the amount of synaptic activation proportionally and the standard volley only recruits MNs 1 to 4. D, By contrast in masseter, steady vibration elicits no presynaptic inhibition of spindle afferents and therefore potentiates the synaptic activation proportionally allowing the standard volley to recruit MNs 1 to 9 (from Desmedt, J.E.: Mechanisms of vibration-induced inhibition or potentiation: tonic vibration reflex and vibration paradox in man. In Motor Control Mechanisms in Health and Disease. Ed. J.E. Desmedt. New York, Raven Press, 1983, p. 671, with permission).

contraction and stretch reflex) is thought to be secondary to a lack of presynaptic inhibition in the masseteric pathway (a state of affairs supported by animal studies).

A tap of the reflex hammer to the brachioradialis tendon may result in brisk contraction of brachioradialis, biceps, and pectoralis. This reflex "spread" in hyperreflexia is familiar to every clinician. Lance views the occurrence of reflex spread in spasticity as dependent on propagation of vibration waves through the limb with consequent spindle activation in remote muscle groups. Reflex contractions of these muscles are thought to ensue because of an increase in central MN excitability.[55]

CLONUS

Clonus is the well-known rhythmic, self-sustaining alternating flexion-extension movement that is most commonly observed in the ankle of spastic subjects. It is more commonly seen in spinal than in "cerebral" spasticity (but is common in both). It may arise spontaneously in association with positional changes of the ankle, or in response to brisk dorsiflexion of the ankle by an examiner. Various cutaneous stimuli (especially cold or noxious stimuli) may give rise to ipsilateral and contralateral clonus in spastic subjects.[57]

Attempts to explain clonus have had to integrate these facts:

1. It tends to have a narrow range of frequencies.
2. It occurs within the context of a hyperreflexive state.
3. Factors which decrease hyperreflexia also tend to decrease clonus.
4. Contractions in clonus are purely alpha-motor in origin and do not appear to be under fusimotor influence.[58]

Various studies have attempted to discriminate between peripheral and central factors controlling clonus. To discern the role of central mechanisms, Dimitrijevic et al.[59] measured physical and electrophysiologic concomitants of clonus in a group with mainly spinal spasticity. Being unable to significantly alter its rate or character by varying physical elements or by introduc-

ing interpolated afferent barrages in the middle of the relaxation phase, they concluded that a central oscillatory mechanism was operative. The central oscillator was postulated to arise from a "transitory functional organization" in the cord which requires periodicity among Ia volleys, coactivation of homologous and synergist MNs, isolation of motor pool reflex arcs from "extraneous volleys," and maintenance of pool excitability.

Rack and associates have recently examined clonus in normal subjects and patients with spasticity.[60] They cited the major prerequisite for clonus as unusually high gain in the stretch reflex circuit. In their normal subjects, this high gain was obtained involuntarily through repetitive cyclical (sinusoidal) joint rotations which facilitated the development of a clonus. In spastic subjects, it seemed as if their reflexes were stuck in the high-gain mode. In them there was a strong, consistent correlation between loading imposed upon the joint during clonus and the frequency and amplitude of the oscillations. They view clonus as a self-sustaining oscillation of a stretch reflex pathway, with the frequency of clonus being determined by physical parameters rather than central mechanisms.

One way of thinking about the neural basis for clonus is to consider two motor neuron pools serving antagonist muscle groups. These pools have been isolated enough from descending control traffic (even if voluntarily) that cortico-α MN links are at least functionally inhibited. Ia afferents are also centrally disinhibited (by pathology in sustained, involuntary clonus) from loss of their supraspinal controls. Either a sudden Ia volley or FRA input causes discharges from one of the hyperexcitable motor pools. The ensuing muscle contraction unloads homonomous spindles even as antagonist muscle (reciprocally inhibited during the agonist contraction) is stretched, resulting in its own roughly proportional afferent Ia barrage which excites the antagonist motor pool. Some form of autogenic inhibition is operating to silence motor pools at the end of their contraction and render them transiently resistant to further positive feedback coming during the end of contraction or early to mid-relaxation phase. While the time course of Renshaw-mediated recurrent inhibition is too short,[61] that of the Ib IN (Golgi tendon organ) system may be a viable candidate. Given the proper externally imposed conditions, sustained clonus results.

THE "CLASP-KNIFE" PHENOMENON

Sherrington did not confine his experimental work to decerebrate cats. He also worked with spinal dogs. He noted a difference in the reactions to passive flexion of their rigidly extended limbs. While the cat hindlimb simply assumed the new position at the end of the stretch (the "lengthening reaction") with resistance throughout the motion, an analogous maneuver in the spinal dog produced sudden loss of resistance during the stretch, after which there was no further resistance.[62] Burke and associates[63] were first to highlight the difference between these separate phenomena, the latter of which they equated with the "clasp-knife" phenomenon seen in human spasticity.

The clasp-knife phenomenon refers to the sudden "give" experienced by an examiner stretching a spastically extended limb. Hypertonia abruptly disappears at a point in the stretch. Although the limb often has to be stretched quickly to elicit spastic hypertonia, the "give" appears to be more length-dependent than velocity-dependent. Lance and Burke[64] found a difference between apparent clasp-knife effects in upper and lower extremities of spastic humans, noting that the purely length-dependent occurrence was more easily observed in the lower limbs. The term "pseudo-clasp-knife reaction" has been used to describe the more velocity-dependent than length-dependent change in resistance to passive stretch in the upper limb of spastic hemiplegics.[65]

The true clasp-knife effect is length-dependent.[66] Its occurrence is predicated upon group II afferent-mediated reflex inhibition of α MNs. The role of Ib tension receptors is unclear, but almost certainly secondary in view of their extreme sensitivity to muscle tension (regardless of length) combined with the fact that Ib-mediated inhibition tends to die out as soon as tension ceases. The fact that a spastic limb *remains* hypotonic after the clasp-knife point is passed argues against such Ib-mediated inhibition.

MECHANICAL ELEMENTS IN GENERATION OF HYPERTONICITY

Muscle-tendon units have intrinsic mechanical properties that contribute significantly to stretch resistance and aid in the recoil at release from stretch. The mechanical model of muscle as spring attempts to account for its passive visco-elastic (or plastic-elastic) properties.

The initial resistance to deformation represents an elastic force arising from the bonds between contractile elements (actin and myosin filaments) that have to be broken during muscle lengthening. Additional elasticity and tendency to "spring back" result from connective tissue elements. Ralston and his colleagues demonstrated that approximately 15% of the resistance to stretch in actively contracting human forearm muscles derives from intrinsic muscle tissue forces, the remainder being provided by active neuromuscular contraction.[67] Houk and his co-workers,[68] examining the relationship between muscle mechanics and the stretch reflex in contracting cat soleus muscle discovered that reflexive responses to stretch versus release were asymmetric in a way which tended to counteract asymmetric intrinsic muscle responses to a set change in length (schematically illustrated in Fig. 2–8). That is, in an isolated soleus preparation subjected to artificial "tonic" innervation, there was an initial resistance to stretch that quickly declined and slowly redeveloped (presumably as actin-myosin bonds were broken and then reformed at the new length). Shortening of the muscle (release from stretch) under the same stimulus conditions resulted in a marked decline in muscle force. When the experiments were repeated in decerebrate cats with intact soleus reflex pathways, much different forces were measured in muscle subjected to standardized changes in length. These additional forces represented reflexive motor activity. These experiments led Houk and his associates to postulate that spindle-mediated autogenic

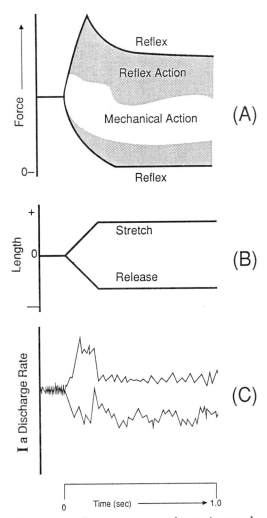

FIG. 2-8. Reflex responses to change in muscle length (B) are balanced in a way that maintains symmetry of muscle force in the face of asymmetric mechanical responses (A). Spindle discharge frequency mirrors the reflex components of muscle response (C) (adapted from Houk, J.C. and Rymer, W.Z.: Neural control of muscle length and tension. In Motor Control. Section 1, vol. 2. Handbook of Physiology. Ed. V.B. Brooks. Bethesda, MD, American Physiological Society, 1981, with permission).

reflexes help to compensate for variations of intrinsic muscular responses to changes in length.

Intrinsic muscular stiffness (resistive force per unit length change) is a dynamic variable. The initial length of a muscle, the degree of length change, and the speed of movement all have a bearing on what intrinsic muscle forces are encountered. Autogenic reflex activity seems to compensate for variations in muscular stiffness during changes of muscle length.[69]

Pathologic states that alter the normal control of limb position and mobility give rise to changes in muscle, tendons, and joints. Such changes have been extensively studied in animals (see Gossman et al.[70] for review) and to a lesser extent in humans. In mammals, fairly consistent age-dependent changes in sarcomeres occur when a limb is fixed in a lengthened state. Young animals adapt by lengthening tendon and correspondingly reducing sarcomere number while adult sarcomeres grow longer under the same conditions. Physiologically, these changes are associated with shifts in length-tension curves without change in basic configuration or slope. On the other hand, fixation in the shortened state in innervated animal preparations causes reversible loss of sarcomeres with increase in fast type 2 fibers and loss of type 1s. Connective tissue elements increase and thicken. Animal models suggest that chronic, imposed shortening of muscle length combined with active contractility gives rise to the greatest reduction in sarcomeres and corresponding increase in stiffness. Because of muscle shortening in contracture, the capacity for development of active tension is less than that normally possible at longer lengths. If a muscle that has undergone contracture is subsequently lengthened, much weakness may then be revealed. Malnutrition and catabolic steroids enhance negative effects of immobility in the shortened state. Reflex activity per se is not required for such changes.[71]

The contribution of passive muscle properties to tone in human spasticity has become clearer as techniques for separating their effects from active or reflex contractions improve. Herman[72] has described the relatively minor, rate-independent stretch resistance offered by atonic, areflexive muscle as a series elastic force. He holds that early spasticity (before any contracture) with its rate-sensitive stretch resistance reflects primarily reflex effect. The contracted spastic muscle shows a decline in reflex activity with emergence of a moderate, rate-sensitive viscous reaction, which Herman viewed as arising from changes in muscle itself.

Recently, Hufschmidt and Mauritz,[73] in controlled studies of the mechanical properties of chronically spastic human muscle, have described velocity-independent elastic and plastic resistive force in both intact and deafferented spastic limbs. In their study, viscous forces were found to be absent within average physiologic rates of movement in spastic limbs. They further divided elastic muscle forces into series and parallel. Short-range, early series forces are attributed to filament cross-bridge breaking, whereas additional longer-range series and parallel forces are attributed to connective tissue elements. Plastic resistance in "spastic" muscles is thought to result from histologic transformation within muscle-involving fibrosis, atrophy, and change in the contractile properties to those of predominantly "tonic" type muscles. Edstrom[74] has demonstrated the selective type 2 fiber atrophy that can be seen in chronic, severe spasticity with relative enlargement of slower type 1 fibers. Changes of this sort in spasticity are thought to be secondary to changes in the quality and frequency of MN discharge.

EXTEROCEPTIVE REFLEXES IN SPASTICITY

Exteroceptive reflexes are mediated by afferents in skin and subcutaneous tissue that subserve primary sensory experiences of touch, pressure, temperature, and pain. These receptors join some of the "enteroceptors" in transmitting information about stimuli arising from intrinsic local tissue changes (such as inflammation or mass lesions). Perhaps best described by "what they are not," nonproprioceptive afferents together comprise the afferent limb of a set of complex, polysynaptic, generally polysegmental reflexes that allow a certain automaticity or efficiency of response to internal or integumentary stimuli. The normal cutaneous reflex is classically exemplified in the short-latency reflex withdrawal of a limb from a noxious (or unanticipated potentially noxious) stimulus while stabilizing

the body through alteration of posture (contralateral extension).

Although not a component of the spasticity syndrome per se as defined in this text (see Chapter 1), exteroceptive hyperreflexia is commonly seen in association with spasticity and is in fact commonly referred to as "spasms." Exteroceptive reflexes are universally altered in clinically complete spinal lesions. So-called flexor reflexes typically emerge as deep tendon reflexes reappear with decline of spinal shock.[75] They are characterized by exaggerated, perverted, and stereotyped responses to cutaneous stimuli. They may be elicited by stimuli that would normally be well below the threshold required to evoke any reflex (e.g, simple light touch or stroke of the foot resulting in marked withdrawal of the leg). Stimuli to one extremity may result in a diffuse, bilateral, and sometimes massive flexor-patterned response with loss of correspondence between the site of stimulation and the propriety or utility of response (i.e., loss of "local sign" normally characteristic of such reflexes). Reflex action is perverted in the sense that the reflexogenic movement fails to accomplish any adaptive purpose and may actually move a limb toward a noxious stimulus instead of away from it (as in Bing's sign, where pin prick to the dorsum of the great toe elicits dorsiflexion toward the pin). Spontaneous flexor spasms commonly seen in spinal injury are most likely a response to occult cutaneous or somatic stimuli. As time passes, there is a tendency in spinal spasticity for flexion responses to yield to or become admixed with cutaneously evoked extensor patterns of movement.[75,76]

Variations on the theme of exteroceptive reflex perversion are also found in association with brainstem and cerebral spastic motor dysfunction. Phenomena such as decerebrate posturing (unilateral or bilateral) to relatively trivial cutaneous stimuli, triple-flexion (i.e., dorsiflexion of great toe and foot with flexion at knee and hip) to stimuli at the distal involved lower extremity in some stroke victims, and incomplete versions of flexor reflexes seen with spinal spasticity are findings familiar to clinicians.

There has been relatively little physiologic study of exteroceptive reflexes in spastic states. Shahani and Young have examined spontaneous and evoked flexor reflex activity in normal subjects and in spinal and cerebral forms of human spasticity (see Chapter 3).[77,78] Their work has shown that normal reflex responses to submaximal electrical stimuli consist of two components. The first is associated with initiation of movement and the second corresponds to gross withdrawal of limb from stimulus. In spinal spasticity, similar stimuli produce a response with a lengthened latency that diminishes as stimulus strength is increased. A two-component response can sometimes be elicited, but generally at higher stimulus amplitudes. In cerebral spasticity, responses are nearly always single and prolonged. Normal recruitment patterns are retained in spontaneous flexor spasms.

Little is known about the physiology of exteroceptive reflexes in man. They are complex and polysynaptic, and involve FRA pathways that are strongly influenced by multiple descending systems. Further investigations of electrophysiology and pharmacology of human flexor reflexes in health and delineation of complex pathways mediating propriospinal and afferent spinal processing in primates should shed light on these interesting reflexes and their sometimes problematic clinical aberrancy.

IMPAIRED MOTOR CONTROL

While numerous pathologic CNS conditions cause loss of motor control without manifesting signs considered components of "spasticity," the states which give rise to spastic hyperreflexia and hypertonia would be considerably less problematic were it not for the attending impairment of willed movements (skilled or gross) or postural set. The spastic limb may or may not demonstrate loss of muscular power. But even the strong spastic limb shows abnormal fatigability and loss of agility or dexterity, while axial musculature displays impaired ability to adjust in accord to the demands of a skilled act or a normally correctible perturbation of balance. Synergies and other primitive motor behaviors may be prominent. Although such features are generally considered components of the "upper motor neuron syndrome" and not of "spasticity" per se, they are the disabling concomitants of lesions with which spasticity is associated (see Chapter 1).

Any attempt to explain the pathophysiology of motor dyscontrol in spasticity would be pretentious at this point. Nevertheless, a number of interesting and important observations have been made regarding relationships between motor function and spasticity in various pathologic or experimental states.

Clinical observations in victims of spastic "paresis" suggest that the final common denominator of motor disability after recovery from early effects of events such as capsular or cortical (and sometimes brainstem) infarction usually involves (at least) performance quality of isolated or fractionated movements, especially distally. What factors contribute to the loss of this ability?

The classic studies by Lawrence and Kuypers of pyramidotomy in rhesus monkeys illustrate the nature of deficit occurring after isolated (and unnatural) lesioning of a main direct corticospinal pathway. After recovery from flaccid paralysis, a striking degree of recovery of motor control occurs. But ability to perform isolated movements of fingers never returns. Such movements are also permanently abolished by ablation of the motor cortical area corresponding to the upper extremity.[79] Experimental ablation of areas 4 and 6 in monkeys yields a combination of effects seen after pyramidotomy along with profound initial flaccidity, which yields after many weeks to a hyperactive state.[80]

There is certainly a tremendous amount of variability in the motor deficits of persons with chronic CNS lesions of similar etiology. One of the factors underlying such individualization of deficit is surely the lack of pathologic homogeneity in nature. Developmental factors related to the age of the patient substantially affect outcome after CNS insult. Individual differences in CNS development within chronological age groups certainly contribute as well. Just as infants establish basic motor skills within a span of time that defines normalcy, individuals establish different levels of motor skills of all types with maturity. There must be neural substrates serving as foundations for such interindividual differences and a corollary should be that roughly equivalent CNS lesions (especially higher level cortical/subcortical ones) might have markedly different manifestations in an individual. One interesting study of cerebral palsy patients undergoing posterior rhizotomy for relief of spasticity assessed responses of dorsal rootlets to stimulation. The study demonstrated that the overall pattern of abnormal evoked motor responses in a given patient was fixed for that patient; i.e., there was a limited motor repertoire in a given individual that presumably reflects reorganization at the spinal level, which leaves some motor neurons accessible to facilitation by way of afferent pathways associated with different segmental levels in a given person.[81]

Veale's studies of Renshaw function in spastic states suggest a way that divorce from cortical (and/or subcortical) control could impair fractionated motor activity.[82] R-cells govern the early part of the MN excitability cycle. In the normal state, their recurrent inhibition allows a focusing of motor excitability on the neurons that are most active at a given time. However, they also mediate an indirect "recurrent facilitation" by inhibition of inhibitory Ia INs. In addition, they exert an inhibitory effect upon each other within adjacent areas, encouraging greater isolation of voluntary motor activity. Veale's work provided evidence that the inhibitory function of R cells is decreased in spasticity while their facilitory impact is increased both temporally and in magnitude. He suggested that R-cell mediated recurrent facilitation might be responsible for abnormal diffusion of activity within MN pools with a corresponding negative effect on fine motor control. Thus, in this view, loss of isolated motor control represents a failure of a motor focusing system.

The notion of hypertonicity masking latent motor control is familiar to anyone who has been involved in application of chemoneurolysis. With regard to spastic phenomena, this area is quite murky. Chemoneurolysis has resulted in improved motor control in Parkinsonism, other states perhaps best characterized as rigidity secondary to CNS lesion, and spasticity (see Chapter 11). Tanaka's work predicts that any therapy decreasing the Ia IN activity of antagonists might improve power within associated agonists. He postulates that in human cerebral spasticity, the release from descending control affects both flexor and extensor systems, but because effects of release are much stronger in physiologic extensor systems, flexor spasticity is masked by Ia IN mediated reciprocal inhibition.[83]

Does severity of clinical weakness correspond in any way with the loss of inhibitory effects that are presumably presynaptically mediated by means of afferents? The controlled study by Iles and Roberts of vibratory inhibition of soleus H reflexes in spastic subjects with residual voluntary function suggests that the loss of inhibitory effects corresponds to the degree of clinical weakness. As stronger voluntary contractions become possible among those with spasticity, however, even as measures of their strength approximate control values, spastic subjects fail to show the decrease in inhibition observed in controls during voluntary contraction.[84]

Such limited insights into motor phenomena related to human conditions associated with spasticity give some (though little) solace to those concerned with the care of afflicted patients. The ultimate measure of our knowledge of motor dyscontrol will be our ability to successfully apply principles derived from research to therapies in the human condition or alternatively to explain why we cannot risk testing potential therapies in humans. Meanwhile, there is an urgent need for cultivation of minds that will be capable (like Brooks[25]) of synthesizing the ever-growing wealth of information on motor control into synopses that form new departure points for future experimentation.

A GLIMPSE OF THE HORIZON

A review of the literature on motor control and the pathophysiology of spasticity suggests that with all that has been learned, we still know little. The position of the physiologist is compromised by the facts that:

1. Animal studies can not be duplicated in humans.
2. Nonprimate animal models of human spasticity may not exist.
3. Animal research in general (in this country) is increasingly threatened by the anti-vivisection movement.
4. Insufficient information precludes development of physiologically based computer models of motor control in humans that could explain spastic phenomena.
5. Diminishing research dollars for increasingly expensive physiologic research combined with absence of fiscal security are contributing to a decline in the numbers of students and clinicians who pursue research-oriented careers.

A potentially rich source of human anatomico-physiologic information does exist and is largely untapped. Collaboration among clinicians, neurophysiologists and neuropathologists could allow vigorous data gathering on cases that subsequently come to neuropathologic study. In vivo electrophysiologic and mechanical/physical studies of people affected by neurologic diseases continue to offer great promise, and well-designed studies along these lines deserve every possible encouragement from the academic and funding communities.

Answers to the following questions (among others) are anxiously awaited by clinicians involved in care of patients with motor disorders:

1. Is there any way to effectively diminish the "experience" of spasticity in a way that can lead to prevention or retardation of associated muscle changes and/or improve recovery of function?
2. How may intact structures and pathways be modified by experience (i.e., therapy), pharmacology, physical/electrical stimulation, or inhibition or surgical ablation to positively influence recovery of function in spastic motor disorder?
3. How, when, and why does chemical neurolysis work in spastic limbs?
4. Are there any physical or pharmacologic methods that might mitigate tissue effects associated with chronic spastic hypertonia?
5. What are beta motor neurons doing in man and what are the likely local and descending influences on them?
6. How do gamma motor neurons fit into the schema of motor learning and motor dyscontrol? What motor "repertoire" is possible among relatively spindle-free motor systems (such as facial muscles) in health and disease?

REFERENCES

1. Sherrington, C.S.: On plastic tonus and proprioceptive reflexes. Q. J. Exp. Neurol. 2:109–156, 1909.
2. Henneman, E.: Skeletal muscle: The servant of the nervous system. In Medical Physiology, ed. V.B. Mountcastle. 14th ed. St. Louis: CV Mosby Co., 1980.
3. Henneman, E.: Recruitment of motoneurons: the size principle. In Motor Unit Types: Recruitment and Plasticity in Health and Disease. Ed. J.E. Desmedt. Prog. Clin. Neurophysiol. 9:26–60, 1981.
4. Edstrom, L.: Relation between spasticity and muscle atrophy pattern in upper motor neurone lesions. Scand. J. Rehabil. Med. 5:170–171, 1973.
5. Emonet-Denand, F., Jami, L., and Laporte, Y.: Histophysiological observations on the skeleto-fusimotor innervation of mammalian spindles. In Spinal and Supraspinal Mechanisms of Voluntary Motor Control and Locomotion. Ed. J.E. Desmedt. Prog. Clin. Neurophysiol., 8:1–11, 1980.
6. Brodal, A.: Neurological Anatomy in Relation to Clinical Medicine. New York, Oxford University Press, 1981, p. 156.
7. Vallbo, A.B., Hagbarth, K.E., Torebjork, H.E., and Wallin, B.G.: Activity in human peripheral nerves. Physiol. Rev. 59:919–957, 1979.
8. Moore, J.C.: The Golgi tendon organ: a review and update. Am J. Occup. Ther. 38:227–236,1984.
9. Carew, T.J.: Spinal cord I: Muscles and mus-

cle receptors. *In* Principles of Neural Science. Ed. E.R. Kandel and J.H. Schwartz. New York, Elsevier/North-Holland, 1981, p. 298.

10. Hultborn, H., Illert, M., and Santini, M.: Convergence on interneurones mediating the reciprocal Ia inhibition of motoneurones. Acta Physiol. Scand. *96*:193–201, 1976.

11. Brooks, V.B.: The Neural Basis of Motor Control. New York, Oxford University Press, 1986, pp. 86–87.

12. Katz, R., and Pierrot-Deseilligny, E.: Recurrent inhibition of motoneurons in patients with upper motor neuron lesions. Brain *105*:103–124, 1982.

13. Eccles, R.M., and Lundberg, A.: Supraspinal control of interneurones mediating spinal reflexes. J. Physiol. *147*:565–584, 1959.

14. Kandel, E.R., and Schwartz, J.H. (eds.): Principles of Neural Science. New York, Elsevier/North-Holland, 1981, p. 302.

15. Jeneskog, T., and Johansson, H.: The rubrospinal path. A descending system known to influence dynamic fusimotor neurones and its interaction with distal cutaneous afferents in the control of flexor reflex afferent pathways. Exp. Brain Res. *27*:161–179, 1977.

16. Oscarsson, O.: Functional organization of spinocerebellar paths. *In* Somatosensory system. Vol. 2. Handbook of Sensory Physiology. Ed. A. Iggo. Berlin, Springer-Verlag, 1973.

17. Lundberg, A.: Function of the ventral spinocerebellar tract. A new hypothesis. Exp. Brain Res. *12*:317–330, 1971.

18. Brooks, V.B., op. cit., 1986, pp. 90–93.

19. Sherrington, C.S.: Decerebrate rigidity and reflex coordination of movements. J. Neurophysiol. (Lond.) *22*:319–332, 1898.

20. Brown, T.G.: The intrinsic factors in the act of progression in the mammal. Proc. R. Soc. Lond. Biol. Soc. *84*:308–319, 1911.

21. Brodal, A., op. cit., 1981, pp. 63–64.

22. La Motte, D.: Distribution of the tract of Lissauer and the dorsal root fibers in the primate spinal cord. J. Comp. Neurol. *172*:529–562, 1977.

23. Loeb, G.E.: The control and responses of mammalian muscle spindles during normally executed motor tasks. Exerc. Sport Sci. Rev. *12*:157–204, 1984.

24. Jankowska, E., Lundberg, A., Roberts, W.J., and Stuart, D.: A long propriospinal system with direct effect on motoneurones and on interneurones in the cat lumbosacral cord. Exp. Brain Res. *21*:169–194, 1974.

25. Brooks, V.B., op cit., 1986, pp. 82–109.

26. Rhines, R. and Magoun, H.W.: Brain stem facilitation of cortical motor responses. J. Neurophysiol. *9*:219–229, 1946.

27. Magoun, H.W., and Rhines, R.: An inhibitory mechanism in the bulbar reticular formation. J. Neurophysiol. *9*:165–171, 1946.

28. Granit, R.: The gamma loop in the mediation of muscle tone. Clin. Pharm. Ther. *5(6)*:837–847, 1964.

29. Pollock, L.J., and Davis, L.: Studies in decerebration, VI. The effect of deafferentiation upon decerebrate rigidity. Am. J. Physiol. *98*:47–49, 1931.

30. Brodal, A., op. cit., 1981, p. 200.

31. Brodal, A., op. cit., 1981, p. 184.

32. Brodal, A., op. cit., 1981, p. 187ff.

33. Evarts, E.V.: Relation of pyramidal tract activity to force exerted during voluntary movement. J. Neurophysiol. *31*:14–27, 1968.

34. Willis, W.D.: The raphe-spinal system. *In* Brainstem Control of Spinal Cord Function. Ed. C.D. Barnes. New York, Academic Press, 1984, pp. 141–214.

35. Fung, S.J., and Barnes, C.D.: Locus coeruleus control of spinal cord activity. *In* Brainstem Control of Spinal Cord Function. Ed. C.D. Barnes. New York, Academic Press, 1984, pp. 215–255.

36. Glaser, G.H., and Higgins, D.C.: Motor stability, stretch responses and the cerebellum. *In* Nobel Symposium I: Neuromuscluar Afferents and Motor Control. Ed. R. Granit, Almqvist and Wiksell, Stockholm. 1966, pp. 121–138.

37. Ebner, T.J., Bloedel, J.R., Vitek, J.L., and Schwartz, A.B.: The effects of stimulation of the stretch reflex in the spastic monkey. Brain *105*:425–442, 1982.

38. Penn, R.D.: Chronic cerebellar stimulation for cerebral palsy: A review. Neurosurg. *10*:116–121, 1982.

39. Adams, J.H., Corsellis, J.A.N., and Duchen, L.W., eds.: Greenfield's Neuropathology. 4th ed. New York, John Wiley and Sons, 1984.

40. Rushworth, G.: Some aspects of the pathophysiology of spasticity and rigidity. Clin. Pharmacol. Ther. *5(6)*:828–836, 1964.

41. Granit, R., op. cit., 1964.

42. Dietrichson, P.: The fusimotor system in relation to spasticity and Parkinsonian rigidity. Scand. J. Rehab. Med. *5*:174–178, 1973.

43. Gilles, J.D., Lance, J.W., Neilson, P.D. and Tassinari, C.A.: Presynaptic inhibition of the monosynaptic reflex by vibration. J. Physiol. (Lond.), *205*:329–339, 1969.

44. Degail, P., Lance, J.W., and Neilson, P.D.: Differential effects on tonic and phasic reflex

mechanisms produced by vibration of muscles in man. J. Neurol. Neurosurg. Psychiatry 29:1–11, 1966.

45. Delwaide, P.J.: Human monosynaptic reflexes and presynaptic inhibition. In New Developments in Electromyography and Clinical Neurophysiology. Ed. J.E. Desmedt. Karger, Basel. 3:508–522, 1973.

46. Ashby, P., and Verrier, M.: Neurophysiologic changes in hemiplegia. Neurology 26:1145–1151, 1976.

47. Ashby, P., Verrier, M., Carleton, S., and Somerville, J.: Vibratory inhibition of the monosynaptic reflex and presynaptic inhibition in man. In Spasticity: Disordered motor control. Ed. R.G. Feldman, R.R. Young, and W.P. Koeller. Chicago, Yearbook, 1980, pp. 335–344.

48. Ashby, P., and Burke, D.: Stretch reflexes in the upper limb of spastic man. J. Neurol. Neurosurg. Psychiatry 34:765–771, 1971.

49. McCouch, G.P., Austin, G.M., Liu, C.N., and Liu, C.Y.: Sprouting as a cause of spasticity. J. Neurophysiol. 21:205–216, 1958.

50. Chambers, W.W., Liu, C.N., and McCouch, G.P.: Anatomical and physiological correlates of plasticity in the nervous system. Brain Behav. Evol. 8:5–26, 1973.

51. Cannon, W.B., and Haimovici, H.: The sensitization of motoneurons by partial denervation. Am. J. Physiol. 126:731–740, 1939.

52. Burke, D.: A reassessment of the muscle spindle contribution to muscle tone in normal and spastic man. In Spasticity: Disordered motor control. Ed. R.G. Feldman, R.R. Young, and W.P. Koeller. Chicago, Yearbook, 1980, pp. 261–285.

53. Burke, D.: Critical examination of the case for or against fusimotor involvement in disorders of muscle tone. In Motor Control Mechanisms in Health and Disease. Ed. J.E. Desmedt, New York, Raven Press, 1983, p. 133.

54. Desmedt, J.E.: Mechanisms of vibration-induced inhibition or potentiation: tonic vibration reflex and vibration paradox in man. In Motor Control Mechanisms in Health and Disease. Ed. J.E. Desmedt. New York, Raven Press, 1983, p. 671

55. Lance, J.W.: Pathophysiology of spasticity and clinical experience with baclofen. In Spasticity: Disordered motor control. Ed. R.G. Feldman, R.R. Young, and W.P. Koeller. Chicago, Yearbook, 1980, pp. 185–203.

57. Dimitrijevic, M.R., Nathan, P.W., and Sherwood, A.M.: Clonus: The role of central mechanisms. J. Neurol. Neurosurg. Psychiatry 43:329, 1980.

58. Hagbarth, K.E., Wallin, G., Lofstedt, L., and Aquilonius, S.M.: Muscle spindle activity in alternating tremor of Parkinsonism and in clonus. J. Neurol. Neurosurg. Psychiatry 38:636–641, 1975.

59. Dimitrijevic, M.R., Nathan, P.W., and Sherwood, A.M., op. cit., 1980, pp. 321–332.

60. Rack, P.M.H., Ross, H.F., and Thilman, A.F.: The ankle stretch reflexes in normal and spastic subjects. Brain 107:637–654, 1984.

61. Veale, J.L., Rees, S., and Mark, R.F.: Renshaw cell activity in normal and spastic man. In Human Reflexes, Pathophysiology of Motor Systems, Methodology of Human Reflexes. Ed. J.E. Desmedt. New Devel. Electromyogr. Clin. Neurophysiol. 3:523–538, 1973.

62. Sherrington, C.S., op. cit., 1947.

63. Burke, D., Knowles, L., Andrews, C., and Ashby, P.: Spasticity, decerebrate rigidity and the clasp-knife phenomenon: An experimental study in the cat. Brain 95:31–48, 1972.

64. Lance, J.W., and Burke, D.: Mechanisms of spasticity. Arch. Phys. Med. Rehabil. 55:332–337, 1974.

65. Herman, R.: The myotatic reflex. Clinicophysiological aspects of spasticity and contracture. Brain 93:273–312, 1970.

66. Burke, D., Andrews, C., and Ashby, P.: Autogenic effects of static muscle stretch in spastic man. Arch. Neurol. 25:367–372, 1971.

67. Ralston, H.J., Inman, V.T., Strait, A., and Shaffarth, M.D.: Mechanics of human isolated muscle. Am. J. Physiol. 151:612–620, 1948.

68. Houk, J.C., and Rymer, W.Z.: Neural control of muscle length and tension. In Motor Control. Section 1, vol. 2. Handbook of Physiology. Ed. V.B. Brooks. Bethesda, MD, American Physiological Society, 1981, pp. 257–323.

69. Nichols, T.R., and Houk, J.C.: Reflex compensation for variations in the mechanical properties of a muscle. Science 131:182–184, 1973.

70. Gossman, M.R., Sahrmann, S.A., and Rose, S.J.: Review of length-associated changes in muscle. Phys. Ther. 62(12):1799–1807, 1982.

71. Gallego, R., Kuno, M., Nunez, R., et al.: Dependence of motorneuron properties on the length of immobilized muscle. J. Physiol. (Lond.) 291:179–189, 1979.

72. Herman, R.: The myotatic reflex. Clinicophysiological aspects of spasticity and contracture. Brain 93:273–312, 1970.

73. Hufschmidt, A., and Mauritz, K.H.: Chronic

transformation of muscle in spasticity: A peripheral contribution to increased tone. J. Neurol. Neurosurg. Psychiatry *48:*676–685, 1985.

74. Edstrom, L., op cit., 1973.

75. Young, R.R., and Shahani, B.T.: Spasticity in spinal cord injured patients. *In* Management of Spinal Cord Injuries. Ed. R.F. Block and A.I. Basbaum. Baltimore, Williams and Wilkins, 1986, pp. 259–263.

76. Kuhn, R.A.: Functional capacity of the isolated human spinal cord. Brain. *73(Pt.1):*1–50, 1950.

77. Shahani, B.T., and Young, R.R.: The flexor reflex in spasticity. *In* spasticity: Disordered motor control. Ed. R.G. Feldman, R.R. Young, and W.P. Koeller. Chicago, Yearbook, 1980, pp. 287–295.

78. Young, R.R., and Shahani, B.T.: A clinical neurophysiological analysis of single motor unit discharge patterns in spasticity. *In* Spasticity: Disordered motor control. Ed. R.G. Feldman, R.R. Young, and W.P. Koeller. Chicago, Yearbook, 1980, pp. 219–231.

79. Passingham, R., Perry, H., and Wilkinson, R.: Failure to develop precision grip in monkeys with unilateral neocortical lesions made in infancy. Brain Res. *145:*410–414, 1978.

80. Lawrence, D.G., and Kuypers, H.: The functional organization of the motor system in the monkey. I. The effects of bilateral pyramidal lesions. II. The effects of lesions of the descending brainstem pathway. Brain *91:*1–14, 15–36, 1976.

81. Barolat-Romana, G., and Davis, R.: Neurophysiological mechanisms in abnormal reflex activities in cerebral palsy and spinal spasticity. J. Neurol. Neurosurg. Psychiatry *43:*333–342, 1980.

82. Veale, J.L., Rees, S., and Mark, R.F.: op. cit., 1973.

83. Tanaka, R.: Reciprocal Ia inhibitory pathway in normal man and in patients with motor disorders. *In* Motor Control Mechanisms in Health and Disease. Ed. J.E. Desmedt. New York, Raven Press, 1983, pp. 433–441.

84. Iles, J.F., and Roberts, R.C.: Presynaptic inhibition of monosynaptic reflexes in the lower limbs of subjects with upper motoneuron disease. J. Neurol. Neurosurg. Psychiatry *49:*937–944, 1986.

3

NEUROPHYSIOLOGIC TESTING IN SPASTICITY

BHAGWAN T. SHAHANI
DIDIER CROS

In strictly physiologic terms, spasticity has been defined as a motor disorder characterized by a velocity-dependent increase in muscle tone, with exaggerated tendon jerks resulting from hyperexcitability of the stretch reflexes, as one component of the upper motor neuron syndrome (see Chapter 1).

This restricted physiologic definition does not include many other features of the upper motor neuron syndrome. These are negative symptoms such as weakness and loss of dexterity, and positive symptoms such as flexor spasms produced by abnormalities of flexor reflexes.

Although most clinical neurophysiologic techniques have been used to document changes in reflexes, there are some techniques that can provide quantitative analysis of negative symptoms produced by the upper motor neuron syndrome. Some of the techniques used to document negative and positive symptoms associated with spasticity and upper motor neuron syndrome are briefly described in this chapter as examples of clinical neurophysiologic methods that can be used in the practice of rehabilitation medicine and quantitative neurology.

EMG ANALYSIS OF NEGATIVE SYMPTOMS ASSOCIATED WITH UPPER MOTOR NEURON SYNDROME

EMG studies of patients with weakness caused by an upper motor neuron lesion show certain characteristic features. The total number of motor units that can be voluntarily recruited is reduced, and, with maximal voluntary effort, the rate of firing of single motor units is slower than that seen in weakness produced by lower motor neuron lesions. In some patients who have severe or complete paralysis of the upper motor neuron type, motor units can be activated only reflexly. For example, if the patient has a foot drop due to an upper motor neuron lesion, it may be possible to recruit more motor units by scratching the sole of the foot rather than by voluntary contraction. This places the lesion in the central nervous system (CNS) rather than in the motor neuron pools controlling the muscles responsible for dorsiflexion of the foot. To confirm that the lesion is in the CNS and not in the lower motor neurons, further studies can be performed to show that normal-size compound muscle action potentials can be recorded in weak or paralyzed

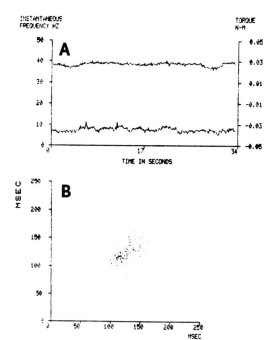

FIG. 3-1. Torque and instantaneous firing frequency (A), joint interval histogram (B) recorded from first dorsal interosseus of normal subject maintaining a constant force. Circular cluster of points reveals a random discharge pattern. Serial correlation coefficient r = −0.04 is statistically insignificant. Mean firing rate 11.7 Hz (Shahani, B.T., and Wierzbicka, M.M.: Electromyographic studies of motor control in humans. Neurologic Clinics 5:541–558, 1987).

dorsiflexors after electrical stimulation of mixed nerves supplying these muscles.

In addition to conventional EMG studies, residual motor capacity in patients with upper motor neuron lesions can also be documented by surface EMG recordings from the tibialis anterior and soleus muscles while the patient flexes and extends the ankle to 45 degrees between two fixed points at the greatest possible speed for 30 seconds.[1] In patients with upper motor neuron lesions, the rate of dorsiflexion and plantar flexion is reduced, whereas the duration of the EMG bursts in both tibialis anterior and soleus muscles is increased. In addition, some patients show evidence of clonus in the soleus muscle when the antagonistic tibialis anterior is being voluntarily activated during dorsiflexion.

Finally, statistical analysis of the behavior of single motor units (SMUs) can be performed using computerized techniques. One method that has proven useful for quantitating changes in the behavior of SMUs is plotting out the joint interval histogram (JIH).[2] In normal individuals, long and short intervals between consecutive discharges of a given motor unit tend to alternate, producing a negative serial correlation (Fig. 3–1); whereas in spastic patients with upper motor neuron lesions, long intervals are followed by long intervals and short intervals by short intervals (Fig. 3–2).[2,3] These trends in patients with upper motor neuron lesions are associated with positive serial correlation in the JIH.

Because of trends in interpotential interval durations, the data points representing SMU firing intervals in spastic patients tend

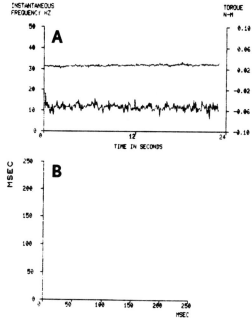

FIG. 3-2. Torque and instantaneous firing frequency (A) and joint interval histogram (B) recorded from first dorsal interosseus of spastic patient. A strong positive serial correlation (r = 0.67) reflects a short-term trend in the discharge pattern. Mean firing rate is 7.9 Hz (Shahani, B.T., and Wierzbicka, M.M.: Electromyographic studies of motor control in humans. Neurologic Clinics 5:541–558, 1987).

to cluster roughly at a 45-degree angle, producing an elongated oval shape rather than the circular one found in normal individuals. Interpotential intervals tend to remain relatively constant at a given time. The fine variations from interval to interval seen in normal people are absent in these patients. In contrast to patients with spasticity, patients with cerebellar ataxia have a rather irregular pattern of SMU firing resulting in a random scatter of dots on the JIH. It must be recognized that, in patients with spasticity, some muscle groups may be more severely affected than others. These changes are appropriately reflected in the behavior of SMUs as studied with the JIH. Not every motor unit in patients with upper motor neuron lesions behaves abnormally. Some units tend to behave like normal units. In some instances, it is possible to drive a slowly discharging motor unit potential to fire at high frequencies by extra voluntary effort with the help of EMG audiovisual feedback.

NEUROPHYSIOLOGIC ANALYSIS OF POSITIVE SYMPTOMS

Clinical neurophysiologic techniques have been used to study hyperreflexia associated with spasticity. Advances in electronic and computer technology have rendered possible the study and quantitation of reflex activity noninvasively in humans. Using these electrophysiologic techniques, one can record most of the reflexes (both proprioceptive and exteroceptive) commonly studied clinically. These studies, in addition to providing better insight into the underlying physiologic mechanisms, furnish an objective quantitative measure of the function of the central and peripheral nervous systems in man.

The application of clinical neurophysiologic techniques using conventional EMG, nerve conduction studies or late responses to evaluate dysfunction of the CNS may appropriately be termed "central EMG."[4] Some of the neurophysiologic approaches used to evaluate abnormalities of different reflexes in spasticity are described in the following sections.

H REFLEX AND F RESPONSE STUDIES

In 1918, Hoffmann[5] demonstrated that the compound muscle action potential associated with ankle and knee jerks was comparable in latency and configuration to that evoked by submaximal electrical stimulation delivered percutaneously to the tibial or femoral nerves, respectively. He concluded that both tendon jerks and electrically induced late responses represented activity in the same kind of stretch reflex. On the basis of his findings, which included abolition of the late response with supramaximal stimulation to the mixed nerve and relatively brief latency of the late response, he concluded that the afferent part of this reflex consisted of fast conducting nerve fibers, and that the central delay was extremely short.

The conclusions from Hoffmann's remarkable experiments were confirmed many years later by Magladery and McDougal,[6] who designated the electrically induced late responses the H reflex after its discoverer. The shorter latency compound muscle action potential (CMAP) evoked by direct electrical stimulation of motor axons was called the M response. In contrast to the large amplitude H reflex, which could be easily recorded in calf muscles following submaximal stimulation, another type of late response was seen in intrinsic muscles of the hands and feet. This late response, which had a latency rather similar to that of the H reflex (but was not reflex), was named the F wave (or F response). F responses, as recorded in the EMG laboratory, are caused by centrifugal discharges from individual motor neurons, each of which is initiated by an action potential propagated antidromically.[7–10] H reflex and F response studies have recently been used to evaluate peripheral nerve function. They have also been used in the evaluation of CNS dysfunction, particularly in patients with upper motor neuron lesions and spasticity.

The most commonly used tests are as follows: (1) Comparison of the maximum amplitude of an H reflex with the maximum amplitude of the compound muscle action potential in the same muscle (H max/M max ratio); (2) Excitability curves of the H reflex; (3) Vibratory inhibition of the H reflex; (4) Comparison of the mean F response with the maximum amplitude of the compound muscle action potential (F mean/FM max ratio); (5) F response persistence.

RATIO OF H MAX TO M MAX. The maximum amplitude of an H reflex is recorded by delivering a series of single electrical stimuli to the tibial nerve at the popliteal fossa. A recording is made by placing surface electrodes over the soleus muscle. The stimulus intensity is adjusted to produce the maximum amplitude H reflex. The maximum amplitude of the compound muscle action potential is obtained in the usual manner by delivering a supramaximal stimulus to the tibial nerve in the popliteal fossa. The H max/M max ratio reflects the percentage of motor neurons in the soleus motor neuron pool that can be reflexly activated by an electrical stimulus delivered to the tibial nerve in the popliteal fossa.

When the excitability of the motor neuron pool is increased, as in upper motor neuron lesions, a great percentage of motor neurons are activated, the amplitude of the H reflex is increased, and the H max/M max ratio is greater than normal. In conditions in which the excitability of the motor neuron pool is decreased, as in spinal shock, it may be impossible to record an H reflex (ratio = 0), or, when the H reflex is recordable, the H max/M max ratio is lower than normal.

EXCITABILITY CURVES. H reflex excitability curves following double stimulation of the tibial nerve at the popliteal fossa have been studied in various neurologic disorders. In these studies, the amplitude of the H reflex elicited by the second test stimulus is plotted as a function of the interval between conditioning and test stimuli. Such curves exhibit characteristic hypo- and hyperexcitable phases in normal subjects.[11,12] The excitability curves are often altered in patients with CNS lesions. It must be emphasized, however, that H reflex excitability curves are particularly affected by such independent variables as the position of the patient

and the amount of ballistic voluntary reflex activity. To obtain reproducible results, the subject must be still, relaxed, and in a comfortable position, and the limb must be rigidly fixed at various joints at appropriate angles to avoid tinges of proprioceptive input. In studies of H reflex excitability curves, it is important to elicit a small preceding M response of constant amplitude and shape from one stimulus to the next, as a proof of the stability of the relationship between the nerve and the stimulating electrode. Some studies have shown that when the two stimuli (conditioning and test stimulus) are delivered at the same site in the nerve, they do not necessarily reflect changes in the central excitability.[13] Local changes in excitability of the peripheral nerve itself can give rise to excitability curves resembling the H reflex recovery curves of patients with CNS lesions. Plotting of H reflex excitability curves elicited by double stimulation at the same site is therefore not recommended. If one wishes to use this technique, it is important that the conditioning stimulus be delivered at a different site along the same nerve or to a different nerve.

VIBRATORY INHIBITION OF THE H REFLEX. When the muscle of a normal individual is vibrated during elicitation of phasic proprioceptive reflexes, the reflexes are significantly inhibited (Fig. 3–3). This vibratory inhibition of the H reflex is diminished in patients with chronic spasticity.[14] It has been suggested that the vibratory suppression of the H reflex may be caused by presynaptic inhibition. Effects of vibration as studied in human subjects, however, are probably more complex (see Chapter 2).

Under standardized conditions, it is possible to calculate an index of vibratory inhibition as follows: H max (vibrated)/H max $\times$ 100.

F RESPONSE AMPLITUDE AND PERSISTENCE. F response studies can provide a measure of the excitability of the spinal motor neurons.[15] In patients with acute CNS lesions, F response occurs with decreased persistence and/or amplitude on the affected side (Fig. 3–4). These abnormalities of F responses corre-

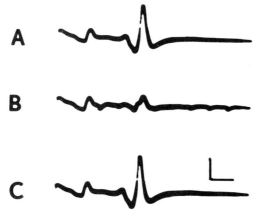

FIG. 3-3. H reflex in the paretic leg before (A), during (B), and after (C) vibration in a patient with a severe motor system deficit studied 3 days after onset of lesion. Note prominent suppression of H reflex by vibration. Calibration: 500 µV and 10 msec (Fisher, M.A., Shahani, B.T., and Young, R.R.: Electrophysiological analysis of the motor system after stroke: the suppressive effect of vibration. Arch. Phys. Med. Rehab. *60*:11–14. 1979, with permission).

late clinically with severe weakness, decreased tone, and depressed tendon reflexes. In patients with chronic spasticity, amplitude and persistence of F responses may be increased in affected muscles.

FLEXOR REFLEXES

One method of assessing human spinal cord function is to study the flexor reflexes recorded electromyographically from the tibialis anterior (TA) in response to electrical stimulation applied to the sole of the foot or directly to the flexor reflex afferents in the tibial nerve at the level of the ankle. Using this method, certain specific physiologic differences can be documented between the reflex behavior underlying spasticity caused by spinal cord lesions and that resulting from hemispheric lesions.

In normal individuals, two EMG components regularly make up the flexor reflex, the first with lower threshold than the second. Detailed studies of SMU behavior have shown that both components arise

from TA and often involve the same motor units. Latency of the first component ranges from 50 to 60 msec, whereas the second component may begin at a latency of 110 to more than 400 msec, depending on stimulus strength. Increasing the stimulus strength decreases the latency and increases the amplitude and duration of both components. Although the latency of the first component may decrease by 10 to 20 msec,[16,17] that of the second component may decrease over a much wider range (more than 100 msec). It is sometimes impossible to see two separate components, especially when supramaximal stimulation is delivered.

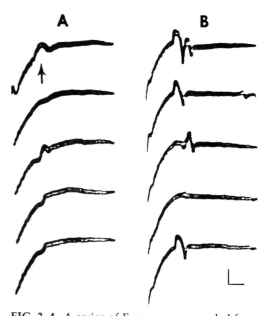

FIG. 3-4. A series of F responses recorded from the thenar eminence following supramaximal stimulation of the median nerve at the wrist. The M response at the rest of each sweep is too high to be photographed at this amplification. The patient had suffered an acute hemiplegia. A is the paralyzed side, B the normal side. The F responses (arrow) on the clinically involved side are considerably less than on the uninvolved side. Calibration 200 µV, 10 msec (Fisher, M.A., Shahani, B.T., and Young, R.R.: Assessing segmental excitability after acute rostral lesions: I. the F response. Neurology *28*:1265–1271, 1978, with permission).

When the two discrete EMG bursts in the flexor muscles are present at submaximal stimulation, simultaneous recording of the mechanogram depicting dorsiflexion of the foot shows that the first component produces a brief, small-amplitude twitch, while the second component is associated with gross withdrawal of the limb. With supramaximal stimulation, however, the time interval between the two reflex components is rather brief, and the mechanogram shows a smooth, continuous movement corresponding to the appropriate withdrawal of the limb.

It appears that the physiologic role of the first component is to initiate the movement quickly, whereas the second component is responsible for continuing and maintaining the withdrawal of the limb from the nociceptive stimulus. It is possible that the strategy used by the CNS to produce stereotyped voluntary ballistic movements during a visual matching task is similar, because EMG components bearing resemblance to the two components of the flexor reflex are regularly seen in those instances.[18,19]

In patients with complete transection of the spinal cord, low-threshold afferent stimulation often produces a flexor reflex with a continuous EMG activity and a latency of 300 to 400 msec. Latency decreases as larger stimuli are delivered, so that a minimum latency of 60 to 80 msec is regularly obtained in different patients. Segmentation of the EMG burst in two components is not seen, however. During the early phase of recovery from spinal shock, a distinct first component with a latency of 50 to 65 msec may be seen. However, the stimulus threshold for evoking the first component of the flexor reflex is always higher than that required for the second component. The first component can also be seen occasionally with supramaximal stimulation in some patients with partial lesions of the spinal cord.[19]

In patients with discrete lesions of the cerebral hemispheres resulting in hemiplegic spasticity, the flexor reflex shows a rather different pattern from that seen in normal persons, with some differences from patients with spinal cord lesions as well. Simultaneous recordings from the flexor and extensor muscles (TA and gastrocnemius-soleus, respectively) show that the electrically elicited flexor reflex in TA often produces a sudden stretch of gastrocnemius-soleus, resulting in clonic activity in that muscle. Each of the EMG bursts in the gastrocnemius-soleus coincides with the transient depletion of activity in TA, suggesting that reciprocal inhibition is preserved in patients with hemisphere lesions. Such reciprocal inhibition is usually not seen in patients with complete transection of the spinal cord. A discrete first component is rarely seen, even in the acute stage, and long, painful trains of stimuli of high intensity produce a prolonged burst rather than the two agonist components seen in normal subjects.[15]

Among the abnormalities of flexor reflexes that have attracted much clinical attention are flexor spasms. When considered from almost any viewpoint, they are extremely variable. The magnitude of the phenomenon varies from activation of an SMU firing at 5 to 10 Hz to that of many units firing together to produce a full recruitment pattern. Studies of the behavior of SMUs show that smaller, lower-threshold units are recruited before larger, higher-threshold units, and the single motor unit that is recruited first is the last to be derecruited. Thus the size principle of recruitment is well-preserved in flexor spasms.[19] Detailed studies of consecutive interpotential intervals are in progress and may help to document differences between normal individuals and patients with lesions at different levels of the neuraxis.

Oral administration of baclofen (30 to 100 mg per day), in addition to being clinically effective, produces significant changes in the electrically evoked flexor reflexes. There are longer intervals between spontaneous flexor spasms, and the apparent threshold, both electrical and mechanical, rises sharply while the patient is receiving this drug. The effect is observed within the first 24 hours after the agent is given by mouth, and equally dramatic results are produced beginning 2 to 3 hours after intravenous injection. The minimal flexor reflex latency (mean of 10 measurements) on supramaximal stimulation of the foot increases from a pretreatment range of 60 to 80 msec to 90 to 120 msec or sometimes even more. In a few patients with partial lesions of the spinal cord, supramaximal stimulation may produce a reflex with two discrete components, giving it the appearance of a normal two-component flexor reflex. On the whole, patients in whom the EMG activity is confined to flexor muscles, and who show release of H reflexes during the flexor spasm, tend to do better with this medication than those who have increased stretch reflexes and do not show these features.

NEUROPHYSIOLOGIC ASSESSMENT OF RECURRENT INHIBITION

Recurrent inhibition, initially studied by Renshaw,[20] is an example of negative feedback whereby a recurrent collateral branch of the alpha motor axon activates a population of interneurons (Renshaw cells), which in turn inhibit neighboring motor neurons (Chapter 2).

This schema must be completed to include more recent information. Renshaw cells inhibit not only alpha motor neurons, but also other Renshaw cells,[22] gamma motor neurons,[23] and the Ia inhibitory interneurons responsible for the disynaptic reciprocal inhibition.[24] This leads to the concept of a spinal functional unit including alpha and gamma motor neurons innervating a muscle as well as the Ia interneurons inhibiting the antagonistic muscle. The components of this system are modulated by parallel control mechanisms, so that the linkage between alpha and gamma motor neurons[25] can be extended to the corresponding Ia interneurons.[26] Because of similarities in the distribution of recurrent inhibition on the three components of this functional unit, there is a possibility that supraspinal centers exert their influence through modulation of Renshaw cell excitability, which would give a crucial role to this descending input in motor control mechanisms.

Haase and colleagues[27] have suggested that decreased recurrent inhibition could be one of the factors leading to decerebrate rigidity in the cat. Similarly, reduction in recurrent inhibition may be responsible for the increased gain of the stretch reflex seen in spasticity. This hypothesis has been tested by an elegant method[28,29] applied to spastic patients.[30]

The method is as follows: the Renshaw cells are activated by a conditioning H reflex (H1) elicited by a conditioning stimulus S1, and the resulting recurrent inhibition assessed by a second H reflex (H2) elicited by a test stimulus (S2). S2 is supramaximal for the alpha motor axons, and therefore, when applied alone, induces an antidromic volley in alpha motor axons that collides with, and cancels, the H reflex elicited by Ia fiber activation. This is not the case when S2 is preceded by a conditioning stimulus (S1) also eliciting an H reflex. In this situation, if the S1-S2 timing is appropriately chosen, an H reflex (H2) will be recordable in response to S2. This reflex represents the activity of motor neurons that have already fired in response to the conditioning stimulus S1. The resulting action potentials have collided with the antidromic action potentials elicited by S2, and these axons are then able to propagate to the periphery the impulses corresponding to the H2, the H reflex elicited by the test stimulus. As the amplitude of H1 increases, there is a progressive decrease in the amplitude of H2, which has been shown to be due to the increase in recurrent inhibition caused by the conditioning reflex.[29]

Ninety-five spastic patients were compared with 31 controls at rest and during motor activities known to change the degree of recurrent inhibition.[30] With patients at rest, no evidence for a decrease in recurrent inhibition was found, but rather an increase was documented in 55 of the 95 patients. The changes in recurrent inhibition known to occur in normal individuals during postural muscular activity or voluntary contraction were not found in spastic patients.

Two conclusions can be drawn from this study. On one hand, decrease in recurrent inhibition is not responsible for the increase in the stretch reflex in spasticity. On the other hand, the lack of modulation of Renshaw cell activity during posture and movement could account for difficulties shown by spastic patients, such as grading the strength of a contraction and regulating reciprocal inhibition during voluntary movements.

CENTRAL CONDUCTION TIME DETERMINATION

In 1980, Merton and Morton[31] described electrical, transcranial stimulation of the human motor cortex. Their method is based on high-voltage electrical stimulation delivered through a pair of stimulating electrodes attached to the scalp. The cathode is placed at the vertex, and the anode over the cortical area to be stimulated. Motor-evoked potentials are readily recordable from distal muscles, and, when central stimulation is combined with peripheral stimulation at the neck encompassing the quasi-total length of the lower motor neuron,[32,33] a central conduction time (CCT) is easily calculated by subtraction (Fig. 3–5).

Barker et al.[34] constructed a magnetic stimulator suitable for studies in humans. This type of stimulator delivers a magnetic pulse of 1.5 to 2.5 teslas. The rapidly varying magnetic field induces an electrical field in volume conductors, including the brain. The current induced within the skin, which is a bad conductor, is low, resulting in a near-painless mode of stimulation adequate for clinical studies, whereas transcranial electrical stimulation is often experienced as quite uncomfortable.

Both methods have been used extensively in several European countries in recent years, and no ill effect of either of the techniques has been reported thus far.

Abnormal central motor conduction times (CMCTs) have been found in several conditions known to often cause spasticity. These include multiple sclerosis,[35,36] amyotrophic lateral sclerosis,[37,38,39] myelopathies caused by cervical spondylosis,[40] and spinal cord trauma.[40] In multiple sclerosis, abnormal CMCTs were found in 72% of 60 patients. Abnormal CMCT correlated well with brisk finger flexor jerks, and was found in 79% of patients with weakness of the abductor muscle of the fifth finger, compared to 54% with a normal muscle.[36] In this series, visual-evoked potentials were abnormal in 67%, somatosensory-evoked potentials abnormal in 59%, and brainstem auditory-evoked potentials abnormal in 39% of those tested. For each of these procedures, more subjects had abnormal CMCTs and normal evoked potentials than the reverse, suggesting that CMCT determination is of value for documenting upper motor neuron lesions in multiple sclerosis.[36]

Abnormal CMCT was also found in amyotrophic lateral sclerosis[37–41] and, on occasion, no recordable response was obtained on cortical stimulation in spite of recordable responses on peripheral stimulation. The factors responsible for these findings are more complex than those responsible for slowing along peripheral

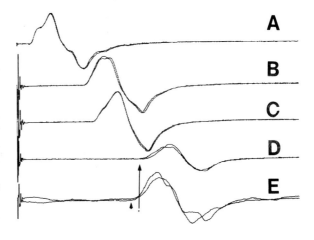

FIG. 3–5. Compound muscle action potential of abductor digiti minimi: electrical stimulation at the wrist (A). Magnetic stimulation at Erb's point (B), cervical spine, 5th cervical vertibra (C), cortical stimulation at the vertex without voluntary contraction (D), cortical stimulation at the vertex with voluntary contraction (E). Arrowhead = onset latency with facilitation; arrow = onset latency without facilitation. Calibration: 10mV and 20 msec.

nerves. They have been discussed in detail recently.[40] Correlation between weakness and spasticity on the one hand, and abnormal CMCT on the other hand, clearly requires additional investigations, but represents a new research avenue in the field.

The neurophysiologic abnormalities described in the preceding paragraphs are helpful in defining alterations in the motor system on the basis of reproducible criteria. It is hoped that these methodologies will lead to better identification of individual components of spasticity and rigidity, which might then be treatable in a relatively specific manner.

REFERENCES

1. Delwaide, P.J.: Contribution of human reflex studies to the understanding and management of the pyramidal syndrome. *In* Central EMG. Ed. B.T. Shahani. Boston, Butterworth, 1984.
2. Young, R.R., and Shahani, B.T.: A clinical neurophysiological analysis of single motor unit discharge patterns in spasticity. *In* Spasticity: Disordered Motor Control. Ed. R.G. Feldman, R.R. Young, and R.R. Koella. Chicago, Yearbook, 1980.
3. Young, R.R., and Wierzbicka, M.: Behavior of single motor units in normal subjects and in patients with spastic paresis. *In* Clinical Neurophysiology of Spasticity. Ed. P.J. Delwaide and R.R. Young. Amsterdam, Elsevier, 1985.
4. Shahani, B.T. (ed.): Electromyography in CNS Disorders: Central EMG. Stoneham, Butterworth, 1984.
5. Hoffman, P.: Über die Beziehungen der Sehnenreflexe zur willkurlichen Bewegung und zum Tonus. Z. Biol. *68*:351–370, 1918.
6. Magladery, J.W., and McDougal, D.B.: Electrophysiological studies of nerve and reflex activity in normal man. 1-Identification of certain reflexes in the electromyogram and the conduction velocity of peripheral nerve fibers. Bull. Johns Hopkins Hosp. *86*:265–282, 1950.
7. Dawson, G.D., and Merton, P.A.: Recurrent discharges from motoneurons. XXth International Physiological Congress, Brussels, 1956.
8. Mayer, R.F., and Feldman, R.G.: Observations on the nature of the F wave in man. Neurology (Minneap.) *17*:147–155, 1967.
9. McLeod, J.G., and Wray, S.H.: An experimental study of the F wave in the baboon. J. Neurol. Neurosurg. Psychiatry *29*:196–202, 1966.
10. Thorne, J.: Central responses to electrical activation of the peripheral nerves supplying the intrinsic hand muscles. J. Neurol. Neurosurg. Psychiatry *28*:482–488, 1965.
11. Paillard, J.: Réflexes et régulations d'origine proprioceptive chez l'homme. Etude neurophysiologique et psychophysiologique. Paris, Arnette, 1955.
12. Taborikova, H., and Sax, D.S.: Conditioning of H reflexes by a preceding subthreshold H reflex stimulus. Brain *92*:203- 227, 1969.
13. Potts, F.A., and Young, R.R.: Long-term poststimulus reduction in axon excitability when tested with submaximal electrical stimulus in vitro and in vivo. Soc. Neurosci. Abstr. *7*:188, 1981.
14. Lance, J.W., De Gail, P., and Neilson, P.D.: Tonic and phasic spinal cord mechanisms in man. J. Neurol. Neurosurg. Psychiatry *29*:535–544, 1966.
15. Fisher, M.A., Shahani, B.T., and Young, R.R.: Electrophysiological analysis of the motor system after stroke: the suppressive effect of vibration. Arch. Phys. Med. Rehabil. *60*:11–14, 1979.
16. Shahani, B.T.: Flexor reflex nerve afferents in man. J. Neurol. Neurosurg. Psychiatry *33*:786–791, 1970.
17. Shahani, B.T., and Young, R.R.: Human flexor reflexes. J. Neurol. Neurosurg. Psychiatry *34*:616–627, 1971.
18. Hallett, M., Shahani, B.T., and Young, R.R.: EMG analysis of stereotyped voluntary movements in man. J. Neurol. Neurosurg. Psychiatry *38*:1154–1162, 1975.
19. Shahani, B.T., and Young, R.R.: The flexor reflex in spasticity. *In*: Spasticity: Disordered Motor Control. Ed. R.G. Feldman, R.R. Young, and R.R. Koella. Baltimore, Yearbook, 1980.
20. Renshaw, B.: Influence of discharge of motoneurones upon discharge of neighboring motoneurones. J. Neurophysiol. *4*:167–183, 1941.
21. Eccles, J.C., Fatt, P., and Koketsu, K.: Cholinergic and inhibitory synapses in a pathway from motor-axons collateral to motoneurones. J. Physiol. (London) *126*:534–562, 1954.

22. Ryall, R.W.: Renshaw cell-mediated inhibition of Renshaw cells: patterns of excitation and inhibition from impulses in motor axon collaterals. J. Neurophysiol. 33:257–270, 1970.

23. Ellaway, P.H.: Recurrent inhibition of fusimotor neurones exhibiting background discharges in the spinal and decerebrate cat. J. Physiol. (London) 216:419–429, 1971.

24. Hultborn, H., Jankowska, E., and Lindstrom, S.: Recurrent inhibition from motor axon collaterals of transmission in the Ia inhibitory pathway to motoneurones. J. Physiol. (London) 215:591–612, 1971.

25. Granit, R.: The Basis of Motor Control. London, Academic Press, 1970.

26. Hultborn, H.: Convergence on interneurones in the reciprocal Ia inhibitory pathway to motoneurones. Acta Physiol. Scand. Suppl. 375:1–42, 1972.

27. Haase, J., Kuckuck, L., and Noth, J.: Disinhibition der Extensor-Motoneurone nach intercollicularer Dezerebrierung. Pflugers Arch. 317:148–158, 1969.

28. Pierrot-Deseilligny, E., and Bussel, B.: Evidence for recurrent inhibition by motoneurons in human subjects. Brain Res. (Amsterdam) 88:105–108, 1975.

29. Bussel, B., and Pierrot-Deseilligny, E.: Inhibition of human motoneurons, probably of Renshaw cell origin, elicited by an orthodromic motor discharge. J. Physiol. (London) 269:319–339, 1977.

30. Katz, R., and Pierrot-Deseilligny, E.: Recurrent inhibition of alpha motoneurons in patients with upper motoneuron lesions. Brain 105:103–124, 1982.

31. Merton, P.A., and Morton, H.B.: Stimulation of the cerebral cortex in the intact human subject. Nature 285:287, 1980.

32. Mills, K.R., and Murray, N.M.F.: Electrical stimulation over the human vertebral column: which neural elements are excited? Electroencephalogr. Clin. Neurophysiol. 63:582–589, 1986.

33. Santamaria, J., King, P.J.L., Cros, D., and Chiappa, K.H.: Cervical magnetic stimulation: Roots or spinal nerves? Neurology 38 (Suppl.):199, 1988.

34. Barker, A.T., Jalinous, R., and Freeston, I.L.: Non-invasive magnetic stimulation of the human motor cortex. Lancet ii:1106–1107, 1985.

35. Cowan, J.M.A., et al.: Abnormalities in central motor pathway conduction in multiple sclerosis. Lancet ii:304–307, 1984.

36. Hess, C.W., Mills, K.R., Murray, N.M.F., and Schriefer, T.N.: Magnetic brain stimulation: Central motor conduction studies in multiple sclerosis. Ann. Neurol. 22:744–752, 1987.

37. Ingram, D.A., and Swash, M.: Central motor conduction is abnormal in motor neuron disease. J. Neurol. Neurosurg. Psychiatry 50:159–166, 1987.

38. Hugon, J., et al.: Central motor conduction in motor neuron disease. Ann. Neurol. 22:544–546, 1987.

39. Schriefer, et al.: Personal communication.

40. Thompson, P.D., et al.: The electrical and electromyographic responses to electrical stimulation of the motor cortex in diseases of the upper motor neurone. J. Neurol. Sci. 80:91–110, 1987.

41. Berardelli, A.: Stimulation of motor tracts in motor neuron disease. J. Neurol. Neurosurg. Psychiatry 50:732–737, 1987.

4 MOTOR LEARNING AND RELEARNING

JOHN WHYTE
JOAN MORRISSEY

Upper motor neuron lesions produce a varied cluster of motor abnormalities, including weakness, loss of coordination, alterations in muscle tone, and alterations in reflex patterns. Although spasticity in itself may be a significant clinical problem, it is usually only one element of impaired motor performance. In other words, upper motor neuron lesions rarely result in the simple addition of spasticity to normal motor behavior. Rather, spasticity appears in conjunction with other motor deficits. It is the sum of all these deficits that causes a given pattern of disability.

Treatment of patients with the upper motor neuron syndrome is generally aimed at maximization of motor performance in general. Thus, it might include attempts to increase strength, improve coordination, alter reflexive patterns, and decrease spasticity. Any treatment intervention, therefore, must be understood in terms of its effects on the motor control system, not simply on spasticity.

Patients without active movement in a spastic limb represent the simplest case of anti-spasticity treatment. Here the issue is not to alter or improve motor control, but rather to decrease disability associated with the positive symptoms of spasticity. Thus, a patient might develop contractures due to persistent limb posturing, injure extremities during flexor or extensor spasms, or suffer from hygiene or skin problems caused by

maceration between adducted limbs or flexed joints. Treatment that decreases abnormal tone in such instances will translate directly into lessened disability.

Many patients with an upper motor neuron syndrome have some residual motor function. Treatment in such cases is more complex. Although spasticity may be a problem in the ways described above, more often the treatment agenda in decreasing spasticity is to improve active movement and optimize motor control. To do this successfully, one must have a sophisticated understanding of normal mechanisms of motor control and an understanding of how spasticity relates to normal or abnormal motor function.

In clinical work, it is common to see patients with significant spasticity in a limb which has only slight active movement. Treatment of such patients might be based on one of three perspectives, simplified here for purposes of illustration:

1. The decreased active movement is *caused by the spasticity* in the sense that the patient is attempting to move against a great resistance. Thus, if spasticity is decreased, active movement automatically increases.
2. The decreased active movement is *caused by other aspects of the upper motor neuron syndrome* (e.g., loss of neural connections subserving voluntary move-

44

ment). Treatments designed to improve strength and coordination, however, are impeded by the presence of spasticity. Thus, if spasticity is decreased, treatment of active movement is facilitated.

3. The decreased active movement is *caused by other aspects of the upper motor neuron syndrome* (as in 2). Moreover, spasticity is a completely irrelevant finding. Thus, the success of treatments designed to improve voluntary movement depends completely on the severity of the impairment in voluntary movement and treatment of spasticity has no effect on motor progress.

These simplified perspectives illustrate the importance of understanding the relationship between spasticity and other aspects of the upper motor neuron syndrome. Such understanding would be expected to allow selection of patients in whom treatment of the spasticity would have significant effects on skilled movement. Along these lines, research on hemiplegics demonstrates a rough correlation between the degree of spasticity and the degree of weakness of the upper extremity. The pattern of EMG activity during active movement, however, is *not* consistent with the hypothesis that spasticity is the obstacle to strength.[1] Rather, it appears that both spasticity and weakness, in this instance, are manifestations of the primary problem: the upper motor neuron syndrome.

NORMAL DEVELOPMENT OF SKILLED MOVEMENT

Motor development is a process of continuous modification caused by neurologic growth and maturation, residual effects of previous experiences, and effects of new motor experiences. Motor development occurs in an ordered sequence, which may provide information about the organization and operation of the systems responsible for skilled motor behavior. The following description of motor development should be kept in mind as various proposed models of skilled motor behavior are subsequently presented.

The first movements and postural responses of the infant are reflexive in character and stimuli result in total body movements (e.g., Moro reflex).[2] As the child progresses, these reflexive responses become more differentiated and subjugated to selective voluntary control. Thus movement begins with multi-joint, multi-muscle responses, which only later become more isolated and selective.

In early stages of development, movement tends to traverse the full joint range. There is an oscillation between extremes of range of motion. As integration occurs, direction and range of movement become more refined. This may serve to allow the child to discover the force relationships among muscle groups throughout their available range.

The sequence of development proceeds as illustrated in Figure 4–1.[2] In general, a child who can maintain a given posture can move in postures from earlier developmental stages. However, a child does not perfect earlier postures until moving on to later ones. This suggests that these developmental stages are not discrete entities which can be perfected in isolation. Rather, the learning about more advanced motor skills contributes in a continuous way to the advancement of prior skills. From a clinical point of view, this also suggests that perfection of lower-level skills may not be a prerequisite for moving on to more challenging tasks.

Development also reveals the intimate connection between the maturation of postural and movement skills. The typical sequence proceeds from mobility to stability to controlled mobility to distal skilled movement with proximal stabilization. Children are able to move their arms, legs, and trunk before being able to maintain a stable posture (e.g., when a standing child reaches for an object and topples over).[3] Although a stable shoulder and trunk are necessary for skilled hand use, and stable lower extremities are necessary for mobile upper extremities, the developmental sequence allows exploration of movement patterns *before* maturation of postural stability. This suggests that postural stability must develop *in relation to* the movement patterns it must support.

The end result of normal development is

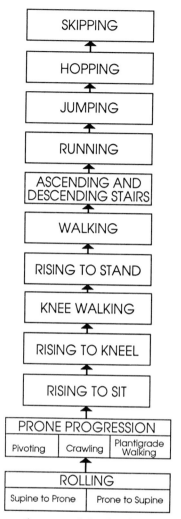

FIG. 4–1. Motor milestones of the developmental sequence.

a vast repertoire of coordinated movements and movement combinations. Examination of the developmental sequence can reveal the natural hierarchy of difficulty within the motor control system (e.g., that control of mass movements is "easier" than isolated control). There is no a priori reason to believe that clinical strategies for the remediation of impaired mobility must recapitulate the normal developmental sequence. To the extent that the same hierarchy of difficulty applies to the damaged nervous system, however, the developmental hierarchy may reveal clinically useful information about the building blocks of skilled movement.

THEORETIC MODELS OF SKILLED MOVEMENT

REQUIREMENTS OF A MOTOR CONTROL SYSTEM

Skilled movement is a remarkable phenomenon, allowing human beings to implement a broad array of plans and goals through the final common pathway of muscle contraction and limb segment motion. Remarkable as this is on the surface, a closer inspection of the requirements of a motor control system highlights the complexity involved. The "simple" act of opening a door requires separate but coordinated rotations at the shoulder, elbow, radioulnar, and wrist joints (ignoring the fingers).[4] The speed and axis of rotation at each joint changes over time. This requires the appropriate activation of 33 muscles, 16 of which operate across more than one joint. Furthermore, an even larger number of muscles stabilizing the legs and trunk and coordinating the fingers must participate. In addition, a door can be opened from different starting angles and at different speeds, each of which will require alterations in the motor program.

Before examining theories of skilled movement, it will be helpful to consider all the performance phenomena for which any such theory must account, as well as the neural machinery which might participate in such a control system. Any motor control theory under consideration must be able to account for the following aspects of skilled movement:

1. Improvement over time (skill development) in the speed, accuracy, and smoothness of a movement.
2. The ability to perform movements under conditions of plentiful or limited sensory feedback.
3. The ability to perform a particular skilled movement under varying environmental conditions (e.g., different angles, speeds, forces).
4. The ability to store the details of a movement program in memory.
5. The ability to perform movements which involve multiple limb segments and multiple limbs at multiple speeds.
6. The ability to specify movement goals at

a general (e.g., "approach a goal via walking, crawling, or running") or specific (e.g., "approach a goal on a bicycle at 30 km/hr on South Street") level

7. The ability to perform skilled movements with relatively little conscious monitoring (automaticity).

CNS COMPONENTS PARTICIPATING IN SKILLED MOVEMENT

Skilled movement involves the participation of many brain systems working in complex coordination. These elements are represented schematically in Figure 4–2. The frontal motor cortex participates in voluntary movement. Movement is elicited by electrical stimulation of its cells and paralysis results from damage to the frontal motor cortex.[5] Each motor hemisphere is capable of controlling proximal movements of either side of the body but distal movements only of the contralateral side.[6] The number of pyramidal cells firing during small, precise movements is larger than during gross movements, suggesting that the averaging of activity of many neurons facilitates precision of control.[7] The distinc-

tion between motor and sensory cortex is graded rather than absolute as evidenced by the ability to elicit movement with electrical stimulation of the sensory cortex at somewhat higher thresholds.[8] Furthermore, the motor cortex receives sensory information directly from dorsal column afferents synapsing in the thalamus, as well as from sensory association fibers from the sensory cortex.[9] The extrapyramidal system is more diffusely organized but involves the participation of the basal ganglia, and a variety of subcortical structures.[10]

The cerebellum and basal ganglia, long known for the coordination of skilled movement, appear to be involved in the initiation of highly practiced movements. The firing of cerebellar and basal ganglia neurons *precedes* the firing of motor cortex cells in skilled movement.[11,12] There are massive neural connections from cortex to cerebellum and basal ganglia and reciprocally from basal ganglia and cerebellum (by way of the thalamus) to the cortex. Furthermore, neither the cerebellum nor the basal ganglia sends fibers to synapse directly in the spinal cord, so their activity must be relayed by way of either the cortex or the brainstem extrapyramidal system.[11]

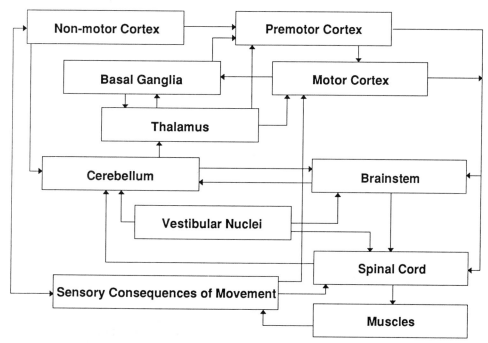

FIG. 4–2. CNS components of skilled movement.

Although these three structures operate as an integrated unit, it appears that the basal ganglia are particularly critical for slow, graded movements, whereas the lateral cerebellum guides rapid ballistic movements, which can be preplanned independently of external feedback.[11,13] The pars intermedia of the cerebellum, in contrast, does participate in feedback-dependent movement by providing continuous corrective outputs.[13,14]

Thalamic and midbrain nuclei are both believed to organize integrated patterns of movement.[15] Electrical stimulation in either region produces a "purposeful" behavior. The particular motor behavior produced by medial thalamic stimulation however, varies with the environmental context, whereas stimulation of midbrain centers produces an invariant behavior regardless of context.

All of the above neural systems must ultimately exert their influence, directly or indirectly, on cells within the spinal cord. Alpha motor neurons are electrically silent in the absence of actual movement. Neurons of the pyramidal tract, however, have tonic and fluctuating activity specifically related to the *intention* to perform a particular movement.[11] The spinal cord is not merely a passive recipient of instructions from above. There are numerous and familiar reflexive patterns organized wholly within the spinal cord (see Chapter 2). Furthermore, there is growing evidence of complex pattern generators within the cord that can produce time-dependent neural outputs to multiple muscle groups. In the decerebrate cat, a central locomotor pattern generator can produce reciprocal limb movements. Severed efferent nerve roots continue to discharge in rhythm. Passive movement of the cat's paralyzed limbs can reset this pattern generator in synchrony with the passive rhythm.[4]

Sensory systems are also critical to motor control. Visual, vestibular, and somesthetic systems provide information which is integrated into slow movements requiring feedback or which provides corrective action when more automatic movements are suddenly disturbed. For example, if a subject is descending stairs and suddenly is placed in free fall by the removal of a step, a burst of EMG activity occurs in the calf muscles as extensor compensation. This burst does not occur in patients without detectable vestibular function.[16]

The sources of proprioceptive feedback are many and varied, including the static and dynamic spindle afferents, the Golgi tendon organs, the joint receptors, and skin afferents.[4] Each source of information is ambiguous in terms of its ability to specify precisely limb position, velocity, or force of movement, and much controversy remains regarding exactly how this afferent information is coherently decoded. Furthermore, proprioceptive, visual, and vestibular systems influence one another's activity, with vision usually playing a dominant calibrating role in humans.

In addition to the familiar motor and sensory systems described above, there are more cognitive aspects of motor control. Any movement, whether novel or practiced, must be initiated. That is, there must be some linkage between motivation, or will, and production of a motor program. There is evidence of prefrontal cortical involvement in this translation of motivation to movement, by way of connections with the basal ganglia and limbic system.[17] In addition, characteristic hippocampal rhythms are associated with certain activity patterns.[15] In animals, rhythmic slow activity (RSA) occurs as a burst with the onset of *any* voluntary activity and continues at a lower amplitude throughout that activity. RSA amplitude is proportional to the intensity of total movement. Large-amplitude irregular activity (LIA), in contrast, occurs at rest *or* during biting, chewing, licking, emotional expression, or pelvic thrusting, suggesting that these motor behaviors are organized quite differently.

Motor memory is also crucial for skilled movement. The benefit of practice in perfecting motor control must be understood in terms of storage of the profits from that practice. It is clear, however, that such storage occurs in at least two quite different spheres. Conscious memory involves the recognition of a familiar situation and the conscious decision to invoke a motor strategy which has been successful in the past. This type of memory is absent in patients with global amnesia due to hippocampal or thalamic damage.[18] In contrast, the ability to perform a specific motor task more rapidly or smoothly with practice can occur in the presence of amnesia, despite the fact that the patient does not recognize ever having performed the task before.[19] This suggests that some aspects of motor (unconscious) memory are intrinsic to the sensory motor system itself.

If one uses a broad definition of motor behavior, virtually the whole central nervous system participates in a coordinated and integrated fashion. Aspects include motivation and goal setting, the selection of certain broad patterns of movement, the precise control of individual muscles, the preparatory and compensatory postural adjustments, the sensory feedback, and the learning and remembering. Because of this highly complex network of interacting systems, damage to the motor control system should not be thought of as damaging one self-contained element of the system. Rather, any CNS damage that affects skilled movement is likely to have broad effects on the entire network of motor control.

THEORIES OF SKILLED MOVEMENT

Having considered the complex phenomena that must be explained by any theory of skilled movement, as well as the neural mechanisms available to control such behavior, it is appropriate to evaluate some representative theories of skilled movement.

AN ADDRESS-SPECIFIC CONTROL MODEL

The most conceptually simple model of skilled movement is predicated on the notion that motor commands, emanating from the motor cortex, descend directly to anterior horn cells in the spinal cord and produce contraction of the desired motor units. In turn, sensory feedback from the periphery informs the cortex about the progress of the movement and allows correction and initiation of the next step. Thus, one could think of a "keyboard" of cortical motor cells "playing" a pattern on the muscular system, as illustrated in Figure 4–3. Each

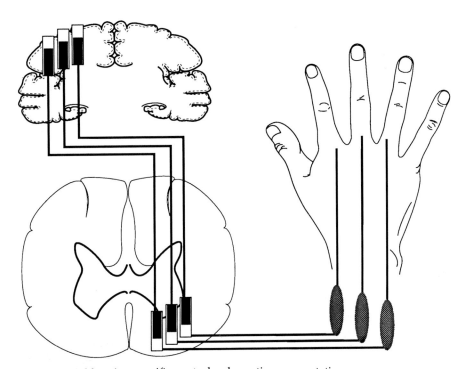

FIG. 4–3. Addressing specific control: schematic representation.

motor unit corresponds to a specific "address" within the motor cortex. No sophisticated student of motor control would accept such a simple model of motor control, but it seems to underlie, unspoken, many clinical notions which stress isolated volitional control of specific motor units in the development of motor skill. Consideration of the strengths and weaknesses of this model will reveal common conceptualizations inherent in clinical thinking.

There is some evidence that direct voluntary control over motor units is possible. There are monosynaptic connections between cells in the motor cortex and anterior horn cells in the spinal cord,[20] and subjects can learn to voluntarily control single motor units in response to feedback from needle EMG signals.[21] Thus, the required circuitry for an address-specific model is present. Furthermore, some relatively novel or slow movements appear to be controlled in a closed-loop fashion, in which sensory information about the course of movement serves to allow continuous correction of the movement in progress, which would be compatible with an address-specific model.[22]

The address-specific model fails to account for a wide range of experimental data, however. Evidence described above suggests that motor development begins with gross multi-segment movements, out of which more discrete movements develop. This is the opposite of what would be expected from address-specific models in which multiple discrete movements would be gradually added together during development. Many rapid and complex movements occur too fast for peripheral feedback at each step to allow production of the next step, indicating that entire movement sequences must be preplanned relatively independently of feedback.[23]

Even in slow movements there is evidence that the available sensory feedback is too ambiguous or gross to provide precise guidance for the continuation of movement. Joint receptors, the least ambiguous source of position information, do not fire informatively throughout the range of motion, and the receptors adapt to a given position so that a specific firing rate does not reliably indicate a specific position.[23] Total joint replacement impairs perception of passive but not active movement.[23] Spindle afferents cannot differentiate position and force information.[24]

If skilled movements cannot effectively be guided by "on-line" sensory feedback, then the address-specific model would have to allow for preprogrammed movement sequences to be stored and executed from the motor cortex. There is, however, much evidence that repetitions of even highly practiced "identical" movements are far from identical. The act of lowering the arm against resistance will be performed with the shoulder adductors, whereas the act of passively lowering the arm slowly against gravity will be performed by the shoulder abductors. Contraction of the hamstrings will flex the knee if the foot is free, but extend the knee if the foot is planted. Similarly, performing the same movement at different speeds can involve quite different motor commands. Abducting the arm slowly may involve fairly isolated and continuous contraction of the shoulder abductors; doing so quickly involves a rapid burst of activity in the abductors followed by a decelerating burst in the adductors and a final burst in the abductors again.

All these examples illustrate the point that each of the minute variations in a common movement requires substantially different motor programs because of differences in movement context. This introduces the need to store different prepared motor programs in memory for each variation, as well as a sophisticated selection mechanism to identify the appropriate variation for the current context.

The degrees of freedom involved in programming even an individual, simple movement represent an additional problem for the address-specific model. Degrees of freedom are all the independent decisions which must be made to specify fully the operation of a system. An analogy from a simpler system, the airplane, may be of help.[25] An airplane has two wing flaps, two tail flaps, and one vertical rudder on the tail, giving it five degrees of freedom. (Fig. 4–4) In reality, each of these flaps can be controlled through a continuous arc rather than in discrete settings, but for the sake of sim-

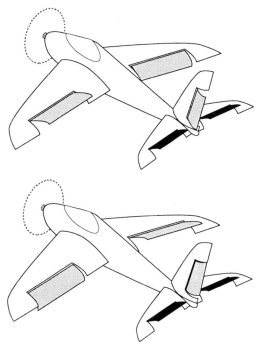

FIG. 4-4. Degrees of freedom and the use of a coordinative structure (adapted with permission from Turvey, M.T., Shaw, R.E., and Mace, W.: Issues in the theory of action: Degrees of freedom, coordinative structures, and coalitions. Requin, J. (Ed.): Attention and Performance VII, Hillsdale, NJ, Lawrence Erlbaum Assoc., 1978, p. 570).

plicity, suppose that each flap can be set in eight different positions. This would mean that there are 8^5 settings of all the plane's flaps, or 32,768 possibilities in controlling the trajectory of the plane. From the pilot's point of view, every change of course involves selecting the one correct setting from the 32,768 options available, a rather formidable task. In the case of the musculoskeletal system, degrees of freedom are great for a number of reasons.

Ball and socket joints can move throughout a path which covers most of the surface of a sphere, depending on which combination of muscles is active across the joint. Therefore all the possible combinations of activity of the relevant muscles must be specified to control the limb segment. Even hinge joints are complicated to control when one considers that many muscles

cross more than one joint. Again, the combination of the activities of all the muscles which cross either joint must be specified.

If each cortical motor cell controls a particular motor unit that can be used in many different movements depending on what other motor units are concurrently active, calculating the precise pattern of activation becomes a computational nightmare. There is, in fact, direct evidence that pyramidal neuron activity reflects which muscle groups are active, not in which direction a joint is moving. Thus, the cortical activity pattern for eccentric elbow extension is comparable to that for elbow flexion, indicating that one neural structure can control different physical activities.[11] In addition, some identical movements can be controlled by completely different neural structures in different contexts. For example, the hemiplegic patient who cannot smile symmetrically on command may do so in response to a humorous event, suggesting that the cortical system is relevant only in the first context.[15]

It is apparent that the address-specific model, which is built on the notion of voluntary control of individual motor units, is unworkable. The relationship between which motor units are active and what movement will occur is complex and highly dependent on contextual factors. Yet the way out of this difficulty, on-line feedback control, is too slow and imprecise to account for the fluidity, flexibility, and speed of skilled movement. It appears, then, that we must think of models which, although conceptually more complex, make fewer computational and feedback demands on the motor control system.

A MOTOR SCHEMA MODEL

Motor schema theory was introduced in an attempt to solve the problem of specifying completely different motor programs for each minor variation of a movement.[26] A motor schema is the specification of a *relationship* between motor commands, environmental contexts, and resulting movements.

Schemas can exist at any level of abstraction or detail. An abstract schema for "approach" could invoke more specific schemas for ambulation, running, crawling, bicycling, etc. In each case, however, the movement is in the same direction (toward the object being approached), and the termination of the movement is the same (when the object is reached). Furthermore, the approach schema can specify the relationship between the movement strategy chosen and the speed of approach (e.g., faster for running than walking). Indeed, there is evidence of movement triggering systems in the hypothalamus which are so general that they lead only to increased or decreased overall motor activity.[15]

Reconsideration of the act of opening a door illustrates a more specific schema. The finger flexion required to grasp a door knob will depend on the knob's size and shape. The arm movements required to open the door depend on the angle at which the door is approached. Schema theory would not require a separate program for every different doorknob and every different angle of approach. Rather, it would specify the *relationship* between degree of finger flexion and doorknob size, or between angle of approach and arm muscle activity. Thus, one schema can subserve all these variations if the environmental circumstances are assessed. Combining schemas at different levels of abstraction/specificity and allowing more abstract schemas to select more specific ones in their service permit complex skills to be controlled.

A particularly attractive feature of schema models, in addition to requiring fewer motor programs, is their ability to cope with movement variations which have never before been experienced. If a doorknob of an unfamiliar size is encountered, address-specific models would have to rely on reverting to feedback-controlled movement. Schema models, however, would be able to take the information about doorknob size and extrapolate the appropriate degree of finger flexion because these models use relationships between instructions and outcomes rather than specific lists of instructions.

There is evidence in support of schema models of motor skill. With practice in a task such as motor tracking, where a subject must control a moving cursor to track a moving target, a schema of the task requirements develops in stages. Initially the subject is in a compensatory phase, constantly seeking to correct the error between the cursor and target. Next the subject is able to predict short portions of the target's trajectory and introduce periodic corrections when the prediction fails. Finally, the subject acquires a complete mental schema of the path of the target and produces an analogous path with the cursor, using feedback only to synchronize the two fully specified patterns.[27]

Practice often involves experimentation with various different motor schemas and variations on them to select the optimal motor strategy. Thus, practice may not produce smooth increments in skill, but may reveal discrete bursts of control from quite distinct motor schemas until one (presumably the most efficient) comes to predominate.[28]

Further evidence for schema models comes from an examination of such tasks as handwriting. One's signature is nearly always written with the dominant hand. Yet one can produce a signature on a blackboard using gross arm movements, in the sand with one's toe, or with a brush held between the teeth. All these signatures will be characteristic of the individual even if performed for the first time.[29] This may be explained by the linkage of an abstract schema for signing one's name, which specifies the *relationship* between vertical (flexion/extension) and horizontal (abduction/adduction) components of movement, with a specific schema for foot or arm control, which specifies the particular muscle groups involved.

Further evidence of the generality of schemas comes from bimanual interference tasks. A subject is asked to perform a specific movement with one hand. Another interfering movement is then performed with either the same or the opposite hand. This movement is interfering in the sense that it prevents the subject from maintaining the characteristics of the original movement in immediate memory. When the subject is asked to reproduce the original movement, it makes no difference whether the interfering movement was made with the same or the opposite hand.[30] This demonstrates that the movement memory is stored not in terms of the specific extremity's muscles but in a more general form applicable to either extremity.

Most motor programs include specifications of movement course (which muscle groups will be activated) and timing (what will be the relationship between activation patterns in different muscles). It is apparent that some motor schemas place course above timing in the control hierarchy (e.g., ambulation involves the same muscle groups controlled at varying speeds) while others place timing above course (e.g., writing involves the same timing relationship among potentially different muscle groups).

There is evidence that practice is more conducive to schema development if it incorporates many task variations. That is, a highly stereotypic practice setting results in a less complete representation of the relationships of interest because few *different* examples of the relationship have been encountered. It might, for example, be predicted that a batter who practices against a pitching machine that pitches identically each time will make less progress than one practicing against a human pitcher. In the latter case, the batter can explore the relationship between the velocity or angle of the pitch, and the optimal swing strategy. Experience with movement variability may also be one of the functions of a child's experimentation with extremes of range of motion. Practicing movements throughout the available range may facilitate the development of the richest motor control schemas.

A great deal of practice may be required to develop a richly elaborated schema capable of directing a complex skill with minimal feedback. A study of workers in a cigar factory illustrates this point. Practice over two years and 3,000,000 instances produces slow but steady improvement in cigar rolling skill.[31] Apparently a great many minor variations in the task (e.g., the size, shape, stiffness, angle of the tobacco leaves) must be experienced before a fully elaborated schema capable of efficiently handling all examples of the task is developed.

Schema theory helps to explain the previously described finding of symmetric facial expressions in emotional situations but not on command in many hemiplegics. Because schemas are not lists of specific muscle contractions, it is possible for two distinct schemas for smiling to exist: one for smiling in response to humor and another for smiling on command. These, in turn, may activate different control structures, one of which is operative and the other impaired.

Address-specific control models make predictions that are clearly disconfirmed by much experimental work in motor skill. Schema theory is much more successful in handling the complexities, flexibility, and variability in skilled movement. Yet schema theory is much less specific about the relationship between the psychology of motor control and the neurophysiology involved. This represents its central weakness. Once a schema for handwriting is developed, where and how is it stored? How does this schema ultimately activate specific motor units in their appropriate relationships? When an abstract schema calls on a more specific one, how does it do so, and how is the particular one selected?

Exploration of the address-specific model has illustrated the fact that simple descending control emanating from the motor cortex is an unworkable means to the execution of skilled movements. But schema theory has largely abdicated the realm of neurophysiology and attempted to describe, at a conceptual level, how movements must be controlled. What remains to be identified is a model that bridges the gap between the psychologic programming requirements of motor skills and their neurophysiologic execution.

COORDINATIVE STRUCTURE MODELS

Every movement involves the regulation of joints and muscles with tremendous numbers of degrees of freedom, as previously discussed. The address-specific model breaks down under the computational load of this problem. The schema models address the problem of degrees of freedom conceptually but do not clarify how the actual degrees of freedom inherent in muscles and joints are handled for the purposes of motor control. The concept of coordinative structures is an attempt to come to terms with the fundamental problem of degrees of freedom in skilled movement. In many ways, the schema and coordinative structure models are similar, differing mainly in semantics and emphasis. Schema theories focus at the level of movement psychology whereas coordinative structure theories focus on movement physiology.

Turvey et al[25] define a coordinative structure as, "a group of muscles, often spanning several joints, constrained to act as a unit." Reconsideration of the airplane analogy (Figure 4–4) will illustrate this concept.

It is possible to link the flaps of the plane into a coordinative structure. Suppose the flaps are linked to each other via cables and these cables are controlled by a single joy stick. In Figure 4–4, the two wing flaps and the vertical tail flap are linked into a single coordinative structure as indicated by the grey shading. The two horizontal tail flaps are linked together into an independent coordinative structure as indicated by the black shading. When the joy stick is moved to the left (as in the top panel), the left wing flap moves up, the right one down, and the vertical tail flap to the left, together resulting in the plane banking to the left. In the bottom panel, the joy stick has been moved to the right in order to bank to the right. Note that in both cases, the horizontal tail flaps are set (independent from the banking coordinative structure) to allow the plane to climb, by moving the joy stick in the vertical axis. This linkage reduces the number of degrees of freedom to 2 (vertical and horizontal stick movements) and, with 8 different positions available in each axis, the number of possible settings is now 2^8 or 64, a much more manageable information load for a pilot.

The notion here is that some amount of flexibility of movement can be exchanged for much greater simplicity of control and decision making, without losing much in the way of skill. At the anatomic level, this can be seen by comparing hinge joints to ball-and-socket joints. The former are much more constrained, but much simpler to control. Most of the time the constraint poses no problems because motion is usually in the plane of the hinge joint. If one wishes to ambulate laterally, however, one must turn one's body rather than revolve one's knees and ankles, which would be possible if they were ball-and-socket joints.

In the case of motor coordinative structures, we are discussing coordinated control, which results from innate neurophysiologic linkage (i.e., a given neural structure controlling two or more muscle groups in a fixed manner), or from learned and less permanent linkage (i.e., learning to control two or more muscle groups in a fixed manner within a specific task), rather than linkages resulting from the physical properties of muscles and joints.

Muscle groups can be linked in different ways at different times and thus participate in more than one coordinative structure. Different coordinative structures are referred to as different *structural* prescriptions for movement, whereas different degrees of activation of a single coordinative structure are referred to as different *metric* prescriptions for movement.[25] The diaphragm and intercostal muscles form a coordinative structure during breathing in that the timing and degree of contraction of the two are innately linked. Fuller inhalation, or inhalation against a greater resistance, increases activity of both muscle groups, but their activity levels remain fixed in ratio. This is referred to as a single structural prescription, which varies in its metric prescription. In another movement, such as lateral trunk bending, however, the intercostal muscles might form a coordinative structure with the paraspinal muscles rather than the diaphragm, resulting in a different structural prescription. Thus, structural prescriptions describe the *relationship* among participating muscles, whereas metric prescriptions describe the *magnitude* of activity within the fixed combination of participating muscles.

There is much evidence for the existence of coordinative structures that are "hardwired," that is, whose common control is related to fixed patterns of innervation. The simplest of these is in the pattern of motor unit recruitment. Even within a single muscle, in theory one could recruit motor units in any order, resulting in a tremendously complex decision about how many and which units to use for each level of force in each task. It is clear, however, that the order of recruitment is fixed (at least in the case of one movement at different intensities) on the basis of neuronal size and sensitivity.[4] A particular muscle, then, is recruited according to a specific structural prescription and its force generation is regulated by a metric prescription. Swallowing is another example of a hard-wired coordinative structure.[32]

There is also much evidence for coordinative structures in ambulation. The central locomotor pattern generator in cats controls the oscillating movements of a variety of muscles according to a common timetable (structural). Its stimulation serves to increase the magnitude and rate of all components in synchrony (metric).[4] Furthermore, stimulation of the motor cortex in freely moving animals has different effects depending on the phase of movement when the stimulation occurs.[25] Thus stimulation cannot be directly controlling movement, but might be stimulating the coordinative structure currently activated.

Movement synergies are also examples of coordinative structures.[4] They suggest relatively rigid patterns of coactivation of multiple muscles, varying in magnitude. It should be noted that a particular muscle may participate in more than one synergy, however, so control of a particular muscle is redundant and can occur through multiple coordinative structures. Similarly, the spinal withdrawal reflex is a coordinative structure organized at the spinal level.[4] Because of the participation of individual muscles in multiple coordinative structures, it is believed that interneurons in the spinal cord and higher centers must be involved in the inhibition of some coordinative structures and facilitation of others.

There is also considerable evidence for the use of coordinative structures in voluntary skilled movements. In manual tasks, the hand generally follows a straight line trajectory to its target.[33] From a geometric point of view, this is surprising because flexion/extension is occurring simultaneously at the shoulder, elbow, and wrist. It appears, however, that the degree of flex-

ion/extension at each of these joints is linked in a coordinative structure in such a way that calculations about the hand's trajectory are simplified.

In speech, articulatory movements occur in coordinative structures. A particular collection of phonemes (the elemental sounds of the language) appears to be linked and controlled as a unit even when the word receives more or less stress.[32] Because different languages involve variations in phonemes and their combinations, it seems likely that these coordinative structures are formed through extensive practice rather than being innately specified.

Many of the tasks discussed within the framework of schema theory can be reinterpreted in terms of coordinative structures. If one develops coordinative structures for flexion/extension and abduction/adduction in each limb segment during development and practice, the task of producing a signature with any limb becomes much simpler, requiring conversion of a shape template into the *metric* prescription which controls the *structural* prescriptions for vertical and horizontal movements.

Research also suggests the use of hard-wired coordinative structures to simplify the control of voluntary movements. Lifting a heavy weight with the wrist extensors is facilitated by turning one's head toward the lifting hand. Lifting the weight with the wrist flexors is facilitated by turning one's head away.[29] Figure 4–5 illustrates this point. A subject is asked to lift a heavy weight repeatedly using either wrist flexors or extensors. The amount of weight lifted on successive bouts (expressed in relation to the amount lifted in the first bout) decreases because of fatigue. The pace of this fatigue, however, is affected by head position, and this effect is reversed depending on whether wrist flexors or extensors are being used. This suggests that the asymmetric tonic neck reflex (an innate coordinative structure) can assist in the performance of voluntary activities.

Athletes appear to discover ways to make use of innate reflexes and coordinative structures. Subjects in the above experiment tended to adopt the most efficient head posture even if not instructed to do so.

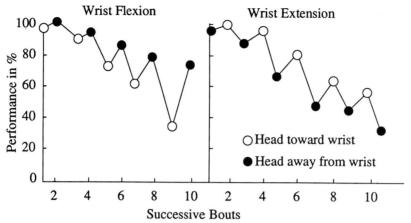

FIG. 4-5. The voluntary use of an innate coordinative structure (reprinted with permission from Keele, S.W.: Behavioral analysis of movement. *In* Brooks, V.B. (vol. Ed.): Handbook of Physiology, Section 1, Volume 2, Bethesda, MD, American Physiological Society, 1981, p. 1410).

Observation of judo postures and baseball pitcher windups suggests that some of the "extraneous" movements seen in athletics serve to activate coordinative structures that are useful for the particular activity.[29] Even in an activity as basic as ambulation, there is evidence that subjects initiate a "trigger movement" that includes contraction of the tibialis anterior. This produces stretch on the plantar flexors, which results in a stretch reflex contraction of the plantar flexors. This, in turn, initiates the gait cycle.[34] Perhaps the most "voluntary" aspect of ambulation is the trigger movement.

Timing and rhythm form the bases for other coordinative structures. There is evidence for rhythm generators in the central nervous system that provide a basis for coordinating the timing of different muscle groups involved in a complex movement.[35,36] In manual movements to a target, the speed of movement is related to the size of the target and its distance from the starting point. Consequently, if a subject is asked to move the two hands to different targets of different sizes and distances, one would predict that the hands would travel independently and arrive at their targets at different times. In reality, however, the hands depart and arrive at their targets simultaneously and reach their peak velocities and accelerations in synchrony, as illustrated in Figure 4–6.[37] Apparently, the anticipated movements of the two hands are formed into a *single* coordinative structure and this composite structure is controlled by a single clock.

The above examples should clarify how the permanent or temporary linkage of muscles into coordinative structures can simplify movement control. Another simplification, heterarchical control, is also important. A hierarchic control system implies that a top level executive system controls a lower system which controls a lower system, and so on. Thus ultimate control always rests with the top component, and no subcomponent ever controls its superordinate. This has been likened to a computer program in which the high-level language calls on subroutines which may, in turn, call on subroutines.[4] Hierarchic systems require that a great deal of information be supplied to the top level controller, leaving little autonomy to the subcomponents, and leaving subcomponents "ignorant" of the activity of other components above or lateral to them.

Turvey and colleagues present another route to simplified control: heterarchies. Heterarchies are flexible control networks in which dominance of control can switch depending on context. Thus the control of a given active movement is partly deter-

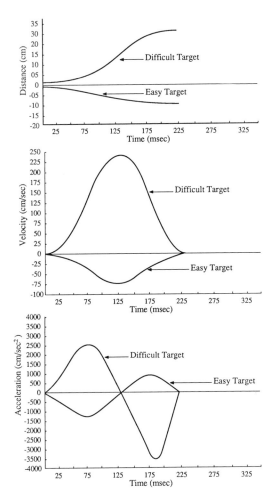

FIG. 4-6. Timing as the basis of movement coordination (reprinted with permission from Kelso, J.A.S., Southard, D.L., and Goodman, D.: On the coordination of two-handed movements. J. Exp. Psychol. (Hum. Percept.) 5(2):229–238, 1979, p. 236).

mined by the state of the postural system preceding it. In turn, the active movement helps to determine the postural state which will follow it. The active movement controls and is controlled by postural factors.[25]

If a subject stands on two platforms that suddenly move up together, the EMG pattern generated in response suggests a bilateral stretch reflex in the plantar flexors. If, however, one platform moves up while the other moves down, the pattern generated appears to derive from the locomotor gen-erator. The type of coordinative structure activated depends on the postural factors which precede it. Combining the notions of coordinative structures and heterarchies allows more powerful models of skilled movement.

Flexion movements of an animal's leg occur differently under the influence of learned conditioning versus cortical stimulation. In the former, lifting the leg is preceded by some extension of the leg, which shifts the center of gravity off the leg, allowing it then to lift safely. Flexion induced by cortical stimulation, in contrast, is not preceded by extension, and often results in the animal falling over its flexed leg.[38] In normal voluntary flexion, therefore, there is heterarchical control between postural mechanisms so that the initial limb extension controls a change in posture which in turn facilitates limb flexion. Developmental evidence, too, supports the interrelatedness of posture and movement. Development of postural stability occurs as the movements that it supports are explored. Further perfection of prior developmental stages occurs even as new stages are active, suggesting that there is a mutual learning cycle between postural and movement development.

Furthermore, there is much evidence that local perturbations in ongoing activities are compensated for at a variety of levels from the spinal stretch reflex to automatic central adjustments, in activities as different as ambulation, manual activities, and speech.[4,39–41] Thus, most voluntary skills allow regulation of different aspects at multiple levels of the nervous system without requiring hierarchic control of all of the compensatory adjustments.

Models of motor skill that include coordinative structures to simplify control and heterarchies to decentralize it can go a long way in addressing the complexities of human motor skill. Many questions, however, remain unanswered. Neurophysiologically, one might postulate that the coordinative structure is, in fact, a set of interneurons that link the motor neurons of the relevant muscles. Thus the structural prescription depends on the ratio of activity of the motor neurons linked by a specific set of interneurons. Metric prescriptions could occur by varying the amount of voluntary activation of the controlling interneuronal network.

This model does not directly answer how these linkages are made. Presumably some are anatomic in nature, such as, for example, the development of a respiratory center with outflow to the appropriate muscles. Others, however, must be acquired through learning and motor experience. How are these linkages made? At what level or levels of the central nervous system are new coordinative structures formed? Do newly learned coordinative structures control motor neurons directly, or simply link lower level coordinative structures into ever more complex patterns?

Perhaps of greatest clinical importance in rehabilitation is the question of how much flexibility exists in acquiring new coordinative structures throughout life and following CNS damage. There is evidence, for example, that there is a critical period for learning the unique sounds of a new language. This might be described as a critical period for forming the relevant articulatory coordinative structures. Is there a similar limitation on the ability to form new coordinative structures following CNS damage?

If the tendons of a salamander's limb flexors and extensors are exchanged, the animal walks in circles indefinitely, suggesting that it has no power to reprogram its coordinative structures.[42] If the same is done to a rodent, it cannot learn to use the limb skillfully again but does learn to lock the joint through cocontraction and walk on it as on a "peg-leg." Primates can actually learn to use flexors as extensors and vice versa, but tend to make errors when distracted or fatigued. It appears that, as one ascends the evolutionary hierarchy, the ability to reshape coordinative structures increases, but it is not clear that this ability is absolute even in humans.

The concept of heterarchies, too, introduces its own need for further specification. Decentralized control certainly facilitates many aspects of skilled performance, allowing error corrections and many other adjustments to occur at multiple levels. If different components of the motor control system can control or be controlled by each other, however, much more needs to be said to explain how the ultimate output remains goal directed and free from chaos.

SUMMARY OF MODELS OF MOTOR SKILL

All of the generic models described above attempt to address the essential requirements of a system for skilled movement detailed at the beginning of this chapter. Any of the models can account for the improvement, with practice, in movement speed, accuracy, and smoothness. This is done by assuming that initial slow and halting movement is due to the constant need to monitor feedback and make moment-to-moment decisions. As motor programs become elaborated (whether as directly stored motor instructions, schemas, or coordinative structures), segments of the movement can occur more smoothly and rapidly.

All the models can deal with performance in the absence of much peripheral feedback in the same way, by assuming the elaboration of a motor program based on prior feedback. As we have seen, however, the address-specific model can profit from practice only when repeating precisely identical movements, a situation which rarely occurs in nature.

Handling realistic environmental variations is the particular strength of the schema theories. Consider again the example of raising one's arm at different speeds and how the schema and coordinative structure views would account for this. The schema theory would note that, at slow speeds, the movement is performed exclusively by shoulder abductors, operating continuously. At fast speeds, the abductors and adductors operate in overlapping fashion. The schema, then, can identify the relationship of speed of movement to the need for one or both muscle groups to be active.

If one assumes that a coordinative structure links the motor neurons of the abductors and adductors in a fixed ratio, that coordinative structure cannot account for the movement at different speeds. It is apparent that these movements differ by structural, not just metric prescription because the adductors are not active at all in slow abduction. Thus, a coordinative structure model would have to mimic a schema at a higher level of control. For example, there could be elementary coordinative structures for shoulder abduction (using the abductors), and "breaking" or "damping" of abduction (using the adductors). Then a higher-level coordinative structure for the whole movement at various speeds could link these simpler coordinative structures appropriately.

Both the schema and coordinative structure models offer benefits in terms of motor memory. They both allow memory to be stored in a form more abstract and economical than a list of actual muscle instructions. Indeed, coordinative structures allow much of movement "memory" to reside in the coordinative structures themselves. This may help to account for the preservation of motor skill learning in amnesia, as discussed above.

In accounting for multi-joint, multi-muscle movements, the coordinative structure model makes the essential contribution of reducing the nearly infinite degrees of movement freedom. The schema theory, although it allows minor variations of movements without wholesale reprogramming, still requires a great many decisions to be made with respect to all the muscles and joints participating.

Both the schema and coordinative structure models allow control of movement at different levels of abstraction. That is, the goal of "approach" can be implemented by either an abstract schema calling on more detailed schemas or a high-level coordinative structure calling on more specific ones. In both cases, it is assumed that the concrete structures or schemas for ambulation, bicycle riding, etc., must be present before they can be called upon by more abstract programs.

Automaticity remains an important phenomenon in skilled performance that none of these models addresses specifically. As motor programs are elaborated that free the individual from monitoring feedback to a large degree, this could explain some of the lessened need for conscious attention and monitoring. Skilled performance, however, is by no means always routine performance. Therefore, many complex movement decisions that cannot be made in advance without feedback must be made during the course of skilled performance, and yet often with hardly a thought (e.g., when to shift a manual transmission automobile when traveling at various speeds). This phenomenon of automaticity remains enigmatic but critically important to clinical work. In particular, it is unclear whether all schemas or coordinative structures are equally amenable to automatic control or if some require more conscious monitoring than others. Unless recovering motor control patterns can become automatic, they are unlikely to be of great use in daily life.

RECOVERY OF SKILLED MOVEMENT

The motor deficit that occurs following an insult to the central nervous system typically undergoes some degree of recovery with time. As with other aspects of recovery of function, the mechanisms responsible for motor recovery are uncertain. Several potential mechanisms have been proposed.[43]

RESOLUTION OF TEMPORARY FACTORS

Some of the initial motor deficit may result from impaired function of neural tissue which is not irreversibly damaged. This impairment might be due to edema, decreased oxygenation or perfusion, effects of medications, etc. As these factors resolve over days or weeks, latent motor function may appear.

REGENERATION AND SPROUTING

There is evidence in various species that severed axons may branch and grow in damaged areas of the CNS in a fashion analogous to that seen in the peripheral nervous system. Intact axons may sprout from nearby synaptic beds and reinnervate sites left vacant due to damage of other neurons. Both these phenomena can be seen histologically, but the evidence that they are responsible for important behavioral changes during recovery is much less clear. Indeed, there is evidence that this regenerative process is sometimes random and dysfunctional.

ALTERATIONS IN SYNAPTIC FUNCTION

Neural impulses are transmitted when neurotransmitters are released from synaptic terminals and bind to postsynaptic receptors, thereby stimulating the distal neuron. When neurons in one region are damaged, the neurons that they normally innervate are left with subnormal stimulation due to less release of the relevant neurotransmitters. Thus, these distal neurons may fail to function although they are not intrinsically damaged. This phenomenon is probably a major mechanism of diaschisis or neural shock.

Over time, the denervated neurons may produce increased numbers of neurotransmitter receptors and, in this and other ways, augment their sensitivity to any neurotransmitter released by remaining afferent fibers. This increased sensitivity may be one mechanism for functional recovery over the weeks and months post-injury, and an explanation for some instances of drug-induced recovery.

VICARIOUS FUNCTION

It has been suggested that neural tissue remains plastic in its organization. In response to neural damage, neighboring intact tissue might reorganize itself to take on the functional characteristics of the damaged region. Thus, after damage to the primary sensory cortex, the neighboring regions that subserve sensory recovery should develop receptive fields similar to the area which was damaged. These new regions should *become* primary sensory areas, a vicarious function.

There is much evidence that neighboring regions of the CNS may be responsible for recovered function. Most of these studies show that, after recovery, lesioning a second area recreates the deficit even though the new area of damage would not have produced that deficit if lesioned alone. It does not appear, however, that the neural tissue subserving the task during recovery alters its normal pattern of organization. Rather, it seems to find ways of altering the task to fit its processing capabilities (see next section, Functional Substitution).

FUNCTIONAL SUBSTITUTION

A paraplegic may regain mobility with the aid of a wheelchair. The function of mobility can be said to have been recovered but is clearly executed by an alternative strategy, which constitutes functional substitution of a physical sort.

If a patient suffers from a visuospatial deficit, he or she might learn to find familiar locations with a verbal list of landmarks. The function, finding one's way about, has recovered. A test of visuospatial function, however, may show continued impairment, suggesting that the task is being mediated by different neural systems (e.g., verbal). This constitutes functional substitution of a cognitive sort.

Recovery of cognitive function or of skilled movement on the basis of functional substitution is evident only if the recovery is imperfect. That is, functional substitution is identified only when the new strategy for performing the task appears different from the normal strategy. The more perfectly functional substitution achieves behavioral goals, the less visible it becomes. Because of this, it is uncertain how broadly this mechanism of recovery applies. Functional substitution can be expected over a broad range of time post-injury, provoked by exposure to tasks in which deficits are experienced and new strategies sought.

LEARNING SPECIFIC TASKS

Even if no general recovery of a cognitive or motor capacity occurs, specific tasks may be recovered by virtue of discovering prosthetic or orthotic adaptations or by learning solutions to a specific instance of the task. For example, although a patient's ambulation may cease improving in terms of strength and coordination, a brace or cane may improve the gait. A patient may not improve in general visuospatial skills but may be taught how to complete one particular drawing with much practice.[44] These mechanisms of recovery may be circumscribed, but can still be of functional importance. This type of recovery can occur at any time post-injury because it requires specific experience.

IMPLICATIONS OF RECOVERY MECHANISMS

The above discussion is meant to point out that there is still much uncertainty about the degree to which the CNS can truly alter its organization during recovery. This question is of central importance to clinicians. It determines whether we are trying to *produce changes* in neural organization and function or to *discover remaining useful patterns of organization* and adapt them to functional needs.

The models of recovery that stress alterations in strategy and specific relearning suggest that efforts should be directed toward discovering and characterizing what remains rather than bringing back what is gone. In the case of skilled movement, specifically, one might inquire whether it is possible to create (or recreate) new patterns of motor organization or if an attempt should be made to identify remaining coordinative structures and find ways of adapting them to the functional tasks of living. Thus, an extensor synergy pattern, although clearly not fully recovered motor function, may be used for standing and transfers.

In some animals, licking behavior is elicited automatically whenever the head and limbs assume a particular position.[15] Thus, assuming the required position activates a coordinative structure for licking. A neural insult might impair drinking if it interfered with assumption of the triggering posture, although the coordinative structure for licking would be intact. If the animal discovers another posture capable of eliciting licking, recovery is observed. "Therapy" for this animal would consist not of retraining in voluntary licking but in identifying remaining strategies capable of eliciting the coordinative structure.

It has been suggested that some of the efficacy of biofeedback in movement retraining may be attributed to the linkage of movement control to new sensory cues.[34] Coordinative structures capable of subserving a given movement may remain, but lack the normal sensory cues to trigger them. Biofeedback may allow those coordinative structures to be related to another set of sensory information.

One study of human hemiplegics showed that maximal voluntary contraction of the paretic quadriceps muscle increased substantially when the relevant sensory dermatome was gently brushed concurrently.[45] Comparable effects were not seen in the knee flexors, although this may have been due to the smaller size of the relevant dermatome available for brushing.

This type of study suggests that a particular type of sensory input facilitates a particular coordinative structure. If, with training, this coordinative structure can be activated without the brushing stimulus, recovery will be promoted. If, on the other hand, we have merely discovered a coordinative structure which is intrinsically dependent on cutaneous stimulation, treatment will be futile, or at best, will prompt us to construct a "brushing orthosis." The fact that the stimulus was ineffective for flexion (if confirmed) highlights the importance of studying which coordinative structures are present and available to be drawn upon.

In clinical practice we have seen many patients who have "discovered" their asymmetric tonic neck reflex and use it to assist functional reaching, or who use an upper extremity extensor synergy to push down their pants in undressing, etc. These are often seen as "the best that can be hoped for" in patients who fail to continue to improve in more normal-appearing movement, but may just be more visible examples of the functional substitution that supports motor recovery in most patients. If so, more energy should be devoted to fostering these strategies intentionally rather than just when all else fails.

If new coordinative structures can be formed through practice, therapeutic energy should be directed to the selection of the most widely useful structures and intensive practice in their use should be given. More information is needed about the optimal teaching strategies for developing smooth performance of newly created coordinative structures.

Whether recovery of skilled movement occurs through discovery of useful coordinative structures that remain, through creation of new ones, or through some combination, alterations in spasticity are particularly relevant to the recovery process. A patient who "discovers" an extensor synergy for weight bearing will need to discover something new if medication or phenol neurolysis inhibits that synergy. A patient learning a new coordinative structure involving a spastic limb will be learning a movement equation that includes that spasticity. An intervention that alters the tone in the limb alters the linkage among muscle groups and thus requires revised learning.

Thus, it can be predicted that interventions that alter spasticity, although potentially helpful in the long run, might require adaptation of other aspects of the motor control system to accommodate to the change in tone (see Chapter 9). A corollary to this is that, following a spasticity-altering intervention, the benefits to skilled movement may not be immediately evident. Learning under the altered conditions may be necessary before a valid assessment can be made. It would even be reasonable to expect some instances of temporary regression in function, as one coordinative structure is inhibited, followed by improved function, as another more efficient structure is discovered or created. At present, it is not known how to predict in advance the short- and long-term effects a given intervention will have on skilled movement.

CLINICAL IMPLICATIONS

Spasticity reduction is rarely a treatment goal in its own right. Although in some instances spasticity reduction may lead directly to greater comfort, hygiene, etc., it is most often undertaken in the hope of improving active movement and related functional activities. As we have seen, the organization of active movement is exceedingly complex in normal individuals. Unfortunately, we understand even less about how skilled movement is disrupted in patients with CNS damage, what role spasticity plays in that disruption, and what the avenues toward recovery of skilled movement are.

CLINICAL PERSPECTIVES ON REMEDIATION OF SKILLED MOVEMENT

Currently there are three major "schools of thought" in clinical movement remediation: Proprioceptive Neuromuscular Facilitation, the Bobath Approach, and the Brunnstrom Approach. A description of the main theories and principles of treatment in each of these approaches allows comparison with the various models of skilled movement previously considered. Their essential similarities and differences are summarized in Table 4–1.

In Proprioceptive Neuromuscular Facilitation (PNF), Knott and Voss[46] advocate the use of the developmental sequence (described earlier in this chapter) as a basis for treatment of patients of all ages. Treatment progresses from prone to sitting to kneeling to standing, etc. In these sequential stages, body patterns incorporating head, neck, trunk, and the four extremities are used. These address ipsilateral, bilateral symmetric, and bilateral asymmetric movements. Muscles are encouraged to contract from the completely lengthened to the completely shortened state.

The patterns used during PNF contain a rotational and diagonal component. This is based on the axes of muscle forces in the musculoskeletal system as opposed to the perpendicular environmental axes. Flexion and extension are the main components of these diagonal patterns. The therapist, when guiding the relevant movement patterns, assumes a position in the same diagonal as the patient and guides the movement through its entire range. Manual contact with the patient is applied over the muscles involved in the movement patterns to facilitate muscle activation.[47]

The principles of PNF emphasize the development of proximal control before distal and total body patterns before isolated movements, analogous to developmental observations. As movement control is acquired, the timing of coordinated movements occurs from distal to proximal (e.g.,

TABLE 4–1. A COMPARISON OF THREE APPROACHES TO MOVEMENT REMEDIATION

Feature	PNF	Bobath	Brunnstrom
Use of the developmental sequence	+	+	0
Use of mass movement patterns	+	−	+
Stimulation of reflexes to elicit movement (i.e., via tapping, quick stretch)	+	0	+
Movement in reflex inhibiting patterns	0	+	−
Emphasis on functional tasks	0	+	+
Use of static reflex inhibiting patterns	0	−	+
Emphasis on work in the seated position	0	+	+
Use of synergies and associated reactions	−	−	+
Use of resistive exercises	+	−	+

+ = Therapeutic approach agrees
− = Therapeutic approach disagrees
0 = Therapeutic approach does not comment

an article is grasped and lifted with a movement that begins at the hand and continues upward to wrist, elbow, shoulder, etc.).

PNF patterns allow transition from movement to posture to movement, emphasising the reciprocal character of movement and posture. These transitions are intended to develop balance reactions. Repeated contractions of weak muscles are used to develop strength. Even these strengthening exercises, however, occur in prescribed movement patterns requiring collaboration of many muscle groups. Transitions between muscle relaxation and isotonic or isometric contractions within the movement pattern occur with increasing strength as recovery ensues.

The use, in PNF, of total body movement patterns before isolated movements is congruent with both developmental research and motor control theories, which emphasize coordinated muscle activation (as opposed to isolated control) as the primary building block of skill. In addition, strengthening within the coordinated movement patterns may be viewed as facilitating schema development for movements in those planes at all forces and positions. The emphasis on transitions from posture to movement is also consistent with the interdependency of these phenomena as previously discussed.

The Bobath Approach[48] emphasizes developing the functional potential of the affected limbs as opposed to teaching compensations. The aim of treatment is to change abnormal movement patterns to normal ones. The Bobaths stress that, during treatment, abnormal movements should not be reinforced by effort involved in strengthening muscles, nor should heavy resistance, irradiation, or associated reactions or synergies be used: ". . . it is impossible to superimpose normal patterns on abnormal ones. We have to suppress the abnormal patterns before more normal ones can be introduced." No specific empirical documentation is provided for this perspective.

Static reflex-inhibiting postures are not recommended because, while they reduce spasticity, they make it impossible for patients to produce voluntary movement and gain control over the abnormal reactions. Movement in reflex-inhibiting postures is recommended because it is believed to facilitate the acquisition of voluntary movement and volitional control over abnormal movements.

The Bobath Approach is similar to PNF in stressing progression through developmental stages, transitions from posture to movement, and its use of manual facilitation by means of contact over muscle bellies.

The theoretical bases of the Bobath Approach are not specified in detail. Thus it is difficult to critique it with respect to psychologic and neurophysiologic theories of skilled movement. It does, however, appear more in line with coordinative structural perspectives than address-specific models, and to draw from developmental observations of motor skill. The notion of suppressing abnormal movements and replacing them with normal ones is not well grounded in the theory or evidence of motor control. It implies that it is possible to recreate skilled movement patterns without drawing on residual movement strategies, which remains a controversial perspective.

Brunnstrom developed an approach that places greater emphasis on functional tasks.[49] Like the previous two approaches, the Brunnstrom approach relies on a progression from mass movements to more isolated control. Unlike the Bobath approach, Brunnstrom does advocate the use of static reflex inhibiting postures, for example, during bed positioning. Treatment begins with passive motion and progresses to resisted exercises, but not in the developmental sequence. Rather, work in the sitting position is begun as soon as possible. This position is chosen to emphasize trunk balance, communication, and functional activities. Brunnstrom makes use of "abnormal" movements such as synergy patterns and associated reactions and incorporates them into functional activities (e.g., using an extensor synergy to stabilize a piece of paper during writing).

The Brunnstrom approach is most consistent with the coordinative structural models of motor skill in suggesting the voluntary use of existing coordinative structures and in placing less stress on the recreation of fully normal coordinative patterns. Although this approach violates the developmental sequence, there is little empiric data to show that the pattern of normal development is essential to recovery in adulthood.

RESEARCH ON THERAPEUTIC EXERCISE

Dickstein et al[50] attempted to compare the efficacy of three therapeutic approaches in recovery from stroke. They assigned sequential patients to PNF, Bobath, or "traditional" treatment (strengthening exercises and compensatory training for functional activities). Testing after 6 weeks of physical therapy revealed few differences among the three groups in Barthel ADL score, muscle tone, isolated control, or ambulation status. Other studies have similarly failed to show substantial advantages of one approach over another.[51,52]

Structured research on the effects of therapeutic exercise on cerebral palsy has been similarly disappointing. In a study of 47 children under 6 years of age with spastic CP, Bobath-based physical therapy for 12 months was compared to no therapy for 6 months followed by Bobath therapy for 6 months and to no physical therapy at all.[53] The outcome measures included indices of cognitive development, motor milestones, and range of motion. No difference was seen among the three treatment groups on any of these measures, although the measures themselves were not very sensitive to change. In a study of 22 children under the age of 18 months with CP, 14 who received neurophysiologically based physical therapy and family training were compared to 8 who received passive range of motion and no family training.[54] Superior gains were seen in the neurophysiological therapy subjects, in terms of physical development, cognitive development, and home management. However, the small sample was extremely heterogeneous in terms of severity and pattern of CP, so that even random assignment may have led to initial differences in the sample. The fact that the smallest difference between groups was seen in home management is particularly troublesome because only the neurophysiologic therapy group received family training.

Perhaps the best-controlled study of physical therapy in CP compared an infant stimulation treatment for 6 months followed by neurodevelopmental training (NDT) for 6 months, to 12 months of NDT.[55] The subjects were 48 children with spastic diplegia between 12 and 19 months of age. Although the sample was relatively small, the subjects were randomly assigned and the pattern of results was rather consistent. The children who received infant stimulation progressed faster than those receiving NDT in both cognitive and motor development. This trend was still present but weaker at the 12-month assessment when both groups had been receiving NDT. Although this study failed to support the efficacy of NDT, the findings suggest a benefit of infant stimulation (or, in theory, a deleterious effect of NDT). Therefore, there may still be productive questions to ask regarding the active ingredients of the stimulation program and the mechanisms for its effects on skilled movement.

All of these studies have focused on the effects of various therapy programs on the pace or level of recovery of skilled movement. A separate question is whether therapeutic exercise can produce temporary improvements in movement quality in a manner analogous to physical modalities. A single subject A-B-A study examined the effects of daily NDT on ankle dorsiflexor EMG activity during equilibrium reactions and on heel contact during standing in a 30-month-old child with CP.[56] The results showed a very consistent increase in both indices during treatment as compared to the pre- and post-treatment baselines. Although temporary gains such as these are less impressive than an effect on the course of movement recovery, they may still have some clinical relevance. Therapy strategies that facilitate positioning, handling, and certain important functional activities may be useful. Furthermore, it will be of interest to see whether interventions such as these, which produce temporary benefits in some patients, will produce long-lasting benefits if they are carried out regularly.

At present, there is little empiric evidence for the notion that any therapeutic exercise approach can facilitate movement recovery. This conclusion must be regarded as tentative, however, because of the sparsity and nature of the research conducted on this topic. In many instances, this research has been poorly controlled and has used rather gross indicators of change. Also, the presence of various abnormal reflexes is extremely variable over time, at least in children with CP, creating considerable "noise" in data regarding motor behavior and therapy-induced progress.[57] In addition, studies may expect too much of the exercise interventions they examine. That is, perhaps certain interventions can produce very specific gains (such as those seen in the single subject study described above) which, although clinically meaningful, are

not evident in such gross indicators as attainment of motor milestones. Thus, research that examines the use of therapeutic exercise to affect very focused movement goals may have a greater chance of success.

Deciding among different therapeutic exercise approaches is difficult, given the lack of clear theoretic or empiric guidelines. There are many possible explanations for the failure to find meaningful differences in outcome from one therapeutic approach to another. The most pessimistic, of course, is that none of them are effective. In other cases, the differences in approach may be more semantic than operational. That is, different authors may have different theoretic perspectives, but the actual physical manipulations carried out by therapists may be similar. Also, all of the major approaches are consistent with one of the principal findings of motor skill research: the fundamental nature of coordinated (rather than isolated) movement. The most important point in need of further clinical study is whether "abnormal" motor patterns should be discouraged and replaced, or incorporated into functional tasks. This would involve a comparison of the Brunnstrom approach with the PNF and Bobath approaches.

SUMMARY

It should be clear by now that spasticity is not simply an obstacle to the skilled operation of an otherwise preserved motor control system. In the upper motor neuron syndromes, the motor control system is disturbed in many ways beyond spasticity.

Whenever spasticity is present in an actively moving limb, it is part of the system that is being controlled. Thus, the calculations of the CNS about the force relationships of various muscles in a coordinative structure, the relationship between muscle activation patterns and movement velocity, etc., must include spasticity as part of the equation. Alterations in spasticity, then, must require recalibration of the system. This, in turn, may require new types of learning and treatment experiences to maximize function under the altered conditions.

Much of the discussion about how alterations in tone might affect immediate performance and subsequent recovery is conjectural. Research is needed to answer the following broad questions:

1. In what circumstances is spasticity a direct impediment to skilled movement, a contributing obstacle, or a functionally irrelevant marker of the upper motor neuron syndrome?
2. What immediate effects do antispasticity interventions have on the imparied motor control system? (e.g., do new coordinative structures appear instantly, do existing coordinative structures vanish, or do the existing coordinative structures simply alter their characteristics as if an external load to which they were accustomed had been removed?)
3. What long-term effects do antispasticity interventions have on the impaired motor control system? (e.g., is it possible to elicit coordinative structures which could not previously be elicited at all, does it become impossible to elicit some which could be elicited previously, or does the system simply adapt to the changed load characteristics?)
4. Is the timing of antispasticity interventions of clinical importance? (e.g., is active movement practice "wasted" if a subsequent intervention alters the system? Should such interventions, when possible, precede retraining efforts?)
5. Under what circumstances should rehabilitation efforts be directed toward creation of coordinative structures which are as normal as possible versus selection of the coordinative structures possessed by the patient which are of most functional use?
6. Are there specific movement rehabilitation strategies that can promote the maximal recovery of skilled movement by applying principles drawn from normal motor control models?
7. Is it important to follow the normal sequence of motor skill development when working with patients with the UMN syndrome, or does the damaged or altered nervous system follow a completely different developmental course?

These would seem to be crucial questions for the clinically oriented researcher if progress is to be made in developing rationally based remediation strategies.

An additional factor often overlooked in rehabilitation therapy is *effort* or its reciprocal, *automaticity*. Any novel task requires considerable conscious monitoring and effort. When first learning to play the piano, one must attend to the placement of each finger individually and its relationship to the corresponding note on the page. With practice, this requires less attention and one becomes able to identify a multi-note chord and translate it into a multi-finger hand posture without reference to each individual movement. Still later, even that level of movement becomes automatic and one is able to attend to phrasing, expression, etc. Indeed, it could be argued that the expressive aspects of piano performance *can occur only* when attention is freed from the concrete movements.

This decrease in effort with practice is what is meant by the development of automaticity. Many patients with CNS lesions appear not only less skilled in their movements but also more effortful. To the extent that simple movements are effortful, the patient is not able to attend to the more abstract or cognitive aspects of tasks, but is occupied with the details of movement execution.

Often a patient with a CVA can clear the toe or hold the flexed arm down at the side during ambulation in therapy. However, if walking while conversing or examining a shop window, such a patient is likely to trip or gradually revert to a flexed arm posture. This indicates that conscious effort is being devoted to the foot or arm position. When that effort is directed elsewhere, the ability fades.

There are several reasons why performance might be less automatic following an upper motor neuron lesion:

1. Because many tasks are being controlled by brain systems not previously responsible for those tasks (functional substitution—see above), they are, in some sense, novel and unpracticed tasks. Thus the patient is an infant with respect to some aspects of movement.

2. Automatic performance generally occurs when the quality of performance is adequate to allow attention to be directed elsewhere. Thus, the development of automaticity may depend on receiving feedback from the environment that performance is "good enough" (e.g., no wrong piano notes).[58] Following CNS lesions, many aspects of performance are never "good enough." Thus, the patient receives constant error feedback and may constantly strive (however unproductively) to improve through conscious monitoring.
3. Some coordinative mechanisms are capable of automatization and others are not. If this were true, innate coordinative structures or innately facilitated structures might be capable of automatization, but others might always require great effort to use.

Clarification of these different views of automaticity is also of clinical importance. Maximal functional recovery occurs when a patient can function smoothly and automatically. The first viewpoint suggests that, while this may require a great deal of time and effort, with sufficient practice it can be achieved. The second viewpoint suggests that the only way to achieve automatic performance is to find movement strategies that are as efficient as their premorbid counterparts in achieving their goals. The third suggests that clinicians might exercise some choice in the movement strategies as they train. A clumsy but automatic movement might serve a patient better in the long run than an exact but effortful one.

CONCLUSION

Research on skilled movement has much still to explain about how everyday skills are programmed and monitored in the central nervous system. Furthermore, there is at present a large gap between what is known of normal motor control and how treatment strategies are designed and implemented for the patient with an upper motor neuron syndrome.

It is hoped that more research on both fronts will eventually form a bridge between the basic science aspects of skilled movement and the therapeutic applications of such knowledge. Until that time, clinicians would do well to remain humble about the complexity of the motor control system we take so much for granted and about the complex relationship between that system when damaged and the phenomenon of spasticity.

REFERENCES

1. Sahrmann, S.A., and Norton, B.J.: The relationship of voluntary movement to spasticity in the upper motor neuron syndrome. Trans. Am. Neurol. Assoc. *102*:108–112, 1977.
2. McGraw, M.B.: The Neuromuscular Maturation of the Human Infant. New York, Hafner Publishing Co., 1962.
3. Charness, A.: Stroke/Head Injury: A Guide to Functional Outcomes in Physical Therapy Management. Maryland, Aspen Publications, 1986.
4. Hasan, Z., Enoka, R.M., and Stuart, D.G.: The interface between biomechanics and neurophysiology in the study of movement: Some recent approaches. Exerc. Sport Sci. Rev. *13*:169–234, 1985.
5. Evarts, E.V.: Role of motor cortex in voluntary movement in primates. *In* Brooks, V.B. (vol. ed.): Handbook of Physiology, sec. 1, vol. 2. Bethesda, MD, Am. Physiol. Soc., 1981.
6. Volpe, B.T., Sidtis, J.J., Holtzman, J.D., et al.: Cortical mechanisms involved in praxis: observations following partial and complete section of the corpus collosum in man. Neurology *32*:645–650, 1982.
7. Siegel, A.: On a possible neural mechanism underlying a finding by Evarts and Fromm. Neurosci. Lett. *14(2–3)*:219–221, 1979.
8. Weisenberger, M.: Organization of secondary motor areas of cerebral cortex. *In* Brooks, V.B. (vol. ed.): Handbook of Physiology, sec. 1, vol. 2. Bethesda, MD, Am. Physiol. Soc., 1981.
9. Asanuma, H., and Arussuan, K.: Experiments on functional role of peripheral input to motor cortex during voluntary move-

ments in monkey. J. Neurophysiol. *52(2):*212–227, 1984.

10. Kitai, S.T.: Electrophysiology of the corpus striatum and brainstem integrating systems. *In* Brooks, V.B. (vol. ed.): Handbook of Physiology, sec. 1, vol. 2. Bethesda, MD, Am. Physiol. Soc., 1981.

11. Evarts, E.V.: Brain mechanisms in motor control. Life Sci. *15(8):*1393–1399, 1974.

12. Meyer-Lohmann, J., Hore, J., Brooks, V.B.: Cerebellar participation in generation of prompt arm movements. J. Neurophysiol. *40(5):*1038–1050, 1977.

13. Kelso, J.A.S.: Motor control mechanisms underlying human movement reproduction. J. Exp. Psychol. (Hum. Percept.) *3(4):*529–543, 1977.

14. Eccles, J.C.: Physiology of motor control in man. Appl. Neurophysiol. *44(1–3):*5–15, 1981.

15. Vanderwolf, C.H.: Limbic-diencephalic mechanisms of voluntary movement. Psychol. Rev. *78(2):*83–113, 1971.

16. Craik, R.L., Cozzens, B.A., and Freedman, W.: The role of sensory conflict on stair descent performance in humans. Exp. Brain Res. *45:*399–409, 1982.

17. Naute, W.J.H.: Some thoughts about thought and movement: An essay based on Hughlings Jackson's notions. Paper presented at Frontiers of Neuroscience, Symposium in honor of W.J.H. Naute, Cambridge, MA, MIT, May 28, 1986.

18. Nissen, M.J.: Neuropsychology of attention and memory. J. Head Trauma Rehabil. *1(3):*13–21, 1986.

19. Granit, R.: Reflections on motricity. Perspect. Biol. Med. *23:*171–178, 1980.

20. Asanuma, H.: The pyramidal tract. *In* Brooks, V.B. (vol. ed.): Handbook of Physiology. sec. 1, vol. 2, Bethesda, MD, Am. Physiol. Soc., 1981.

21. Basmajian, J.V.: Learned control of single motor units. *In* Schwartz, G.E., Beatty, J. (eds.): Biofeedback: Therapy and Research. New York, Academic Press, 1977.

22. Roy, E.A., and Marteniuk, R.G.: Mechanisms of control in motor performance: Closed-loop vs motor programming control. J. Exp. Psychol. *103(5):*985–991, 1974.

23. Kelso, J.A.S.: Joint receptors do not provide a satisfactory basis for motor timing and positioning. Psychol. Rev. *85(5):*474–481, 1978.

24. Roland, P.E.: Sensory feedback to the cerebral cortex during voluntary movement in man. Behav. Brain Sci. *1:*129–171, 1978.

25. Turvey, M.T., Shaw, R.E., and Mace, W.: Issues in the theory of action: degrees of freedom, coordinative structures, and coalitions. *In* Requin, J. (Ed.): Attention and Performance VII, Lawrence Erlbaum Assoc., Hillsdale, NJ, 1978.

26. Schmidt, R.A.: The schema as a solution to some persistent problems in motor learning theory. *In* Stelmach, G.E. (ed.): Motor Control: Issues and Trends, New York, Academic Press, 1976.

27. Krendal, E.S., and McRuer, D.T.: A servomechanisms approach to skill development. J. Franklin Inst. *269(1):*24–42, 1960.

28. Pew, R.W.: Acquisition of hierarchical control over the temporal organization of a skill. J. Exp. Psychol. *71(5):*764–771, 1966.

29. Keele, S.W.: Behavioral analysis of movement. *In* Brooks, V.B. (vol. ed.): Handbook of Physiology, sec. 1, vol. 2, Bethesda, MD, Am. Physiol. Soc., 1981.

30. Trumbo, D., Milone, F., and Noble, M.: Interpolated activity and response mechanisms in motor short-term memory. J. Exp. Psychol. *93:*205–212, 1972.

31. Crossman, E.R.F.W.: A theory of acquisition of speed skill. Ergonomics *2:*153–166, 1959.

32. Kelso, J.A.S., and Stelmach, G.E.: Central and peripheral mechanisms in motor control. *In* Stelmach, G.E. (ed.): Motor Control: Issues and Trends. New York, Academic Press, 1976.

33. Hollerbach, J.M.: Computers, brains and the control of movement. Trends in Neurosci. *5(6):*189–192, 1982.

34. Herman, R.: A therapeutic approach based on theories of motor control. Int. Rehabil. Med. *4(4):*185–189, 1982.

35. Nagasaki, H., Nakamura, R., Taniguchi, R.: Disturbances in rhythm formation in patients with Parkinson's disease. Percept. Mot. Skills *46(1):*79–87, 1978.

36. Delcomyn, F.: Neural basis of rhythmic behavior in animals. Science *210(4469):*492–498, 1980.

37. Kelso, J.A.S., Southard, D.L., and Goodman, D.: On the coordination of two handed movements. J. Exp. Psychol. (Hum. Percept.) *5(2):*229–238, 1979.

38. Ioffe, M.E., Frolov, A.A., Gahery, Y., et al.: Biomechanical study of the mechanisms accompanying learned and induced limb movements in cats and dogs. Acta Neurobiol. Exp. *42(6):*469–482, 1982.

39. Abbs, J.H.M., and Gracco, V.L.: Control of complex motor gestures: Orofacial muscle responses to load perturbations of lip during speech. J. Neurophysiol. *51(4):*705–723, 1984.

40. Cole, K.J., Gracco, V.L., and Abbs, J.H.: Autogenic and nonautogenic sensorimotor actions in the control of multiarticulate hand

movements. Exp. Brain Res. *56(3):*582–585, 1984.

41. Dietz, V., Berger, W.: Spinal coordination of bilateral leg muscle activity during balancing. Exp. Brain Res. *47(2):*172–176, 1982.

42. Gallestel, C.R.: The Organization of Action: A New Synthesis, Chap. 8, Lawrence Erlbaum, Hillsdale, NJ, 1980.

43. Whyte, J.: Mechanisms of recovery of function following central nervous system damage. *In* Rosenthal M, Griffith ER, Bond MR, et al. (eds.): Rehabilitation of the Child and Adult with Traumatic Brain Injury (2nd ed.) Philadelphia, F.A. Davis (1990).

44. Campbell, D.C., and Oxbury, J.M.: Recovery from unilateral visuospatial neglect? Cortex *12:*303–312, 1976.

45. Matyas, T.A., Galea, M.P., and Spicer, S.D.: Facilitation of the maximum voluntary contraction in hemiplegia by concomitant cutaneous stimulation. Am. J. Phys. Med. *65(3):*125–133, 1986.

46. Knott, M., Voss, D.E.: Proprioceptive Neuromuscular Facilitation: Patterns and Techniques (2nd ed.). New York, Harper and Row, 1968.

47. Hagbarth, K.E.: Excitatory and inhibitory skin areas for flexor and extensor motoneurons. Acta Physiol. Scand. 26(suppl. 94):1–58, 1952.

48. Bobath, B.: Adult Hemiplegia: Evaluation and Treatment (2nd ed.). London, Spottiswoode Ballantyne Ltd., 1978.

49. Brunnstrom, S.: Movement Therapy in Hemiplegia: A Neurophysiological Approach. New York, Harper and Row, 1970.

50. Dickstein, R., et al.: Stroke rehabilitation—three exercise therapy approaches. Phys. Ther. *66(8):*1233–1238, 1986.

51. Stern, P.H., et al.: Effects of facilitation exercise techniques in stroke rehabilitation. Arch. Phys. Med. Rehabil. *51:*526–531, 1970.

52. Logigian, M.K., Samuels, M.A., Falconer, J., et al.: Clinical exercise trial for stroke patients. Arch. Phys. Med. Rehabil. *64:*364–367, 1983.

53. Wright, T., and Nicholson, J.: Physiotherapy for the spastic child: an evaluation. Dev. Med. Child Neurol. *15:*146–153, 1973.

54. Scherzer, A.L., Mike, V., and Ilson, J.: Physical therapy as a determinant of change in the cerebral palsied infant. Pediatrics *58(1):*47–52, 1976.

55. Palmer, F.C., Shapiro, B.K., Wachtel, R.C., et al.: The effects of physical therapy on cerebral palsy. N. Engl. J. Med. *318(13):*803–808, 1988.

56. Laskas, C.A., Mullen, S.L., and Nelson, D.L.: Enhancement of two motor functions of the lower extremity in a child with spastic quadriplegia. Phys. Ther. *65(1):*11–16, 1985.

57. Smith, S.L., Gossman, M.R., and Canan, B.L.: Selected primitive reflexes in children with cerebral palsy. Phys. Ther. *62(8):*1115–1120, 1982.

58. Whyte, J.: Automatization of a motor skill: Practice makes perfect. Doctoral dissertation, University of Pennsylvania, 1981.

5 EVALUATION OF SPASTICITY AND ITS EFFECT ON MOTOR FUNCTION

STEPHEN M. HALEY
CONSTANCE A. INACIO

INTRODUCTION

One of the major clinical problems for patients with central nervous system disease is the effect of spasticity on motor function. The purpose of this chapter is to outline procedures for a comprehensive evaluation of the presence and severity of its effects on motor function.

SPASTICITY AND THE UPPER MOTOR NEURON SYNDROME

The presence of spasticity is considered one of the most definitive physical signs of an upper motor neuron (UMN) syndrome.[1] UMN syndrome is a broad term describing abnormal motor function secondary to lesions of cortical, subcortical, or spinal cord structures. Spasticity is a common clinical manifestation in a wide variety of childhood and adult UMN conditions including cerebral palsy, myelomeningocele, spinal cord injury, multiple sclerosis, traumatic brain injury, cerebral vascular accident, and other neurologic diseases.

The evaluation of spasticity is a central element in the motor assessment of the individual with a UMN syndrome. Spasticity may contribute to abnormal control of voluntary movement, alter postural control and alignment, contribute to debilitating contractures, affect hygiene, increase potential for skin breakdown, and restrict the performance of daily functional activities such as ambulation and self-care skills. Posture and movement, however, are often affected adversely by multiple elements of the UMN syndrome, of which spasticity is only one.[2] In patients with a UMN syndrome, spasticity may influence motor dysfunction in several ways:

1. Affect passive movements and static postural alignment.
2. Affect voluntary movement.
3. Coexist with other UMN syndrome deficits and play a minimal, if any, role in motor dysfunction.

Thus, an evaluation of spasticity should be oriented toward assessing the direct influence of spasticity on posture and movement.[3] A series of important clinical outcome variables such as passive movements, postural alignment, and parameters of voluntary movements should be examined in relation to the identified pattern of spasticity.

DEFINITIONS OF SPASTICITY

Unfortunately, the clinical definition of spasticity and the pathophysiology underlying spasticity remain controversial. Spasticity may refer to any of the following abnormal positive signs associated with the

UMN syndrome: hypertonia (often velocity-dependent), increased size of the reflexogenic zones, clonus, and hyperactive tendon reflexes (see Chapter 1). This resistance to passive stretch arises from a combination of changes in the segmental reflex arc and actual changes in the musculotendinous unit.[4] The term spasticity has also been used to signify posturing of extremities, abnormal movement patterns, spasms, flexor reflexes, and stereotypical movement synergies.[1,5–8] Clinically, the term spasticity continues to be used for various phenomena, often according to prevailing clinical viewpoints and perspectives.[2,9] This has led to confusion both in terms of appropriate clinical evaluation and assessment of treatment efficacy.

Many factors have traditionally made quantification and clinical evaluation of spasticity complex and difficult. These include the lack of consistent conceptual definitions of spasticity, the difficulty of reproducing consistent levels of spasticity at rest and during voluntary movements, and the influence of emotional, behavioral, and systemic factors on the clinical manifestations of spasticity.[10] While both conceptual and measurement problems continue to plague the clinical description of spasticity, there is growing recognition that more precise and quantifiable clinical measures of spasticity are needed.[11] More accurate measurement and description will eventually lead to improved understanding and advances in clinical management of the patient with a UMN syndrome.

DETERMINANTS OF MOVEMENT DYSFUNCTION

The ultimate goal in the evaluation of spasticity is to determine its effect on movement dysfunction. In principle, this involves distinguishing the effects of spasticity from those of other positive symptoms of the UMN syndrome (such as nociceptive reflexes); from those of negative symptoms of the UMN syndrome (such as weakness); and from mechanical and elastic changes in the muscle/tendon unit.

The relative importance of spasticity in movement dysfunction, as opposed to these other factors, may differ between passive and active function. In passive restraint, the body part resists movement in the absence of voluntary effort. Although passive restraint may be the result of spasticity, other forms of hypertonia and elastic changes may contribute.

Spasticity is considered an abnormal or positive sign of the UMN syndrome.[7] In the presence of a UMN syndrome, spasticity often coexists with a variety of negative signs, including poor force production, delayed initiation of movement, and the abnormal timing of muscle synergists.[12] These negative performance deficits associated with a UMN syndrome may be even more significant than spasticity in producing voluntary movement dysfunction.[12–15] As in passive movement, other positive symptoms of the UMN syndrome such as rigidity and hyperactive nociceptive reflexes may contribute to voluntary movement dysfunction. In general, the relationships among spasticity, other UMN positive signs, UMN syndrome negative signs, and abnormal movement control are unclear. In many patients with spasticity, therapeutic procedures that decrease spasticity do not necessarily improve voluntary movement control and may even worsen it.[8] Therefore, spasticity should be viewed as one of many possible limiting factors in the development of normal voluntary movement in individuals with UMN disease, and the clinical assessment of spasticity should be conducted with this in mind.

Further complicating matters is the possibility that therapeutic intervention can simultaneously alter spasticity as well as other positive symptoms of the UMN syndrome. For example, baclofen can decrease spasticity as well as flexor spasms, despite the fact that the latter are caused by a nociceptive rather than stretch reflex. This illustrates the fact that a positive treatment response cannot be taken as definitive evidence for a particular form of neuropathology. It is hoped, however, that attempts to distinguish clearly among different manifestations of the UMN syndrome will lead to more rational treatment selection in the future.

Muscle tone is defined clinically as the amount of background activity and tension (that is, resistance to passive stretch) in a muscle.[4,16] The mechanical and elastic characteristics of muscle and the degree of motor unit activity contribute to muscle tone. Thus, hypertonia is a larger phenomenon, of which spasticity is one component. Duncan and Badke[8] presented a model of normal motor control in which muscle tone is described as a supportive element to movement. Normal muscle tone is characterized as facilitating the accuracy and the efficiency of motor control. Parameters such as perception and cognition, range of motion, sensation, and strength are considered equally important components for the development and expression of proper motor control and movement adaptability (see Chapter 4). The objective of an evaluation of spasticity is to selectively identify motor dysfunction that is primarily affected by hypertonia due to spasticity. Additionally, it is also important to determine if spasticity is *not* a predominant factor in dysfunction, but merely coexisting with more debilitating UMN syndrome deficits. The role and importance of abnormalities of muscle tone in movement disorders continue to be of interest in the research and clinical literature.[17–20]

HIERARCHY OF MEASUREMENT VARIABLES

An accurate clinical evaluation of spasticity includes a description of it and an analysis of its effect, as well as the effects of other aspects of the UMN syndrome, on the motor deficits of the individual. The linkage of spasticity with the motor deficits is the key organizing framework for the clinical evaluation of spasticity. Three possible consequences of spasticity to be evaluated in individuals with UMN syndrome are its effects on passive movements, on postural alignment and positional stability, and on selective voluntary movement, which result in decrements in motor performance and daily functional skills. A list of clinical outcome variables that may be affected by spasticity is given in Table 5–1.

The most common method for determining the presence of spasticity is to test for restraint during passive muscle lengthening. A hyperactive stretch reflex characteristically limits passive movement, but other

TABLE 5–1. HIERARCHY OF MEASUREMENT VARIABLES

Passive Movements
  Resistance to passive stretch
  Passive range of motion
  Mechanical (force) output
Postural Alignment
  Postural tone
  Positional stability
  Postural reflexes
Voluntary Movements
  Performance variables
  Active range of motion
  Force
  Motor synergies
  Movement speed
  Movement initiation
  Movement adaptability
Functional Variables
  Balance
  Upper extremity tasks
  ADL skills
  Transfers and mobility
  Gait

forms of hypertonia may also do so. Passive movement restraint may contribute to serious muscle contractures because chronically contracting muscles physically shorten. If it is difficult to move a limb, even passively, hygiene and dressing tasks become difficult and skin maceration may occur. Overactive and spastic antagonists may contribute to stretch weakness because of agonists that are elongated for extended periods.

Postural alignment can be affected negatively by the presence of spasticity as well. Sitting and standing posture can be compromised by the imbalance of spastic muscles about the pelvis and hip. Structural abnormalities such as kyphosis, scoliosis, and hip deformities are common among children and adults with severe spasticity. Spasms induced by movement or tactile input can create instability in sitting and standing positions and lead to injury. In some cases, spasms can be extremely debilitating and painful and may interfere with sleep. Alignment of the head and extremities may influence muscle tone distributions, affecting posture and the stability needed for movement.

Spasticity may also affect or interact with a variety of voluntary movement parameters. These may include force and torque production, rate of torque production, motor synergies, balance, movement adaptability, movement initiation, accuracy, ability to reciprocate movements, movement speed, and movement trajectory. Normal muscle tone is one of the prerequisite components for normal movement. Therefore, disorders of tone, including spasticity, may play a role in impairments in these parameters.

Finally, spasticity can have an important effect on the functional status of the individual.[21,22] Functional skills refer to self-care and mobility activities such as dressing, feeding, transfers, and locomotion. The influence of spasticity on daily functional skills is, for most patients, the most important and relevant question to be addressed in an evaluation. The importance of spasticity may vary among patients as the limiting factor in functional skills. Spasticity may be present and not directly influence the functional ability of the individual. In unusual cases, spasticity may serve to enhance the ability to perform certain functional skills, such as transfers or the ability to maintain upright sitting postures.[23]

Successful clinical trials of spasticity management often utilize a number of levels of the measurement hierarchy to help interpret outcomes. Parke and colleagues[24] examined the long-term results of administering baclofen to severely impaired patients with spinal cord injury and multiple sclerosis. Clinical measures of passive restraint revealed an initial reduction in spasticity. This reduction in passive restraint was maintained and was followed by a gradual improvement over 6 months in the functional status of most of the patients. Although it is always difficult to attribute functional improvement directly to the reduction in spasticity, improvements in performance were strongly correlated to reductions in clinically measured spasticity.

PURPOSES OF SPASTICITY EVALUATION

The specific purpose of the evaluation of spasticity helps determine the variables to be selected for measurement and the focus of the questions addressed. The three major purposes of an evaluation of spasticity are

diagnosis, treatment selection, and evaluation of treatment effects.

Evaluation for the purpose of making a diagnosis concerning the presence of spasticity concentrates on the identification, location, and severity of spasticity. Spasticity can be identified through manual examinations testing passive restraint, and in the observation of stretch-induced spasms and hyperactive tendon jerks. Limitations in either passive or voluntary movements may be caused partly by spasticity. The simplest diagnostic use of the spasticity evaluation is to determine whether a UMN syndrome is present, and to localize it. The presence of spasticity in the right arm and leg in association with other neurologic findings might point to disease in the left cerebral hemisphere, whereas spasticity in both legs usually suggests spinal cord pathology. This type of diagnostic use of the spasticity evaluation plays a small role in rehabilitation, where the disease has usually been identified previously.

A more important diagnostic dilemma in rehabilitation is distinguishing spasticity from other causes of increased stiffness. It may be clear from observation that extending a patient's elbow is difficult, but is this due to spasticity, some other form of hypertonia, or tissue contracture? Little and Merritt[23] described a decision tree to help distinguish factors, including spasticity, that may be responsible for the loss of movement (Fig. 5–1). Although hyperactive reflexes and resulting spasticity may frequently be related to restraint in movement, clinical electromyography can be used to distinguish the presence of spasticity from the other factors limiting movement (such as contracture, central coactivation of antagonistic muscles, or a variety of weakness syndromes).[1] Factors distinguishing spasticity from rigidity, dystonia, primitive motor reflexes, and movement disorders such as athetosis are discussed in Chapter 1.

Evaluation of spasticity for treatment planning and selection assumes that spasticity has already been identified and described. The presence of spasticity alone, however, does not necessarily mean that it is the most important limiting factor in the motor disorder. It is important to determine to what extent spasticity (as opposed to

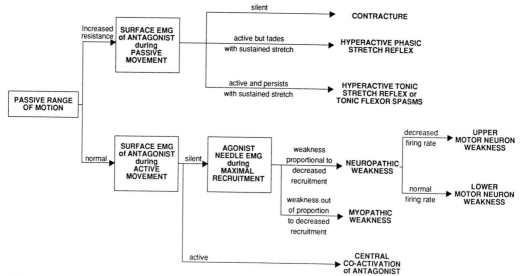

FIG. 5–1. Decision tree of factors that may restrain voluntary movement (with permission from Little, J.W., and Merritt, J.L.: Spasticity and associated abnormalities of muscle tone. *In* Principles and Practice of Rehabilitation Medicine. Ed. J. Delisa, D. Currie, B.M. Gans, P. Gatens, and M. McPhee. Philadelphia, J.B. Lippincott, 1988).

other components of the UMN syndrome) is interfering with passive movement, postural alignment, or aspects of voluntary movement. Answering this question definitively is extremely difficult, particularly in the case of voluntary movement. The process involves an attempt to assess the severity of spasticity and the many other positive and negative symptoms of the UMN syndrome as they relate to the performance requirements of the various tasks of interest. For example, in a patient who finds it difficult to extend the elbow to reach for an object, one would ask the following questions:

1. Is a contracture present that, regardless of other factors, would impede performance?
2. Is the biceps contraction that is palpable during elbow extension caused by activation of the stretch reflex during extension or by central coactivation?
3. Are triceps strength and voluntary control adequate to allow reaching if other obstacles were eliminated?
4. Does the patient have adequate sensation, hand function, and cognition to make use of voluntary reaching if it were facilitated?

Answering these questions will clarify whether successful treatment of spasticity is likely to translate into clinically important gains. At times, however, it may not be entirely possible to distinguish the contribution of spasticity and, for example, the influence of a primitive motor reflex, such as a positive support reaction, on restraint of voluntary movement.

Evaluation of spasticity before and after treatment procedures helps establish the efficacy of various modes of treatment. Evaluation procedures should examine not only the reduction of spasticity, but also the specific changes in passive restraint, postural alignment, and voluntary movement that are associated with the reduction of spasticity. Use of conservative or temporary procedures to reduce spasticity is often helpful in determining the relative influence of spasticity on the motor deficits associated with a UMN syndrome. Pharmacologic agents, physical modalities, local anesthetic nerve blocks, and inhibitive casting are common clinical procedures to help determine if the reduction of spasticity has a motor performance or functional correlate. Reduction of spasticity may allow development of previously restricted movement. The normalization of muscle tone may also facilitate greater adaptability and dexterity of voluntary movements.[8]

Evaluation is part of the continual problem-solving process of measurement, interpretation of findings, treatment, and re-evaluation. An initial evaluation of spasticity should involve not only a plan to obtain an objective baseline measurement of spasticity and related motor abilities, but also a plan to assess the subsequent change in spasticity and the expected change in movement abilities.

CLINICAL MEASUREMENT ISSUES

Quantitative measures of spasticity are needed to describe, objectively and precisely, the severity of spasticity and the extent of associated motor deficits. Clear operational definitions, reliability, and validity are three measurement characteristics that are required for sound and effective clinical measures.

OPERATIONAL DEFINITIONS

An operational definition outlines the specific procedures used in the measurement and provides the set of rules that guides the measurement system.[25] If a fellow clinician describes a patient with severe spasticity, is it readily apparent what he or she means? The clinician may be defining spasticity on the basis of strong clonus, on the basis of the resistance to passive movement, or perhaps from an observation of the patient's voluntary movement. Furthermore, even if the general method of the measurement of spasticity is clear, the specifics of the measurement procedure may not be. For example, a manual examination should specify the patient's positioning, the speed of movement, hand placement, and other factors that may affect the actual measurement. An operational definition should

contain enough specific information that a measurement procedure can be understood and used by people who are similarly trained. Most clinical measures of spasticity do not have adequate operational definitions, and extreme caution must be used in discussing subjective evaluation results.

Clinical measurement requires both consistency and dependability. Reliability is the term used to describe the quality and reproducibility of the measures used in an evaluation. Types of reliability that are reported in the clinical literature are inter-rater reliability (across two or more raters observing the same event), and test-retest reliability (measuring an event on two occasions). One of the most critical questions concerning the quantification of spasticity is the amount of random fluctuation that occurs. The consistency of spasticity across short periods of time is reported to be poor in some patients because of the effects of emotions, positioning, and the difficulty in standardizing test conditions.[10] Rothstein[25] identified three sources of measurement error that may apply to clinical measures of spasticity: flaws in the measuring instrument, lack of consistency of spasticity in specific patient groups, and errors made by those taking the measurements. Some recent reports have highlighted the problems with clinical estimations of spasticity.[26,27]

Validity is a more abstract quality than reliability, and requires an accumulation of evidence from a number of sources. The validity of a measure is related to the usefulness of that measure in making a judgment or inference.[25] Validity is concerned with the application of a measure; measures of spasticity may be valid for some purposes, but not others. For example, the measurement of spasticity by determining the manual resistance to passive stretch of an extremity may be a useful measure of the severity of the neurologic lesion, but may not be useful as an indication of restraint in voluntary movements or as an index of functional loss in ambulation. These are empiric questions that need to be answered before determining the validity of such measures of spasticity. With the current lack of validity information on most measures of spasticity, clinicians must be careful not to make unsubstantiated claims concerning the potential uses of their measures of spasticity. Rothstein[25] describes the numerous types of validity and the procedures by which the validity of clinical measures can be examined.

FRAMEWORK FOR THE EVALUATION OF SPASTICITY

Various measurement strategies can be used to enable the clinician to perform a comprehensive evaluation of spasticity. These strategies may include obtaining a complete history, observation of movement, manual examination, administration of functional or performance measures, and if available, the administration of specialized quantitative tests of spasticity. Table 5–2 outlines five points that provide a framework for the selection and utilization of clinical measurement strategies for a comprehensive spasticity evaluation.

HISTORY

A thorough history is the first step in a comprehensive clinical evaluation of spasticity. It should include basic patient information such as primary and secondary diagnoses, date of injury, level of cognitive functioning, and a chronology of the patient's medical course. Questioning of both

TABLE 5–2. FRAMEWORK FOR THE SELECTION OF MEASUREMENT STRATEGIES

1. What are the distribution and severity of spasticity?
2. Can the spasticity be easily altered or changed? Does spasticity fluctuate because of positioning, modalities, emotions, etc.
3. What is the nature of the resistance to passive stretch? To what extent is the spasticity velocity or position sensitive?
4. How does spasticity affect postural alignment and voluntary movement? Which positions and activities are affected? Is spasticity the limiting factor for these positions or voluntary movements? Is spasticity the limiting factor for functional and self-care activities?
5. What other motor performance factors are likely to be limiting factors in postural alignment, voluntary movements, or functional activities?

TABLE 5–3. PLAN OF INQUIRING FOR HISTORY

Date of onset
Character and severity of spasticity
Location and extent of spasticity
Time relationships
Associated complaints
Aggravating and alleviating factors
Previous treatment and effects
Progress, noting remissions and exacerbations

the patient and the health care team is optimal to provide a more accurate picture of the patient's baseline status. Aronson[28] outlines a plan of inquiry that facilitates appropriate questioning for the evaluating clinician (Table 5–3). Each of these areas is further highlighted in the following paragraphs.

It is important to know if the disease process is static, improving, or progressive because this will shape expectations about the course of spasticity as well as functional abilities. Even in a stable or improving disease, spasticity may be expected to evolve. For example, some diagnoses such as spinal cord injury and cerebral vascular accident (CVA) follow a somewhat predictable time course in the progression or development of spasticity. For this reason, it is crucial to include the date of onset/injury in the history-taking process. These dates should evaluate both the onset of the primary disease entity (e.g., spinal cord injury) and the onset of the specific symptom being assessed (e.g., spasticity). Merritt[29] described such a timetable for traumatic spinal cord injury, beginning with spinal shock characterized by initial flaccidity immediately post-injury. This stage is followed by the development of abnormal muscle tone in specific musculature at predictable times in its recovery. Early development of tone is characterized by mass flexor spasticity, which increases over time. Subsequently, mass extensor spasticity develops and gradually predominates.

The character and severity of the symptoms of UMN syndrome vary from patient to patient. Stolov[30] described some sample questions to investigate these features: "Are there flexor spasms in the lower extremities that are so severe as to compromise wheelchair positioning, transfers and safety? Is clonus so dominant as to interfere with gait or transfers? Is static hypertonus so great that it negatively affects skin and bone integrity or limits voluntary movements of the joint or extremity?" Note that these questions, in addition to assessing the severity and location of spasticity, also establish its functional correlates.

A thorough history includes questions concerning the anatomic distribution of the spasticity.[23] This includes inquiries concerning both the location and extent of spasticity. An important related question is whether spasticity is ever useful for certain transfers and functional skills. The time of day influences the degree or presence of spasticity in some patients. Spasms or hypertonus may be more pronounced in the morning after a relatively inactive sleep period, or for some patients, the dominance of the spasticity may diminish with active movement and proper positioning.

Patients may express associated complaints that indirectly relate to spasticity, such as fatigue caused by increased energy expenditure in walking or activities of daily living.[31] In severe spasticity, pain or generalized stiffness may be a common complaint. It is important to establish what increases or decreases spasticity at any given time. Factors such as fever, infection, stress, a decubitus ulcer, heterotopic ossification, or environmental concerns (e.g., temperature, noise) may influence the severity or frequency of spasms or hypertonus.[29,32] Correct positioning or other measures may help a particular patient to reduce spasticity in certain situations. The history taker should explore the effect of spasticity on functional activities by asking questions such as "In what ways has spasticity interfered with the tasks of daily life?" or "What activities become more difficult when your spasticity is at its worst?"

The history should determine if any previous treatments have been tried (e.g., medications, modalities, positioning, serial casting, phenol blocks), and the long- and short-term effects of the treatment on spasticity and motor function. The examiner should inquire whether any previous treatment that successfully reduced spasticity translated into functional gains. Reports of

previous progress should include remissions and exacerbations of the symptoms during the patient's entire course of rehabilitation. It is important to determine if the patient's perception of progress is consistent with the rehabilitation report.

Obtaining a history for a young child requires a few adaptations to the above interview format. The parents are primarily responsible for reporting how the child's spasticity may interfere with daily functioning and caregiving activities. Parents should be questioned on how the child reacts to handling in bathing, feeding, and dressing activities and in positioning or tone-reducing equipment (prone stander, side-lyer, adaptive seating system, splints or casts).[33]

After a complete history is recorded, the clinician can confirm the history and suspected problems by observing the adult or child and administering a manual examination. Both passive and active manifestations associated with spasticity should be evaluated. Passive issues include problems with passive restraint of a muscle and postural alignment and passive positioning. Issues concerning voluntary movements include problems with motor performance parameters and function. The following sections examine the evaluation of passive and active movement manifestations of spasticity separately.

EVALUATION OF PASSIVE RESTRAINT AND POSTURAL ALIGNMENT

Evaluation of spasticity traditionally has included clinical tests to document passive restraint, and other clinical manifestations that are often associated with spasticity (e.g., clonus, hyperreflexia). Limitations of passive movement include both passive restraint and postural alignment issues. The normal postural control mechanism and tonic postural alignment can also be significantly altered by limitations in passive movement. This section will identify the effects of spasticity on passive restraint and postural alignment and then describe techniques with which to evaluate these effects. Clinical, standardized, and quantitative assessment strategies are reviewed.

EFFECTS ON PASSIVE RESISTANCE AND POSTURAL ALIGNMENT

Passive restraint may lead to fixed postures that can result in contractures and deformities, altered joint osteokinematics due to incorrect tracking of a muscle or tendon at a joint, and difficulty with hygiene and positioning due to limited range of motion.[34] Hypertonia may also influence postural control and postural alignment. It contributes to the inability to express righting, equilibrium, and protective reactions, limits the ability to make transitions between positions, and most importantly, prohibits the normal cocontraction at a joint in weight-bearing positions. All of these postural stabilizing mechanisms are essential prerequisites to more dynamic movement control.[34,35]

Normal muscle tone allows constant interaction between various muscle groups and imparts a readiness to move and react to changes in the environment (internal and external).[36] This provides the individual with the proximal control to hold a given posture against gravity without conscious effort, while allowing voluntary movements to be performed. Development of this stability is considered one of the most important foundations of motor control.[35]

As an infant develops, the emergence of postural control progresses through the acquisition of head control, and the development of sitting and standing. Tonic holding and cocontraction are two phases of the development of stability control. Tonic holding is defined as "the activation of postural muscles in the fully shortened range."[35] Cocontraction is defined as the simultaneous contraction of both the agonist and the antagonist muscles in a weight-bearing position. Hypertonia interferes with ability to develop tonic holding and stability.

Postural reflexes play a dominant role in the regulation of the degree and distribution of muscle tone.[37] Bobath defines the normal postural reflex mechanism as normal tone, integrated primitive reflexes, righting and equilibrium reactions, and protective extension reactions. Most of these mechanisms are stimulated by sensory input to muscles and joints and by the labyrinths (exceptions are the righting reflexes elicited by tactile stimulation of the body and by the semicircular canals). In adults, integrated primitive reflexes are not normally noticeable except after CNS damage. These reflexes are considered pathologic in older children and adults. The tonal changes seen with them are not spasticity, per se, but are part of the larger UMN syndrome. They may be the unfortunate sequelae of traumatic brain injury, CVA, cerebral palsy and demyelinating diseases such as multiple sclerosis. The functional impact of these reflexes can be seen in the resulting problems in postural alignment and specifically in positioning for hygiene, joint integrity, and function (seating and mobility). In evaluating spasticity for therapeutic intervention, it is beneficial to screen for these pathologic reflexes as they often respond to less invasive treatments such as bracing or adaptive positioning and seating. For example, a patient with a seating asymmetry and dominant ATNR may respond to a head positioner, avoiding the need for invasive procedures.

Some stereotypic posturing can also compromise positioning and hygiene and lead to soft tissue contractures. Decerebrate and decorticate posturing are forms of rigidity with specific features that differ from the classic definition of spasticity. Rigidity differs from this definition of spasticity in that it is not associated with hyperreflexia, has no clonus or clasp-knife response, and is not velocity-dependent.[22]

CLINICAL EXAMINATION

The clinical examination will search for passive functional problems and attempt to relate them to spasticity or to other aspects of the UMN syndrome. The examiner will look for asymmetric postures, limitations in range of motion, sites of skin irritation or pressure and attempt to clarify the role of spasticity in their causation.

A complete assessment of range of motion in all joints, passively and actively, is essential to evaluate fully the influence of spasticity on the musculoskeletal system. For some diagnoses, such as CVA, it is predictable which muscle groups are most susceptible to increased tone (e.g., flexors of the upper extremity and extensors of the lower extremity for the hemiplegic side).[32] These are the joints at high risk for loss of motion and require continued accurate joint range of motion measurements to document the need for medical and surgical interventions. If range of motion is extremely limited, problems such as skin breakdown, poor hygiene and structural joint deformities may result. For infants and children it is difficult to measure range of motion using a goniometer, but careful handling of the child will at least highlight obvious range of motion limitations. The postures spontaneously assumed by the patient should also be recorded. Even in the absence of fixed contractures, they may lead to skin and positioning problems.

Once the passive functional problems are identified, an evaluation of spasticity itself is needed. An unmistakable velocity component of the restraint is often seen in passive movements of an extremity with spasticity. The resistance to passive movement increases as the velocity increases, to a certain point (which varies from muscle to muscle), at which time a sudden yielding in the resistance occurs. This clasp-knife phenomenon has been well documented in the literature[1,21,38] and is routinely included in a manual examination of passive restraint. Pedersen[21] has defined mild spasticity as a slight resistance to passive stretching at the end range of a joint, moderate spasticity as early resistance to passive movement with sudden yielding (clasp-knife) and severe spasticity as resistance so severe that it is difficult or impossible to move the extremity.

Hyperreflexia is another feature of the UMN syndrome that is a correlate of passive restraint. Clinically, this is most effectively evaluated by a tendon tap using a reflex hammer. In the spastic muscle, the threshold of the response is significantly decreased or the amplitude of the response is increased.[23] An increase in the reflexogenic zone, a phenomenon often associated with spasticity, may cause irradiation of the reflex. For example, the biceps tendon tap might elicit responses in the wrist and finger musculature of the contralateral or ipsilateral upper extremity.[38]

The testing of the tendon tap should be done with the patient in a relaxed state without active contraction of the muscle because this alters the response of the stretch reflex system.[39] In the upper extremity, muscles to be evaluated for hyperreflexia include the biceps brachii, triceps brachii, brachioradialis, pectoralis major, and long finger flexors. In the lower extremity, the quadriceps femoris, triceps surae, hip adductors, and medial hamstrings should be tested.

Clonus is also associated with spasticity.[40] It can be described as brisk, rhythmic beats in response to sudden passive stretch, especially seen at the ankle, wrist, and fingers.[21,29] The beats may be sustained or unsustained and can vary in their frequency, usually from 5 to 7 Hz.[41] Until recently, it had been widely accepted that the motor unit discharge pattern and rate of clonus can be explained by the stretch reflex mechanism. Some authors have speculated on other systems that may regulate clonus, including the existence of a central pacemaker that cyclically monitors responsiveness of the muscle and its muscle spindle activity.[41] Clonus can be elicited by providing a sudden passive stretch to distal musculature (e.g., ankle, wrist and fingers). The frequency of response and the characteristics of the beats (sustained or waning) should be noted. When present, clonus may lead to skin irritation and loss of position.

Other aspects of the UMN syndrome that may be responsible for impairments in passive function should be differentiated from spasticity. Of critical importance are the tonic and static reflexes that are integrated at the brainstem level and function to maintain posture against gravity. Pathology at this level often results in abnormal responses such as the asymmetric tonic neck reflex, symmetric tonic neck reflex (tonal changes in specific extremities and trunk due to movements of the head), tonic labyrinthine reflex (increased flexor tone/extremity flexion in prone position; increased extensor tone/extremity extension in supine position), positive support reaction (rigid extension of lower extremities with contact of the ball of the foot in upright position), and associated reactions (involuntary movements of a resting extremity as a result of resisted voluntary movement of any body part). The resulting asymmetries at the pelvis, spine, and extremities may lead to poor seating posture, contracture development, and skin breakdown.

The patient with a UMN syndrome may also have delayed or absent responses such as cortical level equilibrium reactions, midbrain righting reactions and automatic movements such as protective extension[39] and may have a Babinski response.[22,23] Spinal level reflexes such as flexor withdrawal, crossed extension and extensor thrust may also significantly impact on the patient's function, again by causing contractures and poor positioning.[11,22] These reflexes are usually triggered by passive movement or volitional effort and also may vary in their intensity and dominance. Clearly, severe flexor withdrawal or crossed extension reflexes would adversely influence the normal postural mechanism, both static and dynamic.

An evaluation of the influence of spasticity on postural tone includes an observation of body position of the patient at rest, noting the ability or inability to attain and maintain correct body alignment in supine and especially in weight-bearing positions. Evaluation should identify abnormal posturing, asymmetry, contractures, and lack of proximal control in weight-bearing positions (e.g. sitting, standing, quadruped). Note whether an abnormal reflex mechanism influences posture and if it interferes with functional positions and activities. This can be done by having the patient actively assume these positions or by assisting the child or adult into the position and evaluating the ability to hold the position against gravity. For example, the asymmetric tonic neck response in the supine position (asymmetric tonic reflex in supine causes the skull side extremities to flex and the face side extremities to extend when the neck is rotated) may prevent rolling due to dominant scapular retraction and/or adduction. In sitting, the hemiplegic patient often displays a thoracic scoliosis with the convexity toward the uninvolved side resulting in pelvic and shoulder girdle asymmetries compromising proximal stability. Unequal weight-bearing in standing is frequently caused by contracture or poor proximal stability and is often reflected in a pelvic obliquity and sometimes a compensatory thoracic curve. If obvious abnormal reflexes are present in the patient, this may warrant formal reflex testing of brainstem, midbrain, and spinal reflexes. Manuals that describe the stimuli and positive and negative reactions for these reflexes are available.[37,42]

As with adults, evaluation of a young child should involve observation of body position at rest and during movement. Abnormal increases in muscle tone interfere with the child's ability to accommodate to passive movements and can delay attainment of gross motor milestones.[43] An abnormal postural reflex mechanism can influence the ability to cross midline during play or in exploring the environment. Excessive extensor dominance, as seen in the symmetric tonic labyrinthine response, can manifest itself in an increased lumbar and/or cervical spinal lordosis that limits the child's ability to roll from supine to side or prone.[33] If the child routinely uses a specialized seating system or other supportive equipment, the need for adjustments which might facilitate more normal positioning for play and function should be evaluated. Oral motor function of the child with UMN syndrome may also be impaired and feeding problems can develop from primitive oral reflexes that have not been integrated.[43]

Hallenborg (see Chapter 6) describes detailed postural alignment evaluations. The assessment provides the clinician with a step-by-step procedure to determine if postural alignment problems are fixed (due to bone and joint deformity) or flexible (abnormal tone and postural reflex mechanism). The results of the evaluation assist in providing appropriate seating and positioning devices.

STANDARDIZED TEST INSTRUMENTS

Ashworth developed a standardized scale to document resistance to passive movement.[44] This system assigns a numeric grade to the amount of resistance felt by the examiner. The original scale included a 5-point rating-scale of tone severity. Since its development, the Ashworth Scale has been widely used clinically and is one of the only

TABLE 5–4. MODIFIED ASHWORTH SCALE*

0	= No increase in muscle tone
1	= Slight increase in muscle tone, manifested by a catch and release or by minimal resistance at the end of the range of motion when the affected part(s) is moved in flexion or extension
1+	= Slight increase in muscle tone, manifested by a catch, followed by minimal resistance throughout the remainder (less than half) of the range of motion
2	= More marked increase in muscle tone through most of the range of motion, but affected part(s) easily moved
3	= Considerable increase in muscle tone, passive movement difficult
4	= Affected part(s) rigid in flexion or extension

*From Bohannon, R.W., Smith, M.B.: Interrater of a modified Ashworth Scale of muscle spasticity. Phys. Ther. 67:206–207, 1986.

standardized tests to measure spasticity. Bohannon states that his previous experience with the Ashworth Scale was that many hemiplegic patients scored at the lower end of the scale rendering grade "1" indiscrete. The addition of the "1 +" level and slightly modified definitions of each grade conformed more precisely to guidelines for ordinal scales. The Modified Ashworth Scale (see Table 5–4) has been shown in recent studies to have good reliability for some but not all muscle groups.[45] It should be noted that at its higher end, the Modified Ashworth Scale measures hypertonia generally and does not specifically distinguish spasticity from other causes of increased tone.

QUANTITATIVE TESTS

The subjectivity of the traditional clinical tools used to evaluate resistance to passive movement has led to research into more quantifiable measurements to document passive restraint in a muscle. These quantitative tests include two major areas, biomechanical tests and electrophysiologic tests. Each of these areas will be briefly reviewed.

The pendulum test named by Wartenburg[46] is one of the most frequently used biomechanical indications of spasticity. The restraint in movement due to pas-

sive stretch has been demonstrated by describing the angular displacement of a limb when it is left to oscillate freely[47] or under controlled speed conditions.[48] Depending on the degree of spasticity and the speed of free oscillations, the spastic limb is characteristically limited in full angular excursions or in the amplitude of oscillation.[49] One of the most common methods of examining this phenomenon is to determine the excursion of a limb as it is released and allowed to swing freely and to record this measurement by an electrogoniometer.

Bajd and Bowman[47] investigated a number of excursion variables during highly controlled pendulum tests of the knee in patients with complete and incomplete spinal cord injury, and developed a mathematic model of movement based on their observations. They identified four causes of fluctuation in resistance noted in their measurement system: the angle from where the limb was released, the position of the subject (supine, sitting) during the test, the number of repetitions of the test, and the velocity of the stretch. All of these factors needed to be controlled to ensure dependable measurements.

Bohannon and Larkin[48] have described a variation of the pendulum test, using an isokinetic dynamometer equipped with an electrogoniometer and a strip recorder to help document the passive elements of spasticity. The Cybex II, because it can control the velocity of the dropping extremity at a maximum speed of 300 degrees per second, does not provide an uncontrolled drop as in most of the previous procedures of the pendulum test. Figure 5–2 compares repeated pendulum tests of a healthy subject to a subject with transverse myelitis in various positions. The healthy subject demonstrated similar goniograms independent of position (A-sitting, B-supine), but the patient with spasticity of the knee extensors demonstrated more knee flexion on the first peak of the goniogram when in sitting position (C) than in the supine position (D). This suggests spasticity of the two-joint rectus femoris. Bohannon and Larkin[48] described a parameter termed the relative angle of reversal (RAR) to quantify the level of passive restraint. The RAR is the angular difference between maximum possible knee

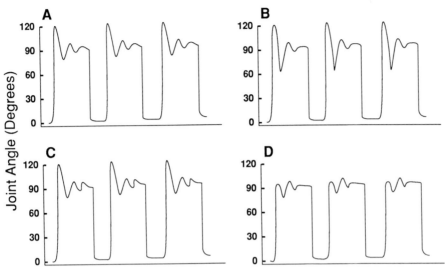

FIG. 5–2. Goniograms from a healthy subject and one with transverse myelitis in sitting, supine (with permission from Bohannon, R.W., and Larkin, P.A.: Cybex II isokinetic dynamometer for documentation of spasticity. Phys. Ther. *65*:46, 1985). See text for description.

flexion and the angle of flexion at which the knee first reversed direction toward extension when dropped. It has been used as an outcome measure for a study on the effect of prolonged stretch and electrical stimulation on knee function in hemiparetic stroke patients.[50] Although much more research needs to be done, it appears that the pendulum test of the knee has potential to be a useful quantitative tool for tracking changes in the passive restraint associated with spasticity. Bohannon reports high reliability among four repeated trials of pendulum testing using the isokinetic dynamometer at one session, but does not comment on its reliability across days or weeks or in other neurologic populations.[51]

Other biomechanical tests focus on the force required to move a spastic limb through the available range manually[52] or through controlled sinusoidal oscillations.[53] Experimental methods have been developed to measure the amount of resistive force to passive movement present in the forearm[54] and the ankle.[53] In a relaxed individual, the joint of an extremity resists movement as a result of inertia of the extremity, the viscoelastic properties of the muscle, gravitational forces, and any muscle contraction of the antagonist evoked by

the stretch reflex.[53] There are several problems to consider when using the force required for passive movement to estimate spastic restraint. These include mechanical oscillations following initiation and termination of movement, a correction procedure for effects of gravity on the extremity, and some large artifacts seen in early phases of fast isokinetic movements.[55,56] These problems can be solved by using an isokinetic dynamometer programmed to control these factors.

Isokinetic force measurements can also be used to quantify changes in velocity and length-dependent reflex activity of patients with spasticity. A protocol for the determination of amount of passive restraint in extremities with spasticity has been described by Knutsson[56] using an isokinetic dynamometer to record this force and the simultaneous torques required to move the limb at different speeds, coupled with the EMG activity in the stretched muscle. The restraint seen in passive movements may vary considerably with the speed of movement, so that the measurement of spasticity should take place across a large range of passive movement speeds. Figure 5–3 displays the torque and EMG responses in passive knee flexion at three velocities in

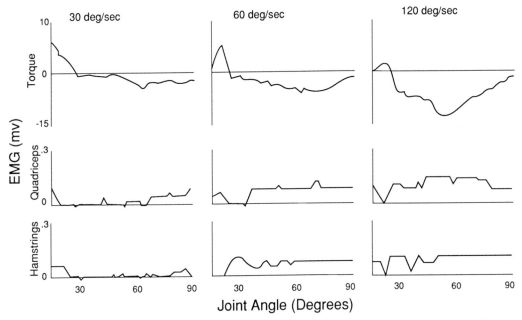

FIG. 5–3. Torque and EMG in passive knee flexion at three velocities in a spastic patient (with permission from Knutsson, E.: Quantification of spasticity. *In* Electromyography and Evoked Potentials. Ed. A. Strappler and A. Weindl. Berlin, Springer-Verlag, 1985).

one patient with spastic paresis. Torque is increased at higher velocities along with an increase in EMG activity of the antagonistic quadriceps. Knutsson's work supports the velocity dependence of spasticity by showing both EMG activity and torque increases with increasing velocities of passive movement.

The measurement of threshold angle has also been used to document passive restraint biomechanically. The threshold angle is defined as the particular angle where torque (or EMG) starts to increase significantly. Katz and Rymer[11] recorded isokinetic torque measurements of spastic hypertonia in the upper extremities of hemiplegic patients. Their results conflict with earlier studies in showing a decrease in the amount of angular displacement necessary to evoke the stretch reflex, rather than an increased velocity dependence in spastic muscles.

Lehmann et al.[57] describe a method to separate viscoelastic changes from reflex changes in spastic muscles because only the latter are likely to respond to drug or phenol block treatments. By measuring torque and evoked EMG activity during controlled oscillations at various velocities, they can determine the overall viscoelastic properties of the limb during passive movement. After lidocaine blocks of agonists and antagonists, the procedure is repeated, demonstrating the viscoelastic properties of the limb without reflex activity. In these studies, although spasticity is the largest determinant of the limb's response, the viscous and elastic properties of the blocked muscles remain abnormal. This suggests early tissue changes even in patients without obvious contractures.

The above measures attempt to assess spasticity by directly examining resistance to passive stretch. Although they have good face validity as indicators of passive restraint, they do not differentiate well among different causes of increased stiffness (e.g., spasticity, rigidity, etc). Electrophysiologic measures have the potential to dissect the increased muscle activity along neurophysiologic lines and thus assist in identifying the precise mechanisms involved in muscle excitability.

Both the H-reflex and the F-wave have

been used to study the excitability of alpha motor neuron in the UMN syndrome. These measures and their use are described in detail in Chapter 3. Although these measures are primarily used for research purposes at present, Delwaide[58] suggests that the analysis of the parameters of the H-reflex can help determine the most appropriate muscle relaxant to prescribe for spasticity.

For many clinical purposes, the H-reflex techniques have limitations. They do not necessarily correspond to the level of clinically defined spasticity[69] and they have considerable variability unless they are tested serially on the same individual.[60] Little and associates[60] reported that serial testing of parameters of the H-reflex did change over time in patients with spinal cord injury, approximately in accordance with the expected appearance of increased flexor reflexes and spasticity. Katz and Rymer[11] also identified methodologic difficulties when studying patients with central nervous system pathology using the H-reflex (e.g., inexact placement of electrodes allowing for gastrocnemius activity to be recorded along with the soleus response). Changes in stimulation frequency, patient relaxation, limb position, or changes in head or neck position can also influence the H-reflex response.

The F-wave requires a supramaximal stimulus and the uncomfortableness of the procedure limits its usefulness as a routine clinical tool.[23] Kimura[61] reports that the F-wave is limited in its clinical uses because of its inherent latency variability from one trial to another. The utility and feasibility of other electrophysiologic measures in the clinical evaluation of spasticity are discussed in detail in Chapter 3. When their technical obstacles are adequately controlled, all these electrophysiologic measures have the advantages of precision, quantifiability, and theoretic significance. They cannot, alone, address the question of treatment outcome, however, because they lack established validity for assessing more functional tasks. A priority in research is to clarify their clinical validity and the degree to which they can be used for selecting patients who will benefit from various treatments.

EVALUATION OF VOLUNTARY MOVEMENTS

Determining the effects of spasticity on voluntary movements involves an analysis of the direct effects of spasticity on the important movement problems of the patient. Direct effects of spasticity cannot always be isolated from other deficits inherent in the UMN syndrome. Hypotheses, however, can be generated and tested through a variety of diagnostic tests and by selective treatment of spasticity to determine if voluntary movement changes occur. Structured clinical evaluations and quantitative tests are used to help determine the influence of spasticity on voluntary movement.

EFFECTS ON VOLUNTARY MOVEMENT

The level of spasticity noted in passive movements may not necessarily coincide with the degree of voluntary movement deficit. Limitations in this assumption will be discussed in the following paragraphs, along with research identifying the conditions under which hyperactive stretch reflexes may impede voluntary movement. Finally, motor performance and motor function deficits commonly associated with the presence of spasticity will be identified.

An important distinction in clinical evaluation procedures should be made concerning the differential influence of spasticity on passive and voluntary movements. A passive movement is performed with the patient relaxed and not using any background stabilization, while active movements have, superimposed upon them, cocontraction of muscles maintaining posture of the trunk and proximal joints.[18] Additionally, synergistic and synkinetic contractions are much greater in active movements than in passive movements. In general, patients with spasticity exhibit a great deal of interindividual variation in the association between passive restraint and voluntary movement dysfunction. Researchers and clinicians have reported cases in which passive movement restraint is relatively strong, yet a corresponding level of voluntary movement dysfunction is not seen.[62,63] Patients with minor spasticity may have severe voluntary movement disorders, but these are largely caused by negative performance deficits of the UMN syndrome rather than spasticity.

Knutsson[64] described a method to evaluate the difference in restraint of passive and voluntary movements of the same range and speed. This method, using an isokinetic dynamometer with surface EMG recordings, is illustrated in Figure 5–4. During passive knee extension, the movement is restrained by reflex contraction of the knee flexors. The passively evoked EMG activity in the flexor muscles increases modestly with increasing movement velocities. During voluntary knee extension, the EMG activity in the antagonistic flexor muscles is not only greater, but increases more dramatically with increased movement velocities.

Although this pattern of greater restraint of voluntary than of passive movements and greater velocity dependence of voluntary restraint is common, it is not universal. The factors that account for the varying patterns of passive and voluntary restraint are unclear. These differences do, however, demonstrate that voluntary restraint cannot be predicted from tests of passive restraint.

Research directed toward identifying the effects of spasticity on voluntary movement has focused on the influence of the stretch reflex. Studies have demonstrated that the hyperactive stretch reflex and the elicitation of clonus can directly affect voluntary movement.[41,65,66] Corcos et al.[20] found the stretch reflex activity was the major factor in restraining movement at the ankle joint in only three of eight patients with spasticity. Stretch reflex contribution to the restraint in movement was determined by the pattern and latencies of the EMG activity of antagonist muscles. The remaining five patients with spasticity demonstrated considerable restraint to active motion that was apparently unrelated to stretch reflex activ-

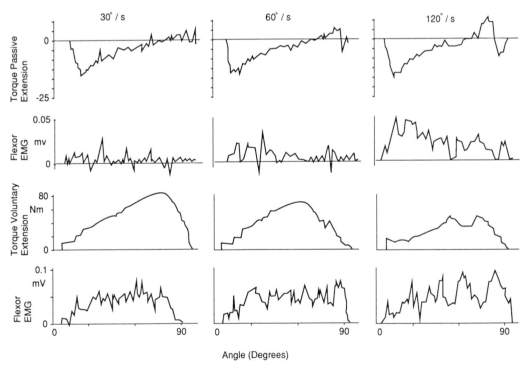

FIG. 5–4. Torque during passive and voluntary knee extension at three speeds of angular rotation in a spastic patient (with permission from Knutsson, E.: Analysis of spastic paresis. *In* Proceedings of Tenth International Congress for Physical Therapy, Sidney, 1987).

ity. The authors listed four conditions that appear to be necessary for stretch reflex activity to influence voluntary movement significantly:

1. The patient must have the ability to initiate rapid voluntary contraction of the agonist muscle and the antagonist must also be able to generate enough force to restrain the movement.
2. The mechanical loading of the joint must not impede the speed of the movement so that the velocity-sensitive reflexes can be elicited.
3. The patient's limb must be moving at relatively fast speeds, because some patients have learned to slow their movements to avoid elicitation of the stretch reflex.
4. The stretch reflex restraint can best be observed in repetitive flexion-extension movements; movements without reciprocal activity may be less affected by abnormal stretch reflex activity.

Other evidence suggests that hyperactive stretch reflexes play a minimal role in restraint of certain movements. Instead, restraint in voluntary movement was attributed to abnormal muscle timing and errors in central coactivation.[17,67–70]

Part of the difficulty in identifying the effect of spasticity on voluntary movement is the variety of other motor disorders that are part of the UMN syndrome. Because spasticity is only one of many factors that may affect voluntary movement, it is often difficult to identify the specific components of motor dysfunction influenced by spasticity. At least three negative symptoms of the UMN syndrome often coexist with spasticity[11]: decreased dexterity, paresis, and muscle timing abnormalities. Part of the task of evaluation, therefore, is to examine the role of these factors, along with spasticity in accounting for observed performance deficits.

Patients with a UMN syndrome often exhibit a significant decrease in the amount of isolated control and dexterity of voluntary movement.[6] Motor patterns available to the patient are often limited and resemble gross synergy movements. Independence from gross synergies and the ability to adapt movement synergies to task demands are

characteristics of the coordination patterns of normal adults. Abnormal synergy patterns have traditionally been linked to the influence of spasticity on voluntary movement and the interruption of dissociated movement patterns.[71–73]

Inadequate force production is a common clinical finding in the presence of the UMN syndrome.[63,74] Patients with UMN syndrome frequently have a substantial fall in single motor unit discharge rate in spastic muscles.[74,75] Knutsson[56] has also documented the loss of force generation in patients with UMN syndrome with an isokinetic dynamometer at different controlled speeds. During concentric voluntary movements, the force produced in patients with UMN syndrome varies with the imposed velocity of movement. In most patients with accompanying spasticity, voluntary torque decreases with increasing speed of movement. Knutsson attributed this pattern largely to the increased activity of the stretch reflex in the spastic antagonist with increased movement velocities, suggesting a direct limiting effect of spasticity.

In addition to the reduced magnitude of force production in patients with UMN syndrome, abnormal timing of muscle contractions affects voluntary movement. Studies have reported a significant delay in force development and a disruption in the normal time interval between reciprocal contractions in patients with the UMN syndrome.[17,76,77] Others have noted that disorders in muscle activity timing patterns lead to delays in the initiation of movement.[68,69,78]

Paresis, loss of dexterity, and improper timing of muscle activation may affect a series of motor control parameters such as movement speed, adaptability and movement initiation. These motor performance deficits, along with spasticity, contribute to the loss or impairment of selected functional skills.

Spasticity is considered an important factor in the loss of functional skills of the patient with UMN syndrome. Spasticity has been reported to affect postural reactions and balance,[1,37] upper extremity tasks,[79,80] transfers, bed mobility,[21,22] and ambulation.[81] Kinematic descriptions of gait of persons with UMN syndrome often report shorter stride lengths, higher cadence, and slower rates of ambulation than in normals[55,82] and poor timing of muscle activity.[81,83-85] In an attempt to distinguish among causes for abnormal gait patterns, Knutsson[81,85] described the presence of three patterns of gait abnormalities in patients with UMN syndrome. They were paresis, exaggerated stretch reflexes that disrupt movement, and exaggerated coactivation. Of these, only the second appears to be a direct effect of spasticity. This restraint of voluntary movement by abnormal reflex activity, when it was present, became more pronounced at higher speeds of ambulation.

CLINICAL EXAMINATION

Clinical evaluation of the effect of spasticity on voluntary movement is a multifaceted process. The key organizing element for the clinical evaluation is to determine the influence of spasticity on many different aspects of voluntary movement. Because voluntary movement can be organized in many different ways, the clinician should use a variety of strategies to assess the influence of spasticity on voluntary movement. General frameworks for conducting an evaluation of the effects of spasticity will be discussed in the following paragraphs, along with motor control variables that may be affected by spasticity. Finally, selected approaches for the evaluation of functional skills will be reviewed.

The performance and execution of voluntary movement have many prerequisites. These range from the conceptualization of movement and motor planning phases to the actual biomechanical execution of the movement[8] (see Chapter 4). Coordination and regulation of muscle tone appear to be important components of all aspects of the control of voluntary movements.

A common clinical framework for the evaluation of a patient with a UMN syndrome is to examine a hierarchy of motor control, including: mobility (freedom of movement, independent of abnormal synergy), stability (ability to maintain a stable alignment against gravity); (see previous section entitled "Evaluation of Spasticity and Its Effect on Motor Dysfunction"), controlled mobility (ability to move between gross motor positions and change positions with control), and skill (discrete motor control of fine movements superimposed on postural stability).[86] O'Sullivan[35] offers a more in-depth discussion of the different clinical evaluation procedures and tasks required to assess each stage of control. For a particular patient, spasticity may differentially affect each level of control.

Clinical checklists and protocols have been established to help organize an evaluation of the qualitative aspects of voluntary movement.[37,39,71,73,87] These clinical checklists of movement components generally contain a comprehensive list of movement activities that assesses increasingly complex levels of isolated movement. Table 5-5 is an example of one such evaluation of voluntary movement described by Brunnstrom[71] and used in the hemiplegic population. Clinical checklists can provide a useful framework for the evaluation of various complex movements. Many of these scales, however, overemphasize the

TABLE 5-5. RECOVERY STAGES AND MOTOR TESTS FOR HEMIPLEGIA

Stage No.	Characteristics
1	No voluntary movement in the affected limb(s) Trunk movements may be fairly well under control
2	Synergies appear as weak associated reactions (flexor synergy before extensor synergy)
3	Synergies or some component are performed voluntarily (flexor, extensor synergy)
4	Movement combinations that deviate from the basic synergy become available: 1. Placing hand behind body (small of back) 2. Elevation of arm to forward-horizontal position 3. Pronation-supination, elbows at 90 degrees
5	Relative independence of basic synergy More difficult movement combinations available: 1. Arm-raising to side-horizontal position 2. Arm raising forward and over head 3. Pronation-supination, elbow extended
6	Isolated joint movements freely performed, movement well coordinated

importance of spasticity as a factor in the loss of voluntary movement control. None of these scales is well standardized, and little technical reliability and validity data have been reported.[88]

A more recent clinical approach has been to assess carefully the direct effect of spasticity on aspects of motor control.[8,89] Emphasis on the motor control approach is to analyze movement requirements of the task. Evaluation should determine whether the movement disorder is related to improper biomechanical factors (limitations in joint range) or to disorders at higher levels of motor control. Evaluative treatments of spasticity, such as physical modalities and local anesthetic nerve blocks, can be used to examine the effects of spasticity on adaptation, errors of speed, limitation of synergistic movements, force generation, control of force production, movement initiation, accuracy, ability to reciprocate movements, response to speed demands, timing, and trajectories of movement. Clinical evaluations of voluntary movements should increasingly take on the form of evaluative treatments, in which motor control parameters are recorded quantitatively and then re-evaluated after reduction of spasticity is achieved through treatment.

An important focus of the evaluation of spasticity is examination of the daily functional activities that appear to be affected by spasticity. Thorough clinical evaluations should cover by observation or report the functional skills of transfers, dressing, feeding, and other self-help skills, wheelchair skills (if applicable), and ambulation. Examination of how these tasks are performed may suggest initial hypotheses regarding what aspects of the UMN syndrome are the major obstacles.

Assessment of gait is particularly important. Observational gait assessments can center upon the qualitative aspects of gait at different cycle points, or upon temporal and distance measures. Observation schemes are available for the systematic observational evaluation of gait,[90] although there is some concern about the reliability of such techniques.[91] Several spatial and temporal methods have also been described, and newer microswitch devices now make it feasible to record both spatial and temporal information simultaneously. Temporal-distance measurements are also used routinely in many clinics.[92,93] None of these gait evaluation systems has been shown to distinguish gait abnormalities caused by spasticity from those related to other aspects of the UMN syndrome. Thus, more research is needed to find ways to identify patients whose gait may benefit from spasticity-reducing intervention.

STANDARDIZED TEST INSTRUMENTS

None of the standardized test instruments used to assess deficits in voluntary movement directly measures spasticity. It is likely that relatively large changes in spasticity are needed before change can be detected in functional scales.[11] Furthermore, it is difficult to attribute functional change directly to spasticity changes. It is important, however, to evaluate the functional problems because they most likely represent the critical issues for the patient. An antispasticity treatment in the mobile patient is unlikely to be successful unless it affects some aspect of function in a positive manner. The functional instruments covered in this selected review are categorized as motor recovery scales, motor performance scales, and motor function scales.

Fugl-Meyer,[72,94] using many of the Brunnstrom[71,95] methods for assessing the interaction of posture and voluntary motor function, developed an evaluation tool based on motor recovery of hemiplegic patients. The evaluation system is comprised of items that assess motor function, balance, sensation, passive range of motion, and joint pain (Table 5–6). The test has been developed within the conceptual framework that the restoration of motor function in hemiplegia follows a definable sequence. The sequence includes initial flaccidity, a recurrence of reflexes and hypertonia, and varying levels of control over selected isolated movements. Reliability data on the Fugl-Meyer Assessment[96] have been reported using a sample of 19 patients with hemiplegia. Intertester and intratester reliability coefficients for the total test were .89 and .99 respectively, with the coefficients of the subscores ranging from .79 to

TABLE 5–6. FUGL-MEYER ASSESSMENT OF
SENSORIMOTOR RECOVERY

Passive joint pain; motion
Sensation: Light touch; proprioception
Movements combining synergies in upper extremity
  and lower extremity: shoulder, forearm, wrist,
  hand function
Supine and sitting lower extremity movements
Grasp patterns (5)
Coordination/speed
Balance:
  Sit without support
  Parachute reaction
  Stand with/without support
  Stand on affected/unaffected side

.99. Researchers have also established the concurrent validity of the test, finding a high correlation between Fugl-Meyer test scores and activities of daily living[94] somatosensory evoked potentials,[97] and organization of postural adjustments.[98] The Fugl-Meyer test is a useful clinical test for the evaluation of motor recovery in patients with hemiplegia. It provides a way to assess whether spasticity-reducing measures are effective during some phases of recovery, and if treatment provides the potential to advance the recovery process.

Motor performance tests have been developed specifically for the assessment of upper extremity function. The Arm Function Test[99] was developed to monitor the recovery of arm function in patients with hemiplegia. This test consists of five measurement dimensions of arm function, including a rating of muscle tone. The items are scored on a dichotomous scale of pass/fail with criteria established for each item. Preliminary reliability of the test has been examined on five patients using six raters, with acceptable reliability in all the dimensions except pain.[100] The Arm Function Test has also been validated by high positive correlations between the test scores and the patient's clinical status as well as on a pursuit tracking task.[100] Other scales with a similar purpose have also been developed.[101,102] Such scales may be useful in measuring whether reduction of spasticity in the upper extremity translates into improved motor control. Because one of the scales of the Arm Function Test assesses tone, however, this scale should be disregarded when measuring influence of tone reduction on other aspects of functioning to avoid circularity.

The Tufts Assessment of Motor Performance (TAMP) is a 32-item standardized, criterion referenced test of motor performance and physical function.[103] The TAMP samples motor performance capabilities in the areas of grasp/release of objects, manipulation tasks, use of fasteners, typing skills, dynamic balance, mat mobility, locomotion and wheelchair skills. Developed for the purpose of detecting motor performance changes during rehabilitation programs, the TAMP is a useful examination for identifying short- and long-term performance effects of spasticity interventions, such as nerve blocks. The TAMP has multiple measurement dimensions including proficiency and time to complete the task. Good intertester reliability data have been reported,[103] and work is now under way to validate the instrument and to further assess its use in clinical trials of spasticity intervention. A pediatric version of the TAMP is also currently being developed. This measure should prove particularly useful in assessing the extent of functionally important changes resulting from antispasticity treatment.

Traditional measures such as the Barthel[104] have provided the means to assess basic physical function of persons with UMN syndrome and accompanying spasticity. Recently, a new consensus measure has been proposed to assess functional skills and is being widely used as a part of a uniform data base in rehabilitation.[105] The Functional Independence Measure samples 18 items and assesses the amount of person and device assistance needed by an individual to accomplish certain daily functional tasks (Table 5–7). These functional tasks are often the focus of intervention in persons with spasticity. Although the Functional Independence Measure is now available only for adults, projects are under way to develop functional measures for pediatric use. Comprehensive reviews of other standardized performance and functional tests for adults[106,107] and children[108] are available. It should be kept in mind that none of these functional measures is likely to show change related to treatment of

TABLE 5–7. THE FUNCTIONAL
INDEPENDENCE MEASURE

1. Feeding
2. Grooming
3. Bathing
4. Dressing: Upper Body
5. Dressing: Lower Body
6. Toileting
7. Bladder Management
8. Bowel Management
9. Transfer: Bed, Chair, Wheelchair
10. Transfer: Toilet
11. Transfer: Tub, Shower
12. Walk/Wheelchair
13. Stairs
14. Communication: Comprehension
15. Comprehension: Expression
16. Social Interaction
17. Problem Solving
18. Memory

**Levels of Assistance for the Functional
Independence Measure**

7. Complete Independence (Timely, Safely)
6. Modified Independence (Device)
5. Modified Dependence: Supervision
4. Minimal Assistance
3. Moderate Assistance
2. Maximal Assistance
1. Total Assistance

spasticity unless that spasticity is a major limiting factor to task performance. Thus, these measures are particularly useful, in both clinical and research contexts, for addressing that question.

QUANTITATIVE TESTS

Most clinical settings do not have available the sophisticated equipment that is often needed to quantify elements of spasticity accurately. Two types of measures, however, are becoming more popular (and economically feasible) in large clinics. These include biomechanical measures during active motion, and kinesiologic studies.

Force production measures of voluntary movements are an important aspect of evaluating the individual with UMN syndrome who also has spasticity. Knutsson[56] discusses the value of examining the torque and EMG of muscle pairs using both concentric (agonist shortens) and eccentric (ag-

onist lengthens) contractions. Concentric and eccentric contractions may be differentially affected by the presence of spasticity, with eccentric contractions actually facilitated by stretch reflex effects because the stretch of the lengthening muscle reflexively augments its activity. (Fig. 5–5). This type of detailed biomechanical analysis can help identify important functional effects of spasticity.

Brown et al.[79] described a thorough clinical neurologic assessment protocol for the study of hand function in children with hemiplegia. They examined the following variables: range of motion, muscle tone, muscle power, speed of movement, fatigability, sensory function, tremor tested by an accelerometer, and the resistance to passive movements with different frequencies using a torque motor. Often a detailed assessment of this kind is necessary to identify the precise contributions of spasticity to the individual's motor dysfunction. In the study of hemiplegic children, spasticity elicited during rapid stretch was found to be more related to dysfunction than spasticity noted during slow, prolonged stretch. Regardless of the degree of spasticity, the performance abilities of distal power and speed correlated most highly with functional hand skills.

Several investigators have developed complex systems of motion analysis coupled with electromyographic (EMG) recordings to study the effect of spasticity on functional skills. Benecke et al.[109] advocated the use of natural complex movements in the analysis of spasticity. They suggest that the movements should have a combination of active innervation and passive lengthening of antagonistic pairs. Gait[55] and bicycling[109] are two of the functional tasks that have been examined by means of this methodology.

The incorporation of kinesiologic EMG with motion analysis is also becoming more clinically feasible because of the ability of microcomputers to analyze the data quickly.[110] EMG coupled with motion analysis has been a useful adjunct to decision-making before orthopedic surgery, and to evaluation of the functional outcome.[111] Many of these studies have shown that the routine clinical observations are inadequate

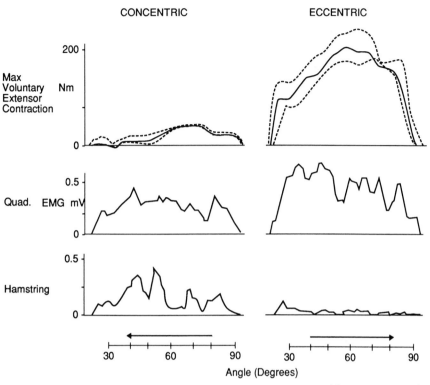

FIG. 5–5. Torque and EMG recording of concentric and eccentric contraction of knee extensors in spastic patient (with permission from Knutsson, E.: Analysis of spastic paresis. *In* Proceedings of Tenth International Congress for Physical Therapy, Sidney, 1987).

to distinguish between dissimilar EMG patterns underlying identical movement pattern problems.[83,112] The ability to differentiate performance deficits related to the stretch reflex from those related to central coactivation can help identify patients likely to benefit from medication, nerve blocks, or surgery. It is clear that there is a high degree of individual variation in disordered movement control associated with a spastic gait. Patterns are so variable and complex that computer-enhanced motion analysis and EMG data are important for clinical decision-making.[81]

There are some limitations in the interpretation of kinesiologic EMG data. Surface EMG data indicate the presence or absence of activity in certain muscles but do not clearly reflect the amount of force or effort generated.[113] There are also serious questions concerning the validity of the normalization and quantification of EMG levels

and patterns of agonist-antagonist timing used to measure coactivation patterns.[62,109] However, this area has great potential to classify patients according to movement pattern pathology, document treatment effectiveness, and determine which treatments are most effective for different clinical manifestations of the UMN syndrome.[111]

SUMMARY

The clinical assessment of spasticity involves using the most appropriate and clinically feasible measurements to make judgments about treatments and patient management. As measurement systems become more precise and informative, our clinical evaluation of spasticity becomes more exact and meaningful. Treatment success is proportional to the degree of understanding of specific effects of spasticity on passive restraint, postural alignment, and voluntary movements.

We have discussed the evaluation of spasticity within the framework of its impact on important movement skills of the patient. Linking our measurements of spasticity to functional problems is the key to the selection of measurement strategies for spasticity. Technology, coupled with skilled clinicians, will continue to provide the field of rehabilitation medicine with updated and more complete clinical procedures for the evaluation of spasticity and its effect on motor function. Clinicians must always direct their evaluations toward the clinical problems created by spasticity or other elements of the UMN syndrome. We must continue to investigate new methods of treatment based on thoughtful and precise evaluation using sound measurement practices.

REFERENCES

1. Landau, W.M.: Spasticity: What is it? What is it not? *In* Spasticity: Disordered Motor Control. Ed. R.G. Feldman, R.R. Young, and W.P. Koela, Chicago, Yearbook Medical Publishers, 1980.
2. Ashby, P., Malibis, A., and Hunter, J.: The evaluation of "Spasticity." Can. J. Neruol. Sci. *14*:497, 1989.
3. Adams, R.D.: Muscular hypertonia—The clinical viewpoint. *In* New Developments in Electromyography and Clinical Neurophysiology. Ed. J.E. Desmedt. Basel Karger, 1973.
4. Wyke, B.: Neurological mechanisms in spasticity. Brief review of some current concepts. Physiother. *62*:316, 1976.
5. Young, R.R., and Shahani, B.T.: Spasticity in spinal cord injured patients. *In* Management of Spinal Cord Injuries. Ed. R.F. Bloch and M. Basbaum. Baltimore, William & Wilkins, 1986.
6. Shahani, B.T., and Young, R.R.: The flexor reflex in spasticity. *In* Spasticity: Disordered Motor Control. Ed. R.G. Feldman, R.R. Young, and W.P. Koela. Chicago, Yearbook Medical Publishers, 1980.
7. Landau, W.M.: Spasticity: The fable of a neurological demon and the emperor's new therapy. Arch. Neurol. *31*:217, 1974.
8. Duncan, P.W., and Badke, M.B.: Determinants of abnormal motor control. *In* Stroke Rehabilitation: The Recovery of Motor Control. Ed. P.W. Duncan and M.B. Badke. Chicago, Year Book Medical Publishers, 1987.
9. Wyn, Jones E., and Mulley, G.P.: The measurement of spasticity. *In* Advances in Stroke Therapy. Ed. F.C. Rose. New York, Raven Press, 1982.
10. Burry, H.C.: Objective measurement of spasticity. Dev. Med. Child. Neurol. *14*:508, 1972.
11. Katz, R.T., and Rymer, W.J.: Spastic hypertonia: Mechanisms and measurement. Arch. Phys. Med. Rehabil. *70*:144, 1989.
12. Lance, J.W.: Symposium synopsis. *In* Spasticity: Disordered Motor Control. Eds. R.G. Feldman, R.R. Young, and W.P. Koela. Chicago, Yearbook Medical Publishers, 1980.
13. Bishop, B.: Spasticity: Its physiology and management. Phys. Ther. *57*:371, 1977.
14. Davidoff, R.A.: Antispasticity drugs mechanisms of action. Am. Neurol. *17*:107, 1985.
15. Young, R.R., and Wierzbicka, M.D.: Behavior of single motor units in normal subjects and in patients with spastic paresis. *In* Clinical Neurophysiology in Spasticity: Contribution to Assessment and Pathophysiology. Ed. P.J. Delwaide and R.R. Young. Amsterdam, Elsevier, 1985.
16. Lance, J.W., and McLeod, J.G.: Disordered muscle tone. *In* Physiological Approach to Clinical Neurology. Ed. J.W. Lance and J.G. McLeod. Boston, Butterworths, 1981.
17. Sahrmann, S.A., and Norton, B.J.: The relationship of voluntary movement to spasticity in the upper motor neuron syndrome. Ann. Neurol. *2*:460, 1977.
18. McLellan, D.L.: Cocontraction and stretch reflexes in spasticity during treatment with baclofen. J. Neurol. Neurosurg. Psychiatry *40*:30, 1977.
19. Van Saint, A.: Designing a definitive clinical study of spasticity. Neurol. Report. *9*:17, 1985.
20. Corcos, D.M., et al.: Movement deficits caused by hyperexcitable stretch reflexes in spastic humans. Brain *109*:1043, 1986.
21. Pedersen, E.: Clinical aspects of spasticity. *In* Spasticity: Mechanisms, Measurement and Management. Springfield, IL, Charles C Thomas, 1969.

22. Griffith, E.R.: Spasticity. *In* Rehabilitation of the Head Injured Adult. Ed. M. Rosenthal, et al. Philadelphia, F.A. Davis Co., 1983.

23. Little, J.W., and Merritt, J.L.: Spasticity and associated abnormalities of muscle tone. *In* Principles and Practice of Rehabilitation Medicine. Ed. J. Delisa, D. Currie, B.M. Gans, P. Gatens, and M. McPhee. Philadelphia, J.B. Lippincott, 1988.

24. Parke, B., Penn, R.D., Savoy, S.M., and Corcos, D.: Functional outcome after delivery of intrathecal baclofen. Arch. Phys. Med. Rehabil. *70:*30, 1989.

25. Rothstein, J.M.: Measurement and clinical practice: Theory and application. *In* Measurement in Physical Therapy. Ed. J.M. Rothstein. New York, Churchill Livingstone, 1985.

26. Katherine, J.E.: Interrater reliability in the assessment of muscle tone of infants and children. Paper presented at the American Physical Therapy Association Combined Sections Meeting, Honululu, HI, 1989.

27. Klassen, L.: The reliability and validity of three methods used to quantify spasticity. Paper presented at the American Physical Therapy Association Annual Meeting, Las Vegas, 1988.

28. Aronson, A.E., et al.: The neurology history. *In* Clinical Examinations in Neurology. Philadelphia, W.B. Saunders Co., 1976.

29. Merritt, J.L.: Management of Spasticity in Spinal Cord Injury. Mayo Clin. Proc. *56:*614, 1981.

30. Stolov, W.C., Cole, T.M., and Tobis, J.S.: Evaluation of the patient. *In* Krusen's Handbook of Physical Medicine and Rehabilitation. Ed. Kottke, F.J., Stillwell, G.K., Lehman, J.F. Philadelphia, W.B. Saunders Co., 1971.

31. Olgiate, R., Burgunder, J.M., and Mumenthaler, M.: Increased energy cost of walking in multiple sclerosis: Effect of spasticity, ataxia, and weakness. Arch. Phys. Med. Rehabil. *69:*846, 1988.

32. Denny-Brown, D.: Preface: Historical aspects of the relation of spasticity to movement. *In* Spasticity: Disordered Motor Control. Ed. R.G. Feldman, R.R. Young, and W.P. Koella, Chicago, Yearbook Medical Publishers, 1980.

33. Scherzer, A.L., and Tscharnuter, I.: Early Diagnosis and Therapy in Cerebral Palsy. New York, Marcel Dekker, Inc., 1982.

34. Charness, A.: Stroke/Head Injury. A Guide to Functional Outcomes in Physical Therapy Management. Rockville, Maryland, Aspen Publications, 1986.

35. O'Sullivan, S.B.: Motor control assessment. *In* Physical Rehabilitation: Assessment and Treatment (2nd ed). Eds. S.B. O'Sullivan and T.J. Schmitz. Philadelphia, F.A. Davis Co., 1988.

36. Ryerson, S.J.: Hemiplegia resulting from vascular insult or disease. *In* Neurological Rehabilitation. Ed. D.A. Umphred, St. Louis, C.V. Mosby Co., 1985.

37. Bobath, B.: Adult Hemiplegia: Evaluation and Treatment. London, William Heinemann Medical Books Ltd., 1978.

38. Bauer, H.J.: Spasticity: Its causes and clinical significance. *In* Spasticity—A Topical Survey. Ed. W. Birkmayer. Switzerland, Hans Huber Publishers, 1972.

39. Nelson, A.J.: Motor assessment. *In* Rehabilitation of the Head Injured Adult. Ed. M. Rosenthal et al. Philadelphia, F.A. Davis Co., 1983.

40. Noel, G.: Clinical changes in muscle tone. *In* New Developments in Electromyography and Clinical Neurophysiology. Ed. J.E. Desmedt. Basel Karger, 1973.

41. Dimitrijevic, M.R., Nathan, P.W., and Sherwood, A.M.: Clonus: the role of central mechanisms. J. Neurol. Neurosurg. Psychiatry *43:*321, 1980.

42. Fiorentino, M.R.: Reflex-testing methods for evaluating CNS development. Springfield, IL, Charles C Thomas Publishers, 1981.

43. Wilson, J.M.: Cerebral Palsy. *In* Pediatric Neurologic Physical Therapy. Ed. O.D. Payton, et al. New York, Churchill Livingstone, 1984.

44. Ashworth, B.: Preliminary trial of carisoprodol in multiple sclerosis. Practitioner *162:*540, 1964.

45. Bohannon, R.W., and Smith, M.B. Interrater reliability of a modified Ashworth Scale of muscle spasticity. Phys. Ther. *67:*206, 1987.

46. Wartenberg, R.: Pendulousness of the legs as a diagnostic test. Neurology *1:*18, 1951.

47. Bajd, T., and Bowman, B.: Testing and modelling of spasticity. J. Biomed. Eng. *4:*90, 1982.

48. Bohannon, R.W., and Larkin, P.A.: Cybex II isokinetic dynamometer for the documentation of spasticity. Phys. Ther. *65:*46, 1985.

49. Bajd, T., and Vodvnik, L.: Pendulum testing of spasticity. J. Biomed. Eng. *6:*9, 1984.

50. Bohannon, R.W.: Result of prolonged stretch and electrical stimulation on knee function in a hemiparetic stroke patient. Neurol. Report *12:*19, 1987.

51. Bohannon, R.W.: Variability and reliability of the pendulum test for spasticity using a

Cybex II isokinetic dynometer. Phys. Ther. *67*:659, 1987.

52. Halpern, D., et al.: Muscular hypertonia: Quantitative analysis. Arch. Phys. Med. Rehabil. *60*:208, 1979.
53. Gottlieb, G.L., Atarwal, G.C., and Penn, R.: Sinusoidal oscillation of the ankle as a means of evaluating the spastic patient. J. Neurol. Neurosurg. Psychiatry *41*:32, 1978.
54. Webster, D.D.: The dynamic quantitation of spasticity with automated intergrals of passive motion resistance. Clin. Pharmacol. & Ther. *5*:900, 1966.
55. Knutsson, E.: Analysis of gait and isokinetic movements for evaluation of antispastic drugs or physical therapies. *In* Motor Control Mechanisms in Health and Disease. Ed. J.E. Desmedt. New York, Raven Press, 1983.
56. Knutsson, E.: Quantification of spasticity. *In* Electromyography and Evoked Potentials. Ed. A. Strappler and A. Weindl. Berlin, Springer-Verlag, 1985.
57. Lehmann, J.F., et al.: Spasticity: Quantitative measurements as a basis for assessing effectiveness of therapeutic intervention. Arch. Phys. Med. Rehabil. *70*:6, 1989.
58. Delwaide, P.J.: Electrophysiological analysis of the mode of action of muscle relaxants in spasticity. Ann. Neurol. *17*:90, 1985.
59. Spira, R.: Contribution of the H-reflex to the study of spasticity in adolescents. Dev. Med. Child Neurol. *16*:150, 1974.
60. Little, J.W., and Halar, E.M.: H-reflex changes following spinal cord injury. Arch. Phys. Med. Rehabil. *66*:19–22, 1985.
61. Kimura, J.: Electrodiagnosis in Diseases of Nerve and Muscle: Principles and Practice. Philadelphia, F.A. Davis, 1983.
62. Knutsson, E., and Martensson, A.: Dynamic motor capacity in spastic paresis and its relation to prime mover dysfunction, spastic reflexes and antagonist co-activation. Scand. J. Rehabil. Med. *12*:93, 1980.
63. Bohannon, R.W., Larkin, P.A., Smith, M.B., and Horton, M.G.: Relationship between static muscle strength deficits and spasticity in stroke patient with hemiparesis. Phys. Ther. *67*:1068, 1987.
64. Knutsson, E.: Analysis of spastic paresis. *In* Proceedings of Tenth International Congress for Physical Therapy, Sidney, 1987.
65. Mizrahi, E.M., and Angel, R.W.: Impairment of voluntary movement by spasticity. Ann. Neurol. *5*:594, 1979.
66. Pierrot-Deseiligny, E., and Mazieres, L.: Spinal mechanisms and underlying spasticity. *In* Clinical Neurophysiology in Spasticity. Ed. P.J. Delwaide and R.R. Young. Amsterdam, Elsevier, 1985.
67. McLellan, D.L., and Hassan, N.H.: The use of electromyograms to assess impaired voluntary movement associated with increased muscle tone. EEG Suppl. *36*:169, 1982.
68. Milner-Brown, H.S., and Penn, R.D.: Pathophysiological mechanisms in cerebral palsy. J. Neurol. Neurosurg. Psychiatry *42*:606, 1979.
69. Neilson, P.: Voluntary control of arm movements in athetotic patients. J. Neurol. Neurosurg. Psychiatry *37*:162, 1974.
70. Nashner, L.M.: A functional approach to understanding spasticity. *In* Electromyography and Evoked Potentials: Theories and Applications. Berlin, Springer-Verlag, 1985.
71. Brunnstrom, S.B.: Movement Therapy in Hemiplegia. Philadelphia, Harper & Row, 1970.
72. Fugl-Meyer, A.R., et al.: The post-stroke hemiplegic patient. I. A method for evaluation of physical performance. Scand. J. Rehabil. Med. *7*:13, 1975.
73. Goff, B.: Grading of spasticity and its effect on voluntary movement. Physiother. *62*:358, 1976.
74. Tang, A., and Rymer, W.Z.: Abnormal force-EMG relations in paretic limbs of hemiparetic human subjects. J. Neurol. Neurosurg. Psychiatry *44*:690, 1981.
75. Rosenflack, A., Andreassen, S.: Impaired regulation of force and firing pattern of single motor units in patients with spasticity. J. Neurol. Neurosurg. Psychiatry *43*:907, 1980.
76. Watkins, M.P., Harris, B.A., and Kozlowski, B.A.: Isokinetic testing in patients with hemiparesis: A pilot study. Phys. Ther. *2*:184, 1984.
77. Chen, W., Pierson, F.M., and Burnett, C.N.: Force-time measurements of knee muscle functions of subjects with multiple sclerosis. Phys. Ther. *67*:934, 1987.
78. Myklebust, B.M., Gottlieb, G.L., Penn, R.D., and Agarwal, G.C.: Reciprocal excitation of antagonistic muscles as a differentiating feature in spasticity. Ann. Neurol. *12*:367, 1982.
79. Brown, J.K., et al.: A neurological study of hand function of hemiplegic children. Dev. Med. Child Neurol. *29*:2-87-304, 1987.
80. McPherson, J.J., Becker, A.J., and Franszczak, N.: Dynamic splint to reduce the passive component of hypertonicity. Arch. Phys. Med. Rehabil. *66*:249, 1985.

81. Knutsson, E.: Gait control in hemiparesis. Scand. J. Rehabil. Med. *13*:101, 1981.
82. Gehlsen, G., et al.: Gait characteristics in multiple sclerosis: Progressive changes and effects of exercise on parameters. Arch. Phys. Med. Rehabil. *67*:536, 1986.
83. Chong, K.C., et al.: The assessment of the internal rotation gait in cerebral palsy. Clin. Orth. *132*:145, 1978.
84. Dimitrijevic, M.R., Faranel, J., Sherwood, A.M., and McKay, W.B.: Activation of paralyzed leg flexors and extensors during gait in patients after stroke. Scand. J. Rehabil. Med. *13*:109, 1981.
85. Knutsson, E., and Richards, C.: Different types of disturbed motor control in gait of hemiplegic patients. Brain *102*:405, 1979.
86. Stockmeyer, S.: An interpretation of the approach of Rood to the treatment of neuromuscular dysfunction. Am. J. Phys. Med. *46*:900, 1967.
87. Clark, B., et al.: A re-evaluation of the Brunstrom assessment of motor recovery of the lower limb. Physiother. Can. *35:4*, 1983.
88. Clopten, S.M.: Reliability of the Modified Brunstrom Assessment. Unpublished Master's Thesis, Massachusetts General Hospital Institute for Health Professions, 1986.
89. Giuliani, C.: Abnormal motor programs: Implications for assessment and treatment. Paper presented at the Combined Sections Meeting, Washington, DC, American Physical Therapy Association, 1988.
90. Craik, R.L., and Oatis, C.A.: Gait assessment in the clinic: Issues and approaches. *In* Measurement in Physical Therapy. Ed. J.M. Rothstein, New York, Churchill Livingstone, 1985.
91. Krebs, D.E., Edelstein, J.E., and Fishman, S.: Reliability of observational kinematic analysis. Phys. Ther. *64*:1027–1033, 1985.
92. Nelson, A.J.: Functional ambulation profile. Phys. Ther. *54*:1059–1062, 1974.
93. Holden, M., Gill, K.M., and Magliozzi, M.R.: Gait assessment for neurologically impaired patients. Phys. Ther. *66*:1530, 1986.
94. Fugl-Meyer, A.R.: Assessment of motor function in hemiplegic patients. *In* Neurophysiologic Aspects of Rehabilitation Medicine. Ed. A.A. Buerger. Springfield, IL, Charles C Thomas, 1976.
95. Brunnstrom, S.: Motor testing procedures in hemiplegia. J. Am. Phys. Ther. Assoc. *46*:357, 1966.
96. Duncan, P.W., Propst, M., and Nelson, S.G.: Reliability of the Fugl-Meyer Assessment of sensorimotor recovery following cerebrovascular accident. Phys. Ther. *63*:1606, 1983.
97. Kusoffsky, A., Wadell, I., and Nilsson, B.Y.: The relationship between sensory impairment and motor recovery in patients with hemiplegia. Scand. J. Rehabil. Med. *14*:27, 1982.
98. Badke, M.B., and Duncan, P.W.: Patterns of rapid motor responses during postural adjustments when standing in health subjects and hemiplegic patients. Phys. Ther. *63*:13, 1983.
99. DeSouza, L., Hewer, R., and Miller, S.: Assessment of recovery of arms control in hemiplegic stroke patients. 1. Arm function tests. Int. Rehab. Med. *2*:3, 1980.
100. DeSouza, L., et al.: Assessment of recovery of arm control in hemiplegic stroke patients. 2. Comparison of arm function tests and pursuit tracking in relation to clinical recovery. Int. Rehabil. Med. *2*:10, 1980.
101. Carroll, D.: A quantitative test of upper extremity function. J. Chron. Dis. *18*:479, 1965.
102. Jebsen, R.H., et al.: Measurement of time in a standardized test of patient mobility. Arch. Phys. Med. Rehabil. *51*:170–175, 1970.
103. Gans, B.M., et al.: Description and interobserver reliability of the Tufts Assessment of Motor Performance. Am. J. Phys. Med. Rehabil. *67*:202, 1988.
104. Mahoney, F.I., and Barthel, D.W.: Functional evaluation: The Barthel Index. Md. Med. J. *14*:61, 1965.
105. Granger, C.V., et al.: Advances in functional assessment for medical rehabilitation. Top. Geriat. Rehabil. *1*:59, 1986.
106. Jette, A.M.: State of the art in functional status assessment. *In* Measurement in Physical Therapy. Ed. J.M. Rothstein. New York, Churchill Livingstone, 1985.
107. Guccione, A.A., Cullen, K.E., and O'Sullivan, S.B.: Functional assessment. *In* Physical Rehabilitation: Assessment and Treatment (2nd ed). Ed. S.B. O'Sullivan and T.J. Schmitz. Philadelphia, F.A. Davis Co., 1988.
108. Haley, S.M., Hallenborg, S.C., and Gans, B.M.: Functional assessment in young children with physical impairments. Topics in Early Childhood Special Education, *9*:106–126, 1989.
109. Benecke, R., Conrad, B., Meinck, H.M., and Hohne, J.: Electromyographic analysis of bicycling on an ergometer for evaluation of spasticity of lower limbs in man. *In* Motor Control Mechanisms in Health and Dis-

ease. Ed. J.E. Desmedt. New York, Raven Press, 1983.

110. Campbell, S.K.: Assessment of the child with CNS dysfunction. *In* Measurement in Physical Therapy. Ed. J.M. Rothstein. New York, Churchill Livingstone, 1985.

111. Campbell, S.K.: Central nervous system dysfunction in children. *In* Pediatric Neurologic Physical Therapy. Ed. S.K. Campbell. New York, Churchill Livingstone, 1984.

112. Holt, K.S.: Facts and fallacies about neuromuscular function in cerebral palsy as revealed by electromyography. Devel. Med. Child Neurol. *8:*255, 1966.

113. Echternach, J.L.: Measurement issues in nerve conduction velocity and electromyographic testing. *In* Measurement in Physical Therapy. Ed. J.M. Rothstein, New York, Churchill Livingstone, 1984.

6

POSITIONING

SUSAN C. HALLENBORG

Changes in general body position can significantly alter muscle tone in persons with upper motor neuron lesions (UMNL). Under normal circumstances, the intact neuromuscular system is designed to bring about automatic changes in muscle tone in response to changes in general body position and/or changes in body part to body part positioning. These changes in muscle tone are necessary to maintain antigravity postures and occur automatically as a result of stimulation of the labyrinths, Golgi tendon organs, and/or joint receptors.

The positions of the developmental sequence create a progressive demand on the neuromuscular system because of decreasing size of the base of support and an increasing number of weight-bearing joints. The tonal changes needed to maintain static and dynamic balance in these positions are brought about by gravitational influence on the neural receptors.

Unfortunately, patients with UMNL may not have the neural connections needed to provide these necessary tonal changes. Thus, depending on the location and extent of central nervous system injury, the patient with a UMNL may need external support (i.e., equipment) to achieve and maintain the positioning changes assumed each day.

The presence of spasticity has an impact on ability to maintain good alignment in a desired position. For example, lower extremity spasms and increased extensor tone can induce loss of position. If the patient is unable to readjust positioning independently, there is a need for a mechanical means to maintain positioning.

The presence of spasticity can also cause loss of available range of motion. Positioning without consideration of repeated spastic patterns will generally result in the development of musculoskeletal deformities which, even when flexible, can be accompanied by pain and skin breakdown. Proper use of positioning aids may be useful in achieving relaxation of muscle tone, thus helping to maintain range of motion and prevent pain and skin breakdown.

POSITIONING PRINCIPLES

Three basic principles apply to the provision of appropriate positioning support for the patient with spasticity. These goals and corresponding aims of treatment are discussed in the following paragraphs.

IMPROVE ALIGNMENT AND SYMMETRY

Providing equipment to obtain improvement in postural alignment and symmetry translates into a method of maintaining range of motion by reversal of flexible postural problems. Consequently, there is also a decreased risk of developing fixed, structural postural problems over time. Proper

97

alignment and symmetry are associated with an improvement in the distribution of the weight-bearing forces, so there is also a reduction in the risk of skin breakdown over the areas of bony prominence.

PROMOTE RELAXATION OF MUSCLE TONE

Many tone-inhibiting positioning techniques can help to achieve relaxation of spasticity and/or avoid the negative effects of involuntary reflexes. Generally speaking, postures opposite to spastic, reflexive patterns can be used to provide a prolonged stretch to spastic musculature to obtain relaxation.[1] For example, a patient who demonstrates a marked increase in flexor tone could be positioned prone for part of each day to provide a period of prolonged stretch to the flexor muscle groups.

Depending on the extent and location of the injury to the central nervous system, various reflex patterns can lead to disruption of desired positioning. For example, brainstem level reflexes such as the asymmetric tonic neck reflex (ATNR) are commonly seen in patients with brain injury, while simple stretch-reflex "spasms" are common among patients with spinal cord injury. Knowledge of the paths of facilitation of any undesirable reflex patterns observed is the first step to finding successful positioning solutions for these problems. In the examples given, a head or neck support that blocks head turning avoids eliciting the ATNR, while proper positioning of the foot on a foot support may help to avoid facilitation of ankle clonus elicited by quick stretch to the gastrocnemius/soleus muscles.

Carefully prescribed equipment can help to achieve a tone-reducing prolonged stretch and/or avoid undesirable intermittent reflex postures. Careful monitoring of patient comfort and skin condition is crucial, however, particularly when resistant materials are used.

IMPROVE FUNCTION

Equipment can also be used to compensate for a loss or absence of function such as inability to sit unsupported in a wheel-chair. Additionally, therapeutic gain can be obtained by supporting the patient into a position which facilitates active contraction of functionally weak muscle groups.

POSITIONING OPTIONS: ADVANTAGES AND PRECAUTIONS

The above principles can be applied to any positioning problem. The remainder of this chapter is focussed on the positions of supine, modified prone, sidelying, sitting, and standing with regard to the advantages and precautions of each position, helpful evaluation procedures, and generic recommendations for commercially available equipment that may be helpful in achieving desired effects.

SUPINE

The supine position is the most common resting position for the patient who spends most of the day upright, sitting or standing. It is also commonly used in providing passive care for hygiene and dressing.

Some patients with brain injury may exhibit a moderate to severe increase in extensor muscle tone when positioned in supine, because this position facilitates the tonic labyrinthine supine reflex (TLSR), which is characterized by an increase in extensor tone. In these cases, it may be desirable to avoid the supine position totally because repeated facilitation of the TLSR may strengthen the response and interfere with voluntary function.

Similarly, those who exhibit a dominant ATNR may have an increased tendency toward windswept posturing when positioned in supine. Windswept posturing is characterized by an asymmetric position of the pelvis and lower extremities in which one hip assumes a posture of flexion, abduction, and external rotation, while the other hip is positioned in adduction and internal rotation. Repeated facilitation of the ATNR and associated windswept deformity is thought to be associated with multiple orthopedic problems including subluxation of the hip on the adducted side.[2]

MODIFIED PRONE

A modified prone position offers several advantages for individuals with UMNLs. When positioned in prone on elbows over a wedge, the patient is given the opportunity to strengthen the back and neck extensors and to experience weight bearing through the upper extremities. This position offers the advantages of improving the scope of the visual field in comparison to supine, and it provides a passive stretch to flexor muscle groups of the hips, abdomen, and chest.

Patients who demonstrate severe flexor spasticity may not tolerate the prone position at all because of the discomfort caused by stretching tight, spastic musculature. If attempts at positioning are preceded by a tone reducing modality such as neutral warmth, however, the patient may adapt to tolerating a prolonged stretch for short periods. Caution must be taken, however, to ensure that the prone position is not facilitating the tonic labyrinthine prone reflex (TLPR), which would increase rather than decrease flexor tone. It is advisable to monitor carefully the patient's response to the prone position by assessing level of comfort, ability to move actively, and the general level of resistance to passive stretch of the flexor muscle groups to ensure that the prone position is not facilitating the TLPR. Facilitation of the TLPR would result in an increase rather than decrease of flexor muscle tone and may be counterproductive to the treatment goals.

SIDELYING

A proper sidelying position can offer particular benefit to the patient with spasticity because both extreme flexor and extensor patterns are avoided. Appropriate positioning in sidelying is characterized by flexion of the hip and knee on the uppermost side of the body and extension of the hip and knee on the lowermost side. The upper extremities should be positioned toward midline to help facilitate development and/or retraining of eye hand coordination.[3] Sidelying also reduces or eliminates many undesirable postures that, if persistent, can lead to loss of functional range of motion and/or risk of skin breakdown due to poor distribution of weight-bearing forces. Common undesirable postures include:

1. Frog-leg position (bilateral hip flexion, abduction and external rotation)
2. Windswept posture (hip flexion, abduction, external rotation on one side and relative hip extension, adduction, internal rotation on the opposite side)[4]
3. Scissored posture (bilateral hip extension, adduction, internal rotation).

The only true disadvantage of the sidelying position is that it is difficult to maintiain without the use of specially designed equipment.

SITTING

The sitting position can offer the advantages of promoting active head and upper trunk control and increasing the scope of the visual field as compared to supine, prone, and sidelying. It can also free the upper extremities for functional activites, if there is any voluntary upper extremity control of which to take advantage. Sitting is the optimal position for feeding for most patients, and it also provides more opportunity for social interaction.[5] As with sidelying, the main disadvantage of the sitting position is that adaptive equipment may be needed to achieve the optimal position.

STANDING

Standing provides the opportunity for active, resisted contraction of the antigravity extensor muscles and/or a passive stretch to the hip flexors, knee flexors, and plantar flexors of the ankle. The standing position may be desirable for functional, social, and emotional reasons. If extensive external support is required, however, standing may not be an appropriate long-term positioning option.

EVALUATION PROCEDURES

Determination of the specific needs of each patient requires a thorough assessment to identify indications and contraindications for positioning.[6] The five major areas to be assessed include medical condition, the musculoskeletal system, the neuromuscular system, functional abilities and inabilities, and any equipment currently being used.

MEDICAL CONDITION

A careful history of the patient's medical condition must be taken to determine if there are any problems related to sitting or other postures. Among the most common problems are postural pain and skin breakdown. For example, poor sitting posture is often characterized by a posterior pelvic tilt, decreased lumbar lordosis, increased thoracic kyphosis, and increased cervical lordosis. This posture may be accompanied by the complaint of neck or low back pain caused by overstretching of the soft tissues in these areas, especially when self-correction cannot be accomplished. In this same example, a report of skin irritation or breakdown over the sacrum is not uncommon because this sitting posture places excessive weight-bearing pressures on the sacral area.

Prognosis for both life expectancy and function are considerations. While positioning goals are unlikely to change if life expectancy is short, the type of equipment to be prescribed may. In some cases, it is more appropriate to rent, rather than purchase, equipment. The higher cost of custom-designed equipment may not be covered by third-party payers. Temporary postural support systems can be constructed by the clinician by using inexpensive materials. Mock-up systems will be further discussed in a later section of this chapter.

Any disability-related issues that may present contraindications to positioning will also need consideration. For example, some patients may experience decreased blood pressure on sitting or standing (orthostatic hypotension), gastroesophageal reflux may be a problem when the patient is supine or prone, and tracheostomy care issues (e.g., the need for frequent suctioning) can present the need for a means of easily changing positions throughout the day. The possible medical problems to be considered are virtually endless. Prescribing equipment on an individual basis ensures that the device will account for any existing medical issues.

MUSCULOSKELETAL ASSESSMENT

Assessment of the musculoskeletal system involves evaluation of flexibility, alignment, and symmetry. It is important to assess available range of motion of the extremities, shoulder girdles, pelvis, and trunk to ensure that flexibility is adequate for optimal positioning. If not, accommodation for any fixed contractures will have to be provided within a positioning system. For example, in cases of fixed kyphosis, the prone position could not be tolerated without accommodating support for the relatively concave posture of the chest and abdomen. Likewise, sitting would be uncomfortable without a supportive contoured or resilient material within the backrest.

Alignment and symmetry should be assessed both with and without external support so that ultimately the minimal possible support can be provided. Once acceptable alignment and symmetry are achieved in the desired position, body measurements must be taken and recorded because these form the basis of the equipment prescription. Positions and special considerations for measurement are outlined in Table 6–1.

Because positioning of proximal parts influences positioning and function of the distal parts,[7] a crucial part of the musculoskeletal assessment is examination of the pelvis, spine, and shoulder girdles. If limitations or problems with alignment or symmetry are discovered, these problems will have to be corrected or accommodation provided within the positioning system. If correction or accommodation is not provided, problems with comfort or function may occur.

The pelvis must be examined to determine any limitation of motion or problem with alignment. Range of motion of the pelvis is assessed for movement in the frontal plane (lateral movement), the sagittal plane (anterior/posterior movement), and the horizontal plane (rotational movement).

TABLE 6–1. SPECIAL CONSIDERATIONS FOR MEASUREMENT

Measurements	Position	Landmarks	Comments
Across hips	Sitting in "ideal" postural alignment	Widest point on pelvis or thighs	Use rigid measure or keep tape taut
Thigh length	Supine on firm mat with hips and knees flexed to 90 degrees	Mat → popliteal fossa	Note if there is "apparent" thigh lengthening resulting from fixed posterior tilt or rotation of pelvis Measure both sides
Leg length	Sitting or supine with hips and knees flexed to 90 degrees	Popliteal fossa → most distal point contacting floor or footrest	Measure both sides Note any fixed plantarflexion contracture → "apparent" leg lengthening

Problems with pelvic alignment include pelvic obliquity, pelvic rotation, and increased anterior or posterior tilt. These are essentially subjective assessments to identify any limitations that would prevent achievement of the postural alignment desired in a given position. Any limitation or asymmetry identified must be accommodated or corrected with the positioning system to ensure maximum comfort and function.

Assessment of the spine requires evaluation of range of motion and general alignment of the spine in the position of interest. For example, unsupported sitting may be characterized by a flexible c-curve scoliosis, but this problem would not be evident if the spine were evaluated in the supine position. Note any increase or decrease in the thoracic kyphosis, increase or decrease in the cervical and lumbar lordoses, or any evidence of a scoliosis.

The shoulder girdle should be examined for limitation in shoulder joint range of motion as well as freedom of scapular movement and scapulohumeral rhythm, again in the position of interest. This assessment provides information on possible limitations of upper extremity function, which could be influenced positively by slight changes in positioning. For example, if range of motion is limited in or around the shoulder caused by an increase in extensor tone resulting from a dominant TLSR, it would be important to ensure that the angle of tilt built into the positioning system does not allow stimulation of the TLSR.

The most important aspect of the musculoskeletal assessment is to determine whether deviations are fixed or flexible. In the final treatment of postural problems, flexible postural problems are treated with corrective measures, while fixed postural problems are accommodated with nonresistant materials. Incorrect treatment of a fixed deformity with resistant materials will result in pain and skin breakdown and must be thoughtfully avoided.

More often than not, postural deviations are somewhat correctable. In these cases, positioning requires a series of successive trials to find the system that provides an optimal degree of correction while comfortably and safely accommodating any deviations that are not correctable. For example, a marked increase in muscle tone is accompanied by limitation of motion of the joints crossed by the spastic muscles. While there may be full passive range of motion when and if tone can be reduced, it may be necessary to treat this situation as a fixed problem in the positioning system by providing accommodation so that skin breakdown and/or pain will not result. It is not always possible to influence muscle tone and associated postural deviations by positioning alone. This is when medical intervention (e.g., blocks, medication) must be considered in conjunction with appropriate positioning options.

NEUROMUSCULAR ASSESSMENT

The neuromuscular assessment involves evaluation of muscle tone, reflex activity, and the influence of positioning changes on tone and reflex activity. This information is needed to predict the patient's tolerance for certain positions and to estimate his/her ability to function within those postures. In addition to general assessment of muscle tone to determine if the patient is hypertonic, hypotonic, or mixed, it is important to note any asymmetry in muscle tone or asymmetry in voluntary motor control. For example, if a patient is more spastic on the right than on the left side of the trunk, a left C-curve scoliosis may result.

This section of the evaluation also involves reflex testing to determine abnormal presence of primitive tonic reflexes such as the ATNR or STNR and/or delay or absence in the higher level righting or equilibrium reactions. Techniques of reflex testing are outlined in detail elsewhere.[8]

Finally, it is necessary to assess muscle tone as it relates to specific positions. For example, if plantar flexor clonus occurs in a patient sitting in a wheelchair, what effect does it have overall on the seated position? What effect, if any, do involuntary reflexes such as coughing and sneezing have on general body positioning? There may be a need to provide a mechanism to block the undesired effects of involuntary reflex activity.

Positioning changes ordinarily alter muscle tone through stimulation of the labyrinths and other neural receptors. Because the presence of a UMNL alters the neural response to positioning changes, it is important to determine what specific effect positioning has on the individual patient.

First, it is important to determine the effect of altering relative alignment of body segments such as introducing hip flexion in supine for the patient with increased extensor tone. Second, one should determine the effect of alterations of body-in-space position. For example, if the patient exhibits a generally kyphotic posture in sitting, tilting back the seating components relative to the horizon will reduce the pull of gravity on the spine, resulting in a more relaxed, neutral trunk position. Some patients, however, may actually exhibit an increase in flexor posturing as a result of this change because of an automatic tendency to right the head to an upright midline position; thus careful monitoring and recording of changes are crucial.

FUNCTIONAL ASSESSMENT

Functional abilities and inabilities must be considered when prescribing a positioning device. Function and independence should never be influenced negatively by altering patient positioning. Among the functional activities to be considered are transfers, dressing, eating, communication, and other activities of daily living that may be performed from the positioning device. Only in this way can one avoid a negative influence on the functional abilities of the patient. Functional issues differ markedly from patient to patient.

PROBLEM SOLVING

Once the assessment process has been completed and positioning problems and needs have been identified, the next step is to decide what type of positioning aid will meet the established positioning goals most appropriately and fully for a particular patient. It is important to establish stated goals to be achieved with the aid of positioning devices because a position change may be different without necessarily resulting in improvement. Some common positioning goals include:

1. Decrease the risk of structural deformity and skin breakdown by improving alignment and symmetry
2. Improve comfort and relaxation
3. Improve functional ability (e.g., improve speed of wheelchair mobility)

Outlined in the following paragraphs are several basic principles involved in developing a prescription for a positioning aid. Each principle is illustrated by a case study featuring clinical problems common among individuals with UMNLs.

PROXIMAL POSITIONING FIRST

All positioning solutions must be worked from proximal to distal in direction regardless of the position in question. Experimentation with external support at the pelvis should be followed by positioning of the trunk and shoulder girdles. Only after satisfactory proximal positioning is achieved should more distal support be provided. Because proximal positioning generally influences the attitude of more distal body parts, strict adherence to this rule can help avoid overtreatment of positioning problems.

Case 1. John, a cervical level 2 quadraplegic, had severe problems with spasticity. When he was seated in a standard recliner wheelchair with a sling style seat and back, it was necessary to strap his pelvis, chest, thighs, legs, feet, elbows and hands to adjacent points on the wheelchair to prevent involuntary spasms from literally "throwing" him from the wheelchair.

The sling seat and back were replaced with a more stable solid seat and back mounted on an inclinable seat/reclining back frame. In this way, a 90-degree angle could be held at the hips while still allowing reclining of the back to provide trunk support. The pelvis was stabilized successfully with a custom molded pelvic belt constructed from orthoplast and webbing. The stability gained with these proximal components significantly reduced his spasticity while sitting in the wheelchair and all distal restraints except heel loops, toe straps, and wrist straps could be eliminated. These solutions markedly reduced the risk of skin breakdown.

MINIMUM SUPPORT FOR MAXIMUM FUNCTION

The second principle is to provide the minimum amount of support needed to maximize active control and function. In other words, the positioning device should be streamlined as much as possible to provide only the amount of support needed. This is another reason for beginning with the proximal segments; one must avoid overtreatment of the problems.

Case 2. Wanda, a 35-year-old woman, had a thoracic level 3 spinal cord injury resulting in spastic paraplegia. Many postural problems were noted when she was seated in a lightweight wheelchair equipped with fabric upholstery and a 2" air-filled cushion. These included posterior pelvic tilt, pelvic obliquity (with the left side lower than the right), minimal kyphoscoliosis with convexity to the left, both hips ad-

ducted and internally rotated. There was evidence of a moderate increase in muscle tone on the right, minimal on the left. Active medical problems included slight skin breakdown on the left side of the sacrum and complaint of shortness of breath by the end of a workday. Functionally, Wanda was independent in all self-care and wheelchair mobility. She was employed full time. She drove a car and wanted to maintain the ability to load her wheelchair into the car.

Wanda's sitting posture was corrected by adapting a commercially available cushion (molded urethane foam base with flolite pad). A pelvic obliquity pad was added to the left side to shift weight bearing toward the right, correcting the flexible pelvic obliquity and achieving some, but not total correction of the kyphoscoliosis. A more neutral alignment of the hips was achieved, although some adduction was still evident. The skin redness and breathing difficulties were resolved. During trials of various possible solutions complete correction of the kyphoscoliosis was achieved. This required a solid seat, back, and lumbar roll, with the seat to back angle at 90 degrees, all tilted back 5 degrees from the horizontal. This solution, however, was rejected to maintain the functional benefits of a lightweight, portable system. Wanda chose the option of daily stretching exercises to help prevent development of a fixed kyphoscoliosis.

CORRECT FLEXIBLE POSTURAL PROBLEMS/ AVOID DEVELOPMENT OF FIXED POSTURAL PROBLEMS

Structurally resistant materials such as wood or plastic coupled with foam protection can be used successfully to counteract the undesirable effects of gravitational pull or increased muscle tone. The positioning system must exert a force on the body greater than or equal to the force of gravity or abnormal muscle tone to achieve correction of flexible postural abnormalities. When the forces of muscle tone cannot be overcome by these corrective techniques, accommodative techniques or medical intervention should be considered.

Case 3. Brian, an 11-year-old boy, had spastic quadriparetic cerebral palsy. Sitting posture was characterized by a posterior pelvic tilt and compensatory lumbar kyphosis. There was also an increase in the thoracic kyphosis and hyperextension of the cervical spine. Because the posterior pelvic tilt and compensatory spinal curves were flexible on examination, this sitting posture was easily corrected by replacing the sling seat and back of the wheelchair with a solid seat and back and the addition of a pelvic belt (which was attached to the lowermost corner of the backrest to achieve a 45-degree angle of contact with the pelvis).

ACCOMMODATE STRUCTURAL POSTURAL PROBLEMS

In contrast, structural or fixed postural problems cannot be treated with resistant materials because pain and skin breakdown will occur. Structural postural problems can result from either soft tissue contracture or a strong increase in resting muscle tone. Surgical and/or nerve block interventions may be helpful in correcting these structural problems, but if positioning is required in the interim, contoured or nonresistant materials such as soft foam can be useful in providing support and comfort while helping to distribute weight-bearing forces over a larger area to avoid skin breakdown.

Case 4. Joseph, a 38-year-old man, had spastic quadriparetic cerebral palsy. Because of his many musculoskeletal problems, including a fixed pelvic obliquity, a fixed S-curve scoliosis, bilateral dislocated hips, and multiple contractures of the joints of the upper and lower extremities, sitting in a wheelchair was not a realistic goal for this patient. At the time of examination, he was positioned on his right side on a foam mattress mounted to a reclining wheelchair frame. The sidelying position was maintained with an array of bed pillows and straps. The chief complaints were general discomfort, the need for constant repositioning of pillows, skin breakdown over the right greater trochanter, and difficulty in activating a single switch that controlled an electronic communication device.

A custom-molded sidelyer was con-structed from ABS plastic and foams and was attached to the reclining wheelchair frame. A socket was cut into the foam to support the communicator controller which the patient could easily activate with his right elbow. This arrangement was successful in providing comfort and support while accommodating his multiple orthopedic problems. Because the weight-bearing forces were now distributed over the entire right side, the trochanters and other bony prominences were successfully protected against skin breakdown.

PROVIDING SOLUTIONS

Once all of the problems have been identified and possible solutions developed, commercially available equipment should be considered to provide the solutions. Because custom design, modifications, and even accessories can be costly, it is important to identify an off-the-shelf solution whenever possible. A knowledgeable durable medical equipment dealer is an essential component in this phase of problem solving. He or she can provide information and ideas about new products on the market and/or suggest creative ways in which generally available equipment can be used. Dealers with extensive rehabilitation experience are most helpful, but still must rely heavily on the information provided by the clinician's complete evaluation. With combining of knowledge bases, clinical problems can be matched with commercially available solutions. The clinician should be prepared to provide the dealer with information about what the device needs to accomplish, in much the same way that goals of hands-on treatment are developed. For example, if the patient has a fixed pelvic obliquity with a skin breakdown on one ischial tuberosity and the goal is upright sitting, the clinician must inform the vendor that the goals are to accommodate the pelvic obliquity, reduce weight bearing on the ischial tuberosity to assist healing, and provide a system that can allow for upright sitting. Once all this information is discussed with the vendor, information exchange can result in some possible solutions for the problem.

When the clinical symptoms are complex, a series of successive trials with proposed solutions may be necessary until the most effective system can be established. If a standard off-the-shelf product is prescribed, a trial period can be arranged through the dealer or manufacturer. Should a totally custom solution be needed, a mock-up can be developed in the clinic. Bergen[7] provides a detailed description of the process of building mock-up positioning devices from triwall cardboard and foam. In some cases, a simple modification or adaptation suffices, and in others an entire positioning system must be custom designed. It is helpful if a commercially available product is used to form the basis of the mock-up. For instance, if a seating system is being prescribed, a basic solid seat and back can provide a base, then cardboard and foam can be added for a custom fit. The definitive seating system would then be ordered to the specifications developed on the mock-up.

An air extraction beanbag like the one pictured in Figure 6–1 can be helpful when considering a custom molded system. It can provide a trial period to determine if the system will be tolerated. It can also be used to estimate the size and configuration needed in the final device.

COMMERCIALLY AVAILABLE EQUIPMENT

SUPINE

The supine position can be maintained by transferring the patient onto a bed or mat. If extensor tone is a problem, however, it may be desirable to avoid excessive extensor patterns by providing a modified supine position with some degree of flexion, abduction, and external rotation of the hips, which can be provided with pillows or rolls. For patients with severe spasticity, more resistance may be necessary. This can be provided with commercially available wedges similar to those shown in Figure 6–2. A wide variety of wedge-shaped pads and supports is available on the commercial market, including those designed for supporting patients while x-rays are being taken.

PRONE

The prone position is usually more easily tolerated if modified with a chest wedge. A mock-up wedge is easily constructed from pillows or foam, but commercially available support is also available. An adaptable wedge system, like that shown above in Figure 6–2, can be arranged to provide anterior as well as posterior support. Some commercially available prone standers can be lowered to a position nearly parallel to the floor for prone positioning while maintaining optimal postural alignment.

SIDELYING

Positioning the patient in sidelying generally requires more than pillows and foam pieces because these can be displaced easily. The two most useful positioning aids for sidelying are beanbag positioners, which utilize vacuum consolidation to provide resistant support (see Fig. 6–1); and

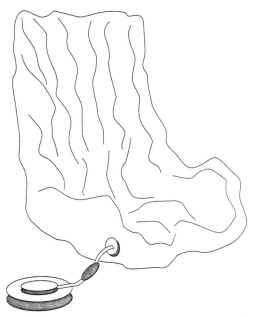

FIG. 6–1. Beanbag positioner can provide adjustable external support during evaluation phase.

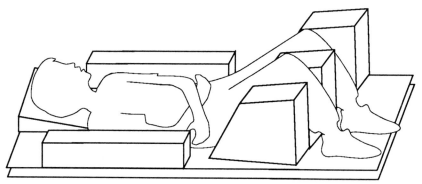

FIG. 6–2. Modular wedges can be combined to provide external support in a variety of positions.

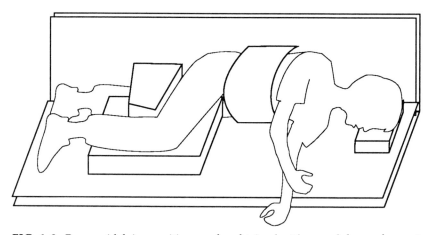

FIG. 6–3. Proper sidelying position can be obtained with a modular wedge system.

specially designed, adjustable wedges that can be arranged to provide a proper side-lying position (Fig. 6–3).

SITTING

The sitting position is one in which most patients with UMNLs spend much of the day. For the patient who has severe problems with spasticity, sitting often requires a significant amount of external support. Seating components can be combined using an eclectic approach to achieve a customized solution. In this approach, various components are chosen from different manufacturers and assembled into a single unit by the dealer. The most important factor for successful design is the dealer's knowledge of compatibility and means of adapting for any incompatibility of different components.

The sitting position outlined in Table 6–2 is considered the "ideal" position because it provides a good stable base of support over which the upper extremities can function. The pelvic position with no lateral tilt, no rotation, and a slight anterior tilt mechanically places the spine into extension and the lower extremities into flexion, slight abduction, and external rotation of the hips. The most important aspect of this posture is extension of the spine because it results in "locking" of the facet joints which is believed to minimize a variety of common seating problems.

The most common positioning problem in sitting is a posture in which there is "un-

TABLE 6–2. "IDEAL" POSTURAL ALIGNMENT IN SITTING

Body Segment	Desired Posture	Benefits
Pelvis	Slight anterior tilt No lateral tilt No rotation	• Results in more stable position of spine • Distributes weight bearing across buttocks/thighs
Hips	Flexion greater than or equal to 90 degrees Slight abduction Slight external rotation	• Helps maintain pelvic posture • Provides wide, stable base of support
Knees	Flexion near 90 degrees	• Minimizes stress on hamstrings
Feet	Neutral, plantargrade	• Maintains functional ROM, comfort
Spine	"Plumb line" posture Slight lumbar lordosis Slight thoracic kyphosis Slight cervical lordosis	• Minimizes stress on trunk musculature • Mechanically stable position for spine
Shoulder	Neutral protraction/retraction	• Minimizes stress to neck and upper back musculature • Functional position for upper extremities
Head	Midline, vertical Eyes horizontal	• Optimizes visual motor and oral motor functions
Upper extremities	Relaxed, on armrests or in lap	• Free for propulsion or other functional task

With permission from Hallenborg, S.C.: Wheelchair needs of the disabled. *In* Therapeutic Considerations for the Elderly. Ed. O.L. Jackson, New York, Churchill Livingstone, Inc., 1987.

locking" of the lumbar facets. The central problem with this posture is a posterior pelvic tilt that results in a lumbar kyphosis. This posture is thought to be associated with the development of scoliosis and pelvic obliquity in patients with weak trunk musculature.[9] The long-term cumulative effects of this sitting posture include uneven loading of weight-bearing pressures,[9-13] an increase in vertebral disk pressures,[14] and a reduction in respiratory capacity.[9,15] This position is further characterized by a hip position of relative extension, adduction, and internal rotation. In short, a posterior pelvic tilt results in an unstable sitting position with a narrow base of support. It takes minimal mechanical advantage of anatomic structures.

In an attempt to correct the posterior pelvic tilt and its associated postural problems (highlighted by "unlocking" of the facet joints), it is necessary to begin positioning changes at the pelvis. The ideal pelvic position can be obtained in most cases by combining commercially available components to meet individual patient needs. As with the three-point pressure system used to correct scoliosis, three points of pressure can be used to obtain a neutral pelvic posi-

tion. Correction is achieved when anterior, inferior and posterior forces (provided by the seat belt, seat, and backrest) are greater than or equal to the forces of gravity or muscle tone that are acting to pull the pelvis into a posterior tilt.

These corrective forces can be obtained by using a firm seat and back (solid plastics and foam, wood and foam, or a taut fabric) and a seat belt positioned below the anterior superior iliac spines of the pelvis. This belt position provides a force in the direction illustrated in Figure 6–4 and, when this force is combined with the forces of the seat and back, correction is achieved.[6]

The lower extremities are the second component of the base of support. An ideal position is generally characterized by 90-degree angles at the hips, knees, and ankles. The hips should be near zero with regard to abduction/adduction, and internal/external rotation. This position minimizes the tendency toward increased extensor tone or flexor tone, and stress on the hamstrings and gastrocnemius muscles is minimal. It is important to observe the effect of stretch on these two-joint muscles. If, for example, there is a marked increase in flexor muscle tone, placement of the feet on

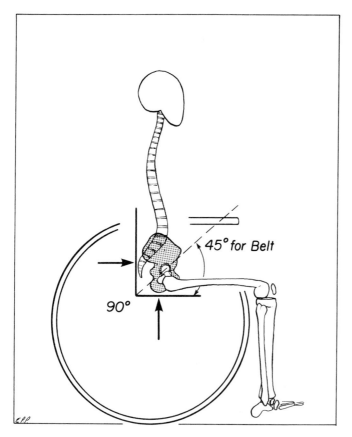

FIG. 6-4. Optimal pelvic alignment achieved with three-point pressure system (with permission from Hallenborg, S.C.: Wheelchair needs of the disabled. *In* Therapeutic Considerations for the Elderly. Ed. O.L. Jackson. New York, Churchill Livingstone, Inc., 1987).

the footplates of a wheelchair can cause a stretch on the hamstrings. A slow, prolonged stretch can result in relaxation of spasticity; however, this is difficult to achieve with wheelchair positioning because it requires complete stabilization of both the hip and the knee joints (because the hamstrings cross both joints). Rather, what usually occur are intermittent quick stretches to the hamstrings which facilitate rather than inhibit an increase in resting muscle tone. Then, when the hamstrings contract, the pelvis may be displaced into a posterior tilt, resulting in all of the complications described above.

Similarly, the gastrocnemius muscle crosses both the ankle and the knee. A facilitatory quick stretch can lead to ankle clonus and displacement of the foot. In more severe cases, displacement of the entire lower extremity can occur.

Some patients need special positioning aids to maintain a neutral lower extremity position in sitting. Most commercially available modular wood and foam systems like that illustrated in Figure 6–5 offer the options of an abductor pommel (blocks adduction), abductor blocks, pelvic blocks, and asymmetric seat depth. Virtually any combination of components can be used to achieve the best possible positioning.

It is best to begin obtaining the best possible pelvic position by applying the three-point pressure system described above. Once that is achieved, observe the posture of the lower extremities. If adduction of the hips is excessive, an abductor pommel may be helpful. This device simply blocks adduction of the hips. Care should be taken to ensure that flexibility is adequate to position the hips in the desired degree of abduction and that placement of the pommel is kept as far distal on the seat as possible to avoid contact with the perineal area. The pommel should be mounted with removable or swing-away hardware so that it will

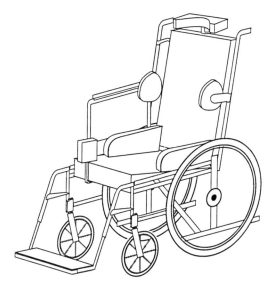

FIG. 6–5. Modular wood and foam systems offer design flexibility and adjustability.

not interfere with transferring in and out of the chair. Swing-away hardware is usually somewhat more expensive but is a better functional choice because there is less chance of loss or improper placement.

The width and shape of the pommel depend on the desired degree of hip abduction. It should align with the top of the thigh (anterior aspect). It may be helpful to sketch the desired shape. This is easily accomplished by placing a piece of paper on a firm sitting surface, preferably the type of seat to which it will attach. Then, while supporting the thighs in the desired position, sketch in a "footprint" of the area to be filled with the pommel. Make a note of the desired height (measure from the seat to the top of the thigh), add the hardware choice, and the prescription has been developed.

Abductor blocks may be needed if there is excessive abduction of one or both hips. These pads are placed along the lateral aspect of the thigh and are designed to block excessive abduction. The height of the pads depends on the size of the patient's thigh. If an abductor pommel is used, the height should be the same for aesthetic purposes. The length is generally the same as the seat depth, but can be made shorter or longer according to individual needs. The thick-

ness of the pad depends on the available space between the patient and the armrest. A snug fit helps to maintain both a good thigh position and a midline pelvic position, but prohibits changes in the weight of clothing needed during season changes. Abductor blocks need to be removable for patients who use a lateral approach to transfer in and out of the wheelchair. Hardware choices include brackets that mount to a solid seat or backrest (removable or permanent) or straps for attachment to the armrests.

Pelvic blocks are similar to abductor blocks except that they are positioned in the pelvic region only. These pads are designed to keep the pelvis in a midline position.

Proper seat depth for each thigh is important to ensure proper pelvic, hip, and knee positioning. If the seat depth is too long, it forces the pelvis into a posterior tilt and applies pressure to the popliteal fossa; this could result in circulatory compromise and/or peripheral nerve damage. If the seat depth is too short, the lower extremities tend to assume a position of hip abduction and external rotation. Additionally, there is excessive weight bearing on the ischial tuberosities and/or sacrum because of failure to distribute weight bearing on the posterior aspect of the thighs.

Knee and leg position depend on pelvic position and seat depth but also on the location of the footrests. Although a 90-degree angle of flexion at the knee is desirable, the location of the casters on most adult-size wheelchairs prevents this optimal positioning. Unless the patient has a particular increase in tone or shortening of the hamstrings, a greater-than-90-degree angle of extension at the knee is generally acceptable. If this positioning does create a problem, however, there are some solutions.

With use of powered or passive mobility devices, the relationship of the upper extremity to rim position is not of concern. It is therefore possible to mount the seating system above the standard position on the frame to position the footrests directly below the front edge of the seat and above the level of the casters to obtain a 90-degree angle of flexion at the knee. Because the floor-to-seat position is higher, however,

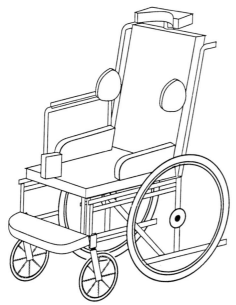

FIG. 6-6. Seating system mounted above the seat rails creates extra clearance needed to allow 90 degrees of flexion at the knee.

there may be difficulty with transfers and with sitting under desks or tables (Fig. 6–6).

The second alternative is illustrated in Figure 6–7. This involves tilting the seating system back on the frame without disrupting the 90-degree seat-to-back angle. In this way, the footrests can still be positioned forward of the casters, but the relative change in thigh position allows positioning of the knees at 90 degrees of flexion. This "solution" creates the same problems as raising the seating system because the knees are elevated. It may also make upper extremity skills more difficult if the patient is weak because gravity must be resisted to obtain a midline position. Furthermore, if there is a dominant TLSR, this position may cause an undesirable increase in extensor tone, or may actually increase a flexor posture because of the automatic tendency to right the head vertically.

Fortunately, ever-increasing alternatives on the commercial market are being developed to help overcome these and other seating problems. For example, most manufacturers of powered wheelchairs offer a power base, as an alternative to a standard wheelchair frame, which permits mounting

of a somewhat wider variety of seating systems as shown in Figure 6–8.

If a manual wheelchair is prescribed, alternative foot placement can be achieved by utilizing 5″ or 6″ versus 8″ casters. Because the radius needed for turning the caster is smaller, the footrests can be positioned closer to the base of the chair. Maneuverability of the wheelchair with 5″ casters is somewhat more difficult than that of the wheelchair with 8″ casters. But when 5″ or 6″ casters are used on lightweight chairs, which are more maneuverable than the heavier chairs of the past, the footrest alternative is now available to persons with a greater range of conditions.

The ideal foot position is one with a 90-degree angle at the ankle and the foot completely supported on the footplate. Some patients with spasticity may require straps to prevent foot displacement during a spasm. It may, however, be necessary to avoid the use of toe straps because these can intermittently stimulate the metatarsal heads and facilitate spinal level reflexes. When straps are needed, a crisscross arrangement around the ankle works well, distributing foot contact more evenly on the footplate. Calf pads, troughs, H-straps, and heel loops are additional accessories that may be helpful in achieving proper foot and leg placement.

Most wheelchair manufacturers offer an

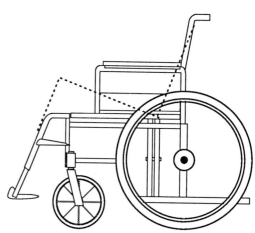

FIG. 6-7. An inclined seat positions the knees at 90-degree angles when standard wheelchair footrests are used.

FIG. 6–8. A modular power base makes available a wider range of seating options.

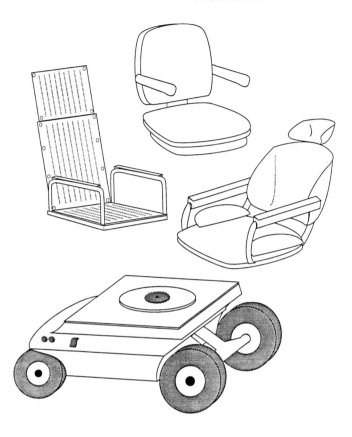

option of elevating leg rests in lieu of footrests. Elevating leg rests offer a range of adjustment between approximately 100 and 180 degrees of knee extension and have the advantage of accommodating a knee extension contracture. In patients with lower extremity spasticity, however, many problems can occur. Unlike standard footrests, the standard calf pads on elevating leg rests often tend to pull the pelvis into a posterior tilt. This is particularly true if hamstring spasticity exists. Also, if extensor spasms are a problem, an involuntary change of knee position can occur.

Once the best position is achieved at the base of support (pelvis and lower extremities), the trunk should be positioned. Again, adhering to a proximal-to-distal direction in problem solving can help avoid overtreatment of seating needs.

Lateral supports are the most common kind of trunk support. They can be used to provide increased lateral stability or can be coupled with pelvic blocks to get some correction and support for a flexible scoliosis (by providing four points of counteracting pressures).

Many styles of lateral support are commercially available. Some are fixed to the chair, some swing away, and others are removable. Most of the models now available are both adjustable and removable. Depending on the size and shape of the pad and the mounting used, some are more supportive than others.

The depth of the pad is the same as the depth of the patient's trunk. If anterior support is required, minimal support can be obtained by using a contoured pad that curves onto the anterior aspect of the trunk. It is essential that this style of lateral support be mounted with swing-away hardware to allow ease of transfers. If more anterior support is needed, it can be achieved by using lateral support pads that are hinged at the anterior border of the chest. An example is shown in Figure 6–9. The anterior pad can be ordered with or without

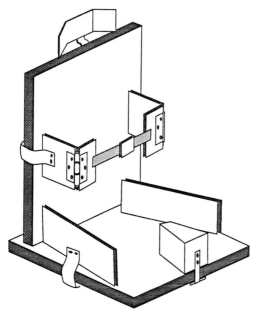

FIG. 6–9. Hinged laterals provide semirigid anterior support.

a connecting strap. The hinge is necessary to permit swing-away of the support for transfers. A simple chest strap connecting lateral support pads may provide sufficient anterior support in some cases. Whenever anterior support is added at the trunk, care should be taken to ensure that the patient is not "hanging" on the strap because skin breakdown, an increase in flexor tone, and generalized discomfort may result.

Another option for providing anterior trunk support is clavicular pads. These generally attach to the posterior/superior aspect of a solid backrest and are made to swing away for transfers. They are preferable to a chest strap when some assistance with head control is needed in addition to trunk stabilization, but again, care must be taken to avoid skin irritation, increased flexor tone, and generalized discomfort.

The length of the lateral trunk support depends on the amount of support needed and the length of the patient's trunk. If a flexible scoliosis is being corrected by the lateral support pads, the forces provided by these pads must be greater than or equal to the forces of gravity or muscle tone that are pulling the trunk into a scoliotic posture. It is usually necessary to experiment with different sizes and shapes of pads to locate the combination that works most effectively.

Lateral support pads should be kept as thin as possible so that they do not interfere with upper extremity positioning and function. Likewise, the placement of the lateral support pad with relationship to the axilla is crucial because placing it too high can result in impingement of the axillary nerves and blood vessels, while placing it too low can result in ineffective correction of the curve.

When lateral support pads are being used to support a collapsing spine against the forces of strong spasticity, it may be necessary to use heavy duty metal mounting brackets, or breakage can be a problem. In severe cases, it may not be possible to use removable or swing-away hardware because these adjustment points provide a point of loosening or breakage. Although transfers in and out of the chair will be more difficult, this problem has to be balanced against the need to achieve correction of poor spinal alignment, which often causes pain and skin problems.

In most cases of extreme spasticity and/or in heavy patients, spinal correction cannot be adequately achieved with lateral supports. In these cases, it is best to consult an orthotist for possible orthotic correction and support.

A lumbar roll is another type of trunk support, used to increase and maintain a lumbar lordosis. These rolls must be used with caution and coupled with an anterior counteracting force or a tilted seat. Otherwise, they tend to push the patient forward in the chair without affecting the position of the lumbar spine.[13]

An increase in lumbar lordosis can also be achieved with a lumbar orthosis. A simple elastic corset with a molded plastic insert may work for some, but if greater force is required, a more extensive corset with metal stays will be needed. The disadvantages of a corset are difficulty in putting it on and taking it off and its tendency to slide upward on patients who are seated most of the time.

Seating components have not been shown to prevent progression of any spinal deformity; thus, if there is a progressive scoliosis, kyphosis, and/or a significant amount of growth remains, a body jacket should be considered.

As soon as trunk position is satisfactory, the need for head and neck support should be evaluated. In general, it is best to avoid direct pressure on the occiput because this may increase extensor tone. This can be done by using a neckrest versus a headrest, providing support below the occipital level. This may not be effective in some patients, however. If extension over the top of the neckrest is observed, a fully contoured head and neckrest may be helpful.

Forward flexion can be blocked with a halo that is generally attached to the posterior aspect of the headrest, but this must be used with caution. If increased muscle tone is the cause of the forward flexion, the use of a halo, against which the patient can continually contract the flexor muscles, will increase the strength in these muscles. When this problem exists, it is preferable to tilt the seating system backward in space to allow relaxation against the headrest for at least part of the day.

The most difficult positioning problem at the head and neck is controlling a tendency to turn or bend the neck laterally. There is no cosmetically pleasing means of solving this problem. A bicycle helmet with a chin strap mounted to the headrest may be helpful in some patients. A lower profile support can be constructed with heat-sensitive plastics. If the clinician is able to achieve a relaxed position of the head and neck by handling the patient's head, a moulded plastic "orthosis" can be designed to duplicate the control provided by the clinician's hands. The orthosis must be flexible enough to allow application and removal but rigid enough to block undesirable patterns. It may still be necessary to tilt the seating system back in space to achieve sufficient relaxation and tolerance.

The upper extremities are the last to be positioned. A tray provides the most support, but weight bearing through the upper extremities to achieve extension of the trunk should be avoided. Proximal control is preferred because the upper extremities are needed for functional use. Nonfunctional upper extremities are simply supported on a tray or trough. Blocks can be added to the surface of the tray to prevent undesirable involuntary postures such as excessive shoulder extension or internal rotation. When stabilizing an upper extremity, however, observe the effect on the trunk. For example, hemiplegic patients who demonstrate the tendency to pull into a typical position of elbow flexion, shoulder adduction, and internal rotation, may benefit from neutral alignment of the upper extremity on an arm support. Straps or foam blocks can be used to prevent loss of positioning when spasms occur, but in the presence of a marked increase in muscle tone, the patient may simply rotate the trunk toward the spastic upper extremity, causing a disruption of total body positioning. It is just as important to refer back to proximal parts when positioning distal parts as it was to begin with proximal positioning.

ALTERNATIVE SEATING DEVICES

Many other types of sitting supports are commercially available. Devices such as bolsters, floor sitters, and feeding seats are used primarily with children and are very useful aids to hands-on treatment. A standard classroom desk chair can be adapted to provide the proximal support needed to enhance the fine motor skills needed in the classroom. This allows the child to sit in a chair similar to those used by able-bodied peers, and is important for the child's socialization.

The developing child needs to experience time out of the primary seating device (usually the wheelchair) so that potential voluntary motor development can be facilitated. Devices similar to the posture chair shown in Figure 6–10 provide significantly less support than a wheelchair seating system. The hands-on therapy program can be enhanced by providing some proximal support with good alignment while calling for some dynamic control of the trunk and upper extremities.

Additional seating devices are used less commonly with the adult population because the advantage of the wheelchair is that it provides a mechanism for mobility as well as positioning.

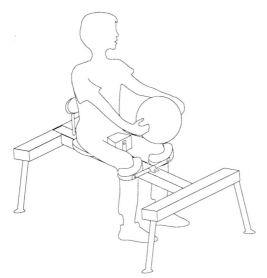

FIG. 6-10. Dynamic control is facilitated with this adjustable seat.

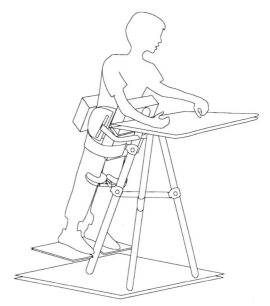

FIG. 6-11. Prone standers can provide the external support needed for standing.

STANDING

If standing is a positioning goal, different styles of frames and tables may be used. Prone standers (Fig. 6-11), supine standers,[16] and standing frames (Fig. 6-12) are the most commonly prescribed standing aids. Like alternative seating, these devices are used more commonly with children to aid development of bone growth, spatial awareness, and socialization, and simply to provide an alternative to sitting.

Recently available on the commercial market are wheelchairs that give both children and adults an option of standing. An example is shown in Figure 6-13. These may be beneficial for social reasons, and have an additional functional benefit of allowing the user to reach previously inaccessible areas of the environment. The difficulty in prescribing this option is the relative lack of evidence for the medical necessity of standing; hence, medical insurers rarely cover the cost of this accessory.

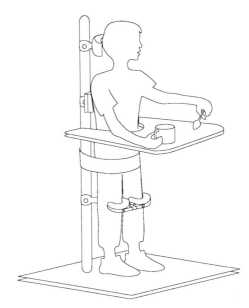

FIG. 6-12. Standing frames require intact postural control in the upper trunk.

STRUCTURAL PROBLEMS IN POSITIONING

There are special considerations for fixed or structural problems, but just as with flexible orthopedic problems, each patient needs to be carefully assessed, and all of the same principles apply. The major difference is that, rather than correcting postural problems, the positioning system must be designed to accommodate and support fixed deformities and to equalize weight-bearing

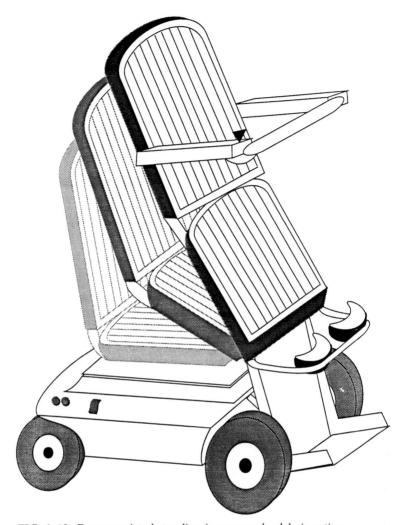

FIG. 6–13. Power-assisted standing is now a wheelchair option.

forces to achieve comfort and skin protection.

Almost any positioning aid can be adapted with wood and foam pads to provide accommodation for minimal to moderate fixed deformities. There has been a recent surge of products for this purpose on the commercial seating market. These products can be mixed and matched to develop solutions for patients who have fixed orthopedic problems that preclude safe or comfortable use of a standard seating system. The components of these systems can be used to adapt seating, sidelying, standing, or other positioning devices to meet individual patient needs.

To ensure successful accommodation, the positioning device should be adapted through a series of successive trials with mock-up materials. In this way the most comfortable and supportive system can be provided. Mock-up systems should be carefully measured and illustrated to ensure accuracy of the final product. Some manufacturers do custom work to modify a device before delivery to the local dealer, while others rely on the technical staff of the dealer to provide this service. It is more common to find manufacturers of seating systems that will provide a custom fit than the other devices described, but this is changing with an increasing market demand.

Manufacturers of modular seating sys-

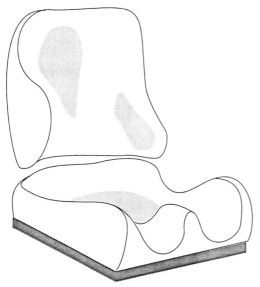

FIG. 6–14. A custom-molded system may be needed to accommodate severe orthopedic deformities.

ticularly for patients who depend on more than one caregiver.

Patients with multiple, severe orthopedic deformities generally require a custom-molded positioning system[17,18] similar to that pictured in Figure 6–14. Construction of these systems begins with a plaster mold taken with the patient in the desired position, whether seated, sidelying, supine, or other. Once the best possible alignment, comfort, and distribution of weight-bearing forces is achieved, a mold is taken. The final version of the positioning system is constructed from foams and mounted on a plastic, metal, or wood base. Manufacturers generally provide adjustment and modification as needed on the positioning system itself, while the local dealer assumes the responsibility for long-term servicing for minor adjustments and repairs.

tems like that shown in Figure 6–5 offer a wide range of alternatives in densities of foam, size, and shape. A variety of hardware choices makes nearly any configuration possible. An additional advantage of modular systems is that parts can be replaced as needed without the need to replace the entire seating system. A disadvantage is that removable and adjustable parts are not always an appropriate solution, par-

SUMMARY

When prescribing any positioning aid, whether it is a wheelchair, a prone stander, or a sidelying device, a structured, orderly approach helps to ensure that any equipment provided will meet the medical, musculoskeletal, neuromuscular, and functional needs of the patient.

The success of any positioning aid depends on proper fit and design, both initially and in the long term. Because people grow and change, it is necessary to set up a mechanism for follow-up and alteration based on individual patient needs.

REFERENCES

1. Eldred, E.: Peripheral receptors: Their excitation and relation to reflex patterns. Am. J. Phys. Med. Rehabil. 46(1):69, 1967.
2. Letts, M., Shapiro, L., Mulden, K., and Klassen, O.: The windblown hip syndrome in total body cerebral palsy. J. Pediatr. January 4, 55, 1984.
3. Bergen, A.F.: Sidelyer with positioning blocks. Phys. Ther. 59:301, 1979.
4. Brown, J.K., and Fulford, G.E.: Position as a cause of deformity in children with cerebral palsy. Dev. Med. Child. Neurol. 18:305, 1976.
5. Hulme, J.B., Poor, R., Schulein, M., and Pez-

zino, J.: Perceived behavioral changes observed with adaptive seating devices and training programs for multiply handicapped, developmentally delayed individuals. Phys. Ther. 63:204, 1983.
6. Hallenborg, S.C.: Wheelchair needs of the disabled. In Therapeutic Considerations for the Elderly. Ed. O.L. Jackson. New York, Churchill Livingstone, Inc., 1987.
7. Bergen, A.F.: Positioning the Client with Central Nervous System Deficits. 2nd Ed. Valhalla, NY, Valhalla Rehabilitation Publications, Ltd., 1985.
8. Fiorentino, M.R.: Reflex Testing Methods for

Evaluating CNS Development. Springfield, Ill, Charles C Thomas, 1963.

9. Morimoto, S.: Effect of sitting posture on the human body. Bull. Tokyo Med. Dent. Univ. *20(1)*:19, 1973.

10. Zacharkow, D.: Wheelchair Posture and Pressure Sores. Springfield, IL, Charles C Thomas, 1984.

11. Koreska, J., Gibson, D.A., and Albisser, A.M.: International Series on Biomechanics: Structural Support System for Unstable Spine. Baltimore, MD, University Park Press, 1976.

12. Minns, R.J., and Sutton, R.A.: Pressures under the ischium detected by pedobarograph. Eng. Med. *11(3)*:111, 1982.

13. Shields, R.K., and Cook, T.M.: Effect of seat angle and lumbar support on seated buttock pressure. Phys. Ther. *68(11)*:1682, 1988.

14. Anderson, B.J.G., Ortengren, R., Nachemson, A.L., et al.: The sitting posture: An electromyographic and discometric study. Orthop. Clin. North Am. *6*:105, 1975.

15. Bunch, W.H., and Keagy, R.D.: Principles of Orthotic Treatment. St. Louis, C.V. Mosby Co., 1976.

16. Ivey, A., et al.: Supine standing for severely handicapped children. Phys. Ther. *61*:525, 1981.

17. Seeger, B.R., and Sutherland, A.D.: Modular seating for paralytic scoliosis: Design and initial experience. Prosthetics and Orthotics International *5*:121, 1981.

18. Hobson, D., Driver, K.O., and Hanks, S.: Foam in place seating for the severely disabled. Proceedings: Fifth Annual Conference on Systems and Devices for the Disabled, 153, 1978.

7

PHYSICAL MODALITIES

KAREN B. GIEBLER

A modality is defined by Dorland as "a method of application of, or the employment of, any therapeutic agent; limited usually to physical agents."[1] Physical agents include light, heat, cold, water, electricity, and mechanical apparatus. Modalities can be used effectively as adjuncts to a therapeutic exercise program. They can be of benefit in decreasing spasticity, allowing an increase in range of motion and comfort. Achieving a decrease in spasticity before, or in conjunction with, exercise may permit work on voluntary control, normal movement patterns, and strengthening. Most modalities are time-effective, meaning that the time required to apply or administer them is justified by the results achieved. Many can be used at the same time as functional skills are being taught. Most are noninvasive, and few have significant side effects or contraindications.

Care must be taken to apply the modality appropriately and correctly. A treatment time that is too short or selection of the wrong parameters can reverse the desired effect. For example, ice applied by quickly stroking for less than 2 minutes has a facilitatory effect. When applied in a stationary manner for 20 minutes, it has an inhibitory effect. High-frequency vibration has a facilitatory effect, whereas low-frequency vibration has an inhibitory effect.

There are three general modes of action of physical modalities in decreasing spasticity:

1. Facilitation of the antagonist of a spastic muscle to relax the spastic muscle by reciprocal inhibition.
2. Relaxation, inhibition, or fatigue of the spastic muscle directly.
3. Generalized relaxation.

Relief of pain may also be relevant to the decrease of spasticity. It is known that pain can increase muscle contraction in normal individuals. Noxious input increases the activity of the reflex arc even if there is no connection to supraspinal centers, such as when tight jeans increase spasticity in a quadriplegic patient. Intrathecal morphine has been shown to decrease spasticity, as well as pain, possibly by decreasing the transmission of noxious input in the spinal cord.[2]

One proposed mechanism for local inhibition is counterirritation, also called hyperstimulation analgesia.[3] Modalities may influence pain perception by providing a counterirritant to the painful stimuli. According to the "gate" theory of Melzack and Wall, the perception of pain is influenced by the amount of competing sensory stimulation.[4] If the sensory system is flooded with sensory input, the perception of pain will be reduced. This sensory input can be from a physical agent such as heat or cold. In addition, it can come from monotonously repetitive mechanical skin stimulation such as massage. Whatever the method, bombarding the sensory system may close the "gate" that controls the activity of the reflex arc. The different afferent nerves may inhibit each other at the presynaptic level.[5] The "gate" may be closed by increasing the amount of input from large, fast conducting fibers or by decreasing the amount of small fiber input.[4]

Decreased muscle tone is seen with the administration of some types and levels of general anesthesia.[6] Spasticity can be observed clinically to decrease during sleep. The relaxation induced by a modality will probably not approach that reached under anesthesia, but on a continuum from hyperactivity to relaxation, may be able to shift the level of muscle tone toward the relaxed end.

Pain-relieving modalities may help decrease spasticity, especially if pain is present. It is possible that pain-relieving modalities might decrease spasticity even in patients without pain. Using the framework just described, it is proposed that modalities that decrease pain may decrease spasticity by local inhibition or by generalized relaxation.

The objective of treatment with a modality is not merely a reduction in spasticity. Rather, the goal may be to improve function, to increase passive range of motion, or to increase comfort. The treatment approach applied, including the use of modalities, depends on many factors, including the extent and severity of the spasticity, the overall medical condition of the patient, the environment, and the immediate treatment goals. A particular modality may be considered for its mode of action, availability, ease of application, length of carryover, or other factors. It is difficult, if not impossible, to make guarantees about the specific effects of a modality on an individual. Response to many of the modalities varies widely even among normal individuals. Therefore, the effectiveness of a modality must be individually assessed, especially initially. The modality used to decrease spasticity should generally not adversely affect voluntary control or decrease strength. Functional training should be the focus of treatment whenever possible.

COLD

Cold can inhibit a spastic muscle directly or may do so indirectly by facilitating the antagonist of the spastic muscle. The length of time that the cold is applied, and thus the extent of tissue cooling, may be the primary determining factor.

SUSTAINED LOCAL COLD

Sustained local cold provides direct inhibition of the spastic muscle. Several mechanisms for this effect have been proposed. Lowering of skin temperature inhibits the skin receptors, which decreases the amount of small fiber input and closes the "gate." Cooling the skin to below 10 degrees Celsius (10°C) reduces skin receptor sensitivity. At that temperature, most of the mechanoreceptors stop responding to mechanical stimulation. Responses can usually be elicited, however, by increasing the strength of the stimulus. Many receptors continue to have reduced sensitivity long after the skin temperature has returned to the control value.[7] Thus, when cutaneous input is involved in the generation of hypertonia, cooling of skin receptors may be therapeutic.

Sustained cold may also inhibit the monosynaptic stretch reflex by decreasing spindle sensitivity. Knutsson and Mattsson applied a Hydrocollator Colpac to the triceps surae muscles of 15 normal individuals. Temperature was measured by thermistors in thin flexible catheters. Application of the cold pack dropped the subcutaneous temperature to 20 to 25°C within a few minutes. They found that the average amplitude of the Achilles reflex was significantly decreased after sustained cold. The mean decrease was 34% after 20 minutes.[8] Bell and Lehmann also found a significant decrease in T-reflex amplitude after a 20-minute application of an ice/water pack to the calf muscles of 16 normal subjects. They found no change in the H-reflex, indicating decreased spindle afferent firing as the cause of the decrease.[9] A decrease in the T-reflex has also been observed in patients with spasticity. Miglietta found a decrease of 34% in the magnitude of the patellar

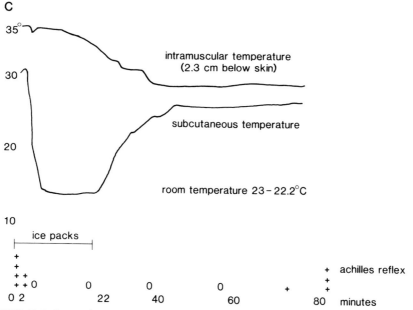

FIG. 7-1. Ice packs on gastrocnemius muscle (adapted with permission from Hartviksen, K.: Ice therapy in spasticity. Acta Neurol. Scandinav. *38*:82, 1962).

stretch reflex after cold application in a study of 10 patients with quadriceps spasticity.[10] Hartviksen studied 10 patients with spastic paresis of the lower extremities. The Achilles reflex was absent 3 minutes after cold was applied to the triceps surae. The treatment lasted 20 minutes. The Achilles reflex usually did not return for 30 to 60 minutes after the cold pack was removed. Clonus did not return for another hour (Fig. 7-1).[11] Eldred et al. investigated the effects of local cooling on cat muscle spindles that were under moderate tension. They found that the spindle afferents fire more slowly when cooled. The firing rate from primary endings was decreased more than that from secondary endings.[12]

Nerve conduction velocity has been shown to be decreased by the application of sustained cold.[13,14] Although there is an initial superficial vasoconstriction followed by a superficial vasodilation, a study by Lee et al. found no correlation between skin temperature changes and the nerve conduction velocity changes. They found that the nerve conduction velocity began to rise after the ice was removed, but remained below the initial velocity 30 minutes after removal.[14]

Decreased blood circulation to the cooled area may slow the rewarming process and thus contribute to the prolonged relaxation of spasticity seen with sustained cold.[15]

The decrease in spasticity noted with the application of sustained cold appears to be caused initially by the cooled skin receptors. This effect occurs after approximately 2 to 3 minutes. After sustained cold for 10 minutes, there is a decrease in the rate of firing of the muscle spindle afferents and slowed conduction velocity in motor and sensory nerves.

Sustained cold can have significant effects on voluntary movement and on neurophysiologic parameters. Knutsson did a study of patients with upper motor neuron lesions who had limited active range of motion secondary to spasticity. Commercial cold packs were applied to the spastic muscle for 15 to 20 minutes. In 8 of 12 patients studied, voluntary range of motion increased an average of 35° after sustained cold.[16] In a study of 12 children with spasticity and contracture, Kelly found a significant increase in range of motion when an exercise program was preceded by sustained local cold to the spastic muscles for

8 minutes 5 times a week for 4 months. The cold packs consisted of towels dipped in ice chips and water. The towel was changed after 4 minutes.[17] The children served as their own controls, receiving the same exercise program for 8 months, but with the cold packs added only in either the first 4 months or the last 4 months.

Knutsson reports that the strength of the antagonist of a spastic muscle increased by more than 50% in 11 of 29 cases following sustained cold to the spastic muscle. The patients all had pronounced spasticity secondary to CVA, MS, or SCI. Strength was measured with a strain gauge transducer. This increase was attributed to the release of the influence of the spastic agonist.[16]

Sustained local cold is applied to the length of the spastic muscle. It can be applied in several ways, using a commercial refrigerated cold pack, a plastic bag of crushed ice, or an envelope of toweling filled with ice cubes. A damp, warm towel placed on the skin, followed by the cold pack, allows gradual cooling, which enhances comfort.[15] Another alternative is to use a towel that has been dipped in a mixture of ice chips and water. The towel is then wrung out and placed on the spastic muscle. It must be replaced during the treatment to maintain the cold level.[11] The process of replacing towels may provide cutaneous input and thus decrease the inhibitory effect of the cold. In addition, the towels may drip, and the client may find this annoying; therefore the desired effect will be counteracted.

The usual treatment time for sustained cold is 20 minutes. It may be shorter for thin individuals and longer for heavy individuals.[18] A useful technique to decrease spasticity in the lateral neck muscles is to apply sustained cold to the spastic neck muscles while maintained stretch is applied to those muscles with the patient in a side-lying position.

It has been recommended that the body temperature be maintained during any application of cold to avoid shivering and a resultant increase in hypertonia.[15,19] Cold is not tolerated well by all patients. Hartviksen states that he has observed three cases of hypersensitivity to cold during hundreds of applications, exhibited by temporary redness and swelling where the cold pack had been applied.[11] There is a report in the literature of a patient with left hemiplegia and known coronary disease who showed significant electrocardiographic changes after application of a cold pack to the shoulder.[20]

The spastic muscle may be inhibited for 30 minutes or more after 20 minutes of sustained cold. Therefore active exercises, stretching exercises, and/or functional activities should follow the sustained cold application.

GENERALIZED COOLING

Generalized cooling has been recommended primarily to decrease spasticity and increase function in patients with multiple sclerosis. Several case reports suggest that 10–20 minutes in a 26.7°C tub or whirlpool may improve function.[21,22] No objective studies were located on this technique.

QUICK ICING

There is some evidence that the initial response of some thermoreceptors and mechanoreceptors in the skin to cold application is an increased rate of firing.[8] This response may be elicited by the movement of the ice across the skin and/or by the passage of the skin receptors through a critical temperature range. Knutsson and Mattsson found an increase in the amplitude of the H-reflex during the first few minutes of cold application, indicating stimulation of the Group Ia afferent fibers.[8] Bell and Lehmann, however, found no significant changes in H-reflex amplitudes during cold applications to normal subjects.[9] Neither of these studies used movement of the ice, but in a study by Clendenin and Szumski that did so, it was found that single motor unit activity increased with 1 to 2 minutes of icing over the biceps in normal individuals. The facilitatory effect generally lasted 5 to 10 minutes. Facilitation of the motor unit was seen during light stroking with ice in 60% of the subjects who were able to isolate single motor units using biofeedback. This facilitation was shown by increased firing of the unit.[23] However, no control stroking without ice was used, so it is difficult to tell whether the cold or the mechanical stimulation was the active treatment.

Quick ice is applied to the antagonist of the spastic muscle. It may relax the spastic muscle by reciprocal inhibition. Quick icing involves stroking the skin over the antagonist with an ice cube or popsicle. The stroking must be brief. This technique seems to be most effective when it is accompanied by attempted active contraction of the stimulated muscle by the patient.

It has been said that quick icing produces unpredictable results, may result in a "rebound" phenomenon, and should never be done above the level of the lips.[24] Objective evidence for these precautions has not been found.

EVAPORATIVE COOLING SPRAY

Evaporative cooling spray has been found to rapidly decrease skin temperature to below 10°C. Skin receptors have been shown to be less sensitive to mechanical stimulation when the skin cooling caused by evaporative cooling spray persists longer than 2 minutes.[7] Thus, it appears that in the first 2 minutes after evaporative cooling spray has been applied, the effects are similar to those observed with sustained cold during the period when it has been on the skin for 3 to 10 minutes. The skin temperatures are similar at these times. Skin temperature during quick icing never drops to 20°C because of the short application time. Quick ice may increase the firing of the skin mechanoreceptors due to its application in a stroking motion. Evaporative cooling spray may act more by decreasing the temperature of the skin receptors and subsequently decreasing their responsiveness.

A study of the tonic reflexes of the foot by Duncan found that ethyl chloride spray did not decrease the temperature of the subcutaneous tissues. Four reflexes on the sole of the foot elicited by vibration were abolished by the application of ethyl chloride spray. These reflexes were similarly abolished by a local infiltration of procaine. It seems then that evaporative cooling spray blocks the skin rather than the muscle receptors.[25] Travell comments that certain muscle groups, namely, the iliopsoas, scaleni, and "elbow muscles," respond poorly.[26]

Although it is generally used to decrease muscle spasm, evaporative cooling spray has also been applied to spastic muscles. Its efficacy in decreasing spasticity has not been objectively documented. One study in normal individuals found that spraying the hamstrings in conjunction with static passive stretch produced a significant increase in passive hip flexion over that of their control group, which received static passive stretch.[27] Because it has been shown to decrease tonic reflexes and at least one study shows an increase in range of motion in normal individuals, evaporative cooling sprays may have a use in local inhibition of spasticity. Unfortunately, a recent commentary asserts that these products are implicated in the destruction of the ozone layer.[28]

In evaporative cooling, Gebauer FluoriMethane* or ethyl chloride is applied along the length of a spastic muscle. Ethyl chloride is flammable and, therefore, chlorofluoromethanes are more commonly used. Travell recommends that the muscle be sprayed 6 times in 5-second sweeps, with 3 seconds between sweeps. It is sprayed from proximal to distal at about 4 inches per second. The stream is pointed at an angle to the body, not perpendicular. The face should be protected and kept higher than the area sprayed because the vapor is heavy and tends to fall. Travell recommends stretching the muscle gently while spraying, going only to the point of pain.[26]

TOPICAL ANESTHESIA

Topical anesthesia has been proposed as a method to decrease spasticity. One study on five patients with spasticity used a 20% benzocaine spray for 15 seconds to the entire leg below the knee or including the thigh. The patients were of mixed diagnoses. Two had CVAs, two MS, and one head

---

*Gebauer Chemical Co., 9410 St. Catherine Ave., Cleveland, OH 44104

injury. A decrease in spasticity was found that lasted 3 to 4 hours. Improvements were seen in both active and passive range of motion and a more normal gait pattern was observed as assessed in a gait laboratory. Improvements began 10 minutes after the application.[29] Although the observed clinical effects indicate a decrease in spasticity, one of the underlying neurophysiologic tests was in the opposite direction. The H-reflex increased in amplitude by 29% after 30 minutes and then decreased gradually.[29] This implies facilitation of the alpha motoneuron pool. Tendon reflexes showed no significant change.[29] It must be noted that this study was not blind, did not have a control group, and was limited to five patients. A different clinical result was obtained in a study performed by Inacio et al.,[30] using a double-blind design. Nine patients with spasticity secondary to head injury received either a 20% benzocaine ointment applied to a spastic extremity or a placebo preparation. The study was performed on 4 successive days with random assignment of the placebo or the benzocaine in either ABAB or BABA order. Patients served as their own controls. Decreased spasticity was defined as an increase in active range of motion. Two testers measured three trials of passive range of motion and three trials of active range of motion on each subject with a standard goniometer. The test position, tester, and verbal commands remained constant for each subject. Ointments were applied quickly to reduce the possible massage effects. Each tester wore examination gloves to prevent contact with the ointments. Both ointments were similar in texture and smell. Subjects relaxed for 15 minutes after ointment application, and then three repeated trials of passive and three trials of active range of motion were measured. No difference was found in either active or passive range of motion between the benzocaine trials and the placebo trials. Of interest, however, is the observation that there was a significant increase in range of motion between the first measurement of each patient and the third. This appears to support the use of exercise, but not topical anesthesia, to decrease spasticity.[29] The discrepancy between these two studies may be related to a placebo effect in the first, differences in diagnostic groups, or different operational measures of spasticity.

Ease of application, availability, and lack of side effects make this an attractive modality if it is effective in decreasing spasticity. Further research in this area is warranted. Benzocaine or xylocaine preparations can be applied topically to an extremity. Over-the-counter sunburn relief medication can be obtained in spray, foam, ointment, or lotion form with various concentrations of the active ingredient.

HEAT

Heat is used for both local relaxation of a spastic muscle and generalized relaxation. Heat modalities are usually divided into superficial and deep heat.[31] All the methods included here are superficial except ultrasound.[31] Heat has been shown to increase blood flow, relieve muscle spasm, increase tendon extensibility, provide pain relief,[31] and decrease fusimotor efferent activity.[32]

NEUTRAL WARMTH

Fischer and Solomon found that covering the thigh with a blanket in a comfortable-temperature room raised the skin temperature from 33 to 36°C.[32] It is thought that heating the skin produces relaxation of skeletal muscles by a reflex action.[31] Neutral warmth, therefore, is a method to provide direct relaxation of spastic muscle.[24,33]

Wells found that the optimum temperature for relief of pain by heating was a temperature of the skin equal to the temperature of the blood and deep tissues.[34] Thus, if spasticity is influenced by noxious input, neutral warmth may be able to decrease spasticity. Rood speculated that neutral warmth to the trunk over the area innervated by the posterior rami reduces sympathetic outflow[35] for general relaxation.[24,36]

There are several ways to apply neutral warmth. An extremity can be covered with a pillow or wrapped in a towel, or the trunk can be wrapped in a blanket. Neutral warmth is usually administered for 10 to 20 minutes.[33] The effect is of short duration.[31]

HYDROCOLLATOR PACK

A hydrocollator pack to the thigh has been found to increase the temperature of the skin 11 to 42.5°C in 8 minutes. At the depth of the muscle, the temperature rises approximately 3°C from 34 to 37°C in 20 minutes.[37] The firing rate of muscle spindle afferents has been shown to decrease at 42°C,[38] but because the muscle temperature does not reach 42°C by the application of a hot pack, firing rates of spindle afferents are probably not the cause of the observed relaxation.

The soothing effect of heat has often been attributed to the increased blood flow. Wells, however, found that complete interruption of the blood flow did not change the ability of heat to decrease pain. He created moderate pain by attaching a spring-type artery clamp to the web of a finger. Warming the hand and the clamp in air or water lessened or abolished the pain. Stopping blood flow to the arm did not change this effect.[34] A hot pack may therefore decrease spasticity by counterirritation.[39]

The hydrocollator pack is wrapped in 4 to 8 layers of terry cloth and applied to the spastic muscle for 20 minutes. The skin should be checked frequently when the patient has decreased sensation, is unable to communicate, or is elderly. The relaxation effect generally lasts only until the temperature returns to baseline.[31] Therefore, if spasticity reduction is desired to gain range of motion, stretching exercises need to be started in conjunction with the heat treatment or immediately following.

PARAFFIN

Paraffin can increase subcutaneous tissue temperature 4.4°C using the dip method.[40] A rise of 4.5°C has been found in hand muscles.[41] This heat produces muscle relaxation, increases tendon extensibility,[31] and decreases pain.[32] Paraffin is an effective[41] but short-term[31] means of delivering heat for localized spasticity of the hand or foot.

The temperature of the paraffin bath is maintained at 52 to 54°C.[31] For the dip method, the hand or foot is submerged seven to twelve times, put in a plastic bag, and then wrapped with a towel. The paraffin is peeled off after 20 minutes. The immersion method, which has been recommended for greater heat absorption,[40] is often difficult to accomplish with the spastic limb because of problems in positioning. Stretching exercises, joint mobilization techniques, or splint application should immediately follow the paraffin treatment to obtain any prolonged benefit.

FLUIDOTHERAPY

Borrell et al. found a temperature rise of 5.27°C in the hand muscles with Fluidotherapy.*[41] Fluidotherapy is advertised as a dry whirlpool that can be tolerated at temperatures of 46 to 49°C.[42] Theoretically, it combines the effects of a light stroking massage by its monotonously repetitive mechanical skin stimulation[43] with the benefits of superficial heat.

Positioning and maintaining the spastic limb in the standard unit (10″ × 29″ × 34″) can be difficult. The larger, bed size tank (21″ × 58″ × 47″) was reported by Alcorn et al. to relieve pain and increase range of motion in clients with sickle cell anemia.[44] Research is needed to see if this tank could have a generalized relaxation effect on spasticity.

WHIRLPOOL

Whirlpool combines superficial heat and massage action[45] to relax muscles, decrease pain, and sedate.[32,46] The Hubbard tank (Fig. 7–2) or large whirlpool can be used to provide generalized relaxation. Including the neck in the treatment may decrease fusimotor activity, resulting in diminished muscle spindle excitability,[32] apparently because of stimulation of some skin reflexes in the upper thoracic and neck region.[48] As heated blood returns to the general circulation (assuming that the water is warm

*Fluidotherapy, Henley International/Neuromedics Inc., 104 Industrial Blvd., Sugar Land, TX 77478

FIG. 7-2. Hubbard tank.

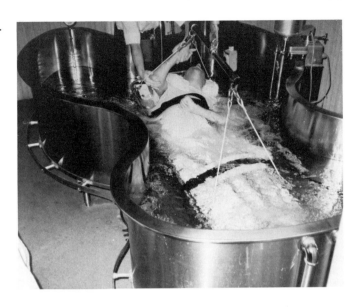

enough to actually heat the blood) during a Hubbard tank treatment, it stimulates the hypothalmus to decrease arousal and fusimotor activity. This decreases the spindle afferent activity at a constant level of muscle stretch. In a study on cats and rabbits in which the hypothalmus was directly heated, fusimotor activity was found to be inhibited.[48] For full body immersion, the water temperature should be maintained from 37 to 40°C. Improved spasticity reduction is usually noted at the higher portion of the temperature range. The oral temperature should be monitored when the water temperature is above 37.8°C.[47] Whirlpool treatment of an extremity has more of a local inhibitory effect on the spastic muscles. A rise of 4.3°C was found in hand muscles after 20 minutes in a 38.89°C whirlpool.[41] The usual treatment time is 20 minutes.

The relaxation effects of whirlpool treatment can last from 30 minutes to 12 hours.[49] Patients may be able to move more easily while in the water, possibly allowing some carryover in voluntary control. Heat, however, has been shown to decrease strength,[38] which may be counterproductive. The client may be initially anxious. Therefore, it may take several treatments to judge whether whirlpool treatment will have a positive effect on spasticity.

ULTRASOUND

Ultrasound is applied to the spastic agonist to relax the muscle.[32] Ultrasound increases tendon extensibility through its heating effects.[47] It also increases blood flow, increases tissue metabolism, and elevates the pain threshold.[31] The temperature elevation achieved may decrease fusimotor activity, thus decreasing the sensitivity of the muscle spindle to stretch.[31,50] Lehmann et al. found that a dosage of 1.5 w/cm^2 caused a temperature increase of 4.5°C in the anterior thigh.[51] A small study of three subjects by Stillwell and Gersten found a significant decrease in spasticity that lasted 10 to 15 minutes when ultrasound was applied at 1.9 w/cm^2, but an increase in spasticity at a dose of .76 w/cm^2.[50]

Continuous ultrasound delivered in a stroking manner is the recommended technique.[31] The usual treatment time is 5 to 10 minutes, but this depends on the size of the area.[31] Shunt tubing and areas of plastic implants should be avoided because of their possible absorption of heat.[47,50] The area over the carotid sinus should also be avoided. Significantly greater residual elongation was achieved with low load stretching when a rat's tail was heated first.[52] Thus ultrasound may help in spasticity control by allowing an increase in muscle/tendon length as well as through reflex inhibition. Because joint limitation is a major complication of spasticity, ultrasound can be of benefit in its treatment. The optimal treatment combines heat and stretch.[31,52,53] Ultrasound can be combined with stretch by positioning the patient with spastic gastrocnemius and soleus muscles on a prone stander or standing with the muscles on a stretch while the ultrasound is applied. A knee flexion contracture can be treated by applying ultrasound to the spastic muscles, tendons, and the posterior joint capsule. This can be performed in conjunction with sustained stretch with weights while the patient is positioned prone or followed by Buck's traction while the patient is supine. Serial casting can be preceded by several days of ultrasound treatments.

ELECTRICAL STIMULATION

Electrical stimulation can be used in several ways to decrease spasticity.[54,55] The stimulation is most often applied to the antagonist to achieve reciprocal inhibition of the spastic muscle.[54,56] The stimulation can be applied directly to the spastic muscle to inhibit, relax, or fatigue it.[54,57] The stimulation may also be performed to achieve a generalized relaxation effect.[55]

Electrical stimulation is available in various waveforms and stimulation parameters. The terms used to describe the stimulation generators are numerous and often overlap. Some of the choices available are functional electrical stimulation (FES), transcutaneous electrical nerve stimulation (TENS), medium frequency, high voltage, low voltage,

TABLE 7–1. PARAMETERS OF ELECTRICAL STIMULATION DEVICES AND TECHNIQUES USED TO DECREASE SPASTICITY

Devices/ Techniques	Pulse Frequency (rate)	Pulse Duration (width)	Intensity
FES NMES Low voltage current	0 – 150 pps 35 pps most common	100 – 700 μsec 300 μsec most common	0 – 100mA
Medium frequency "Russian" stimulation	1000 – 100,000 Hz 2500 Hz modulated at 50 bursts per second most common	N/A	0 – 100mA
High voltage pulsed current HVPGS	1 – 120 twin pulses per second 50 pps most common	5 – 200 μsec 20 μsec most common	0 – 2500mA
High rate TENS Conventional TENS Electroanalgesia	40 – 150 pps 85 pps most common	40 – 300 μsec 75 μsec most common	0 – 50mA
Low rate TENS Acupucture–like TENS Electroanalgesia	1 – 25 pps 2 pps most common	40 – 250 μsec 220 μsec most common	0 – 100mA

and neuromuscular electrical stimulation (NMES). Table 7–1 shows the parameters of some of these devices/techniques. The waveforms and other parameters available may differ among various units and manufacturers.

There are a few contraindications to the use of electrical stimulation. It should not be used when a muscle contraction is not desirable, such as around an unstable fracture. It should probably not be used on the chest or arm if the patient has a demand pacemaker or cardiac arrhythmias.[54] Obesity may be a contraindication because of the poor conductance of fat.[54] There is potential for skin irritation[54,59] and for burns.[57,59]

STIMULATION OF THE ANTAGONIST

Stimulation of the antagonist of the spastic muscle decreases spasticity by reciprocal inhibition.[54,56] Alfieri found that 10 minutes of electrical stimulation to the antagonist of a spastic muscle achieved an immediate decrease in spasticity. This decrease lasted from 10 to 15 minutes to 2 to 3 hours, with an average of about one hour. He studied 115 hemiplegic patients, using the Ashworth scale to grade the degree of spasticity. One examiner was used throughout. Figure 7–3 illustrates the change in spasticity of wrist and finger flexors in a single representative subject in this study. Grading was done before treatment (b), during treatment (d), after treatment (a), after one hour (1h), and after about 23 hours (23h) from the first treatment session.[56]

The following parameters are suggested for beginning FES to the antagonist of a spastic muscle:

Pulse rate	35–50 pps (pulses per second)
Pulse duration	300 μsec
Rise time	4 sec
Fall time	2 sec
On/off time	12 sec/18 sec
Intensity	Increase gradually to achieve the strongest contraction tolerated well by the patient

These are only suggestions for initial settings. The rise time may need to be increased further to avoid eliciting a stretch reflex in the antagonist muscle.[54] Stimulation can be performed before or in conjunction with a functional activity.[54] The sessions should last only as long as a contraction is obtained. Initially this period may be short because a muscle that has been inhibited for a significant time by a spastic antagonist may fatigue quite rapidly. A general rule to start is that the peak "on" time should be a third of the "off" time.[54] The "on" time includes the rise, the peak "on" time, and the fall (Fig. 7–4). Over a period of time the peak "on" time can be extended. The goal is for the on/off time to approach normal movement times. A heel switch may be available that allows timing of the stimulus to coincide with the swing phase of gait so that the anterior tibialis muscle is stimulated when pressure is taken off the sole of the foot.

Treatment time can be gradually extended. The recommended length of a treatment session in the literature varies from 10 minutes[56] to as much as 8 hours for some uses.[54] The relaxation effect may last only the duration of the stimulation or may

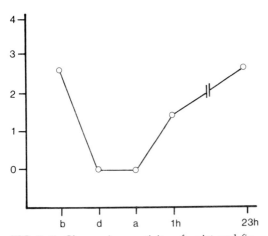

FIG. 7–3. Change in spasticity of wrist and finger flexors with electrical stimulation to the extensors (with permission from Alfieri, V.: Electrical treatment of spasticity. Scand. J. Rehabil. Med. *14*:179, 1982). See text for explanation.

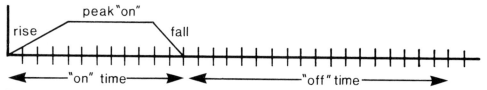

FIG. 7–4. On and off time. See text for explanation.

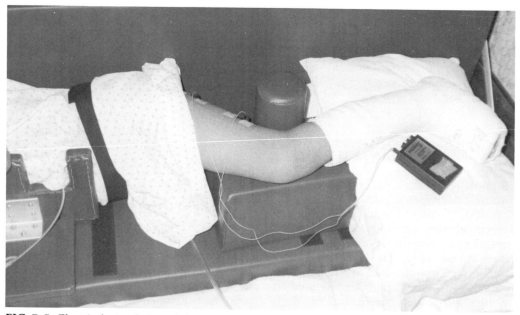

FIG. 7–5. Electrical stimulation of the hamstrings to decrease quadriceps spasticity while patient is in a sidelyer.

extend for 2 to 3 hours.[56] Post-tetanic potentiation may account for the longer-lasting effects.[54,60] Post-tetanic potentiation is the increased muscle response to a stimulus that is felt to be related to an increase in transmitters at the synapse following a short burst of stimulation.[60] Because spasticity usually decreases as the patient gains active control and strength,[54] the possibility exists that the treatments will lead to a more long-lasting effect.

This type of stimulation has benefits other than the reciprocal inhibition of spasticity. Range of motion has been shown to be improved.[61] Treatment must last at least 1 hour per day to overcome a contracture and requires at least 1 to 2 weeks of treatment.[54] Figure 7–5 demonstrates the use of electrical stimulation to gain knee flexion in a child who was admitted with a 15-degree hyperextension contracture of the knee secondary to quadriceps spasticity. Stimulation in conjunction with a dropout cast is particularly effective in gaining range of motion[62] (Fig. 7–6). FES can be used as an orthotic substitute. In addition to its use for ankle dorsiflexion, it can substitute for a sling.[63] Electrical stimulation of the deltoid, in addition to improving the painful hemiplegic shoulder, will decrease spasticity in the pectoralis major and facilitate wrist and finger extension.[56] FES provides a biofeedback effect. The patient can see the muscle contraction, and sensory feedback is obtained.[54,56] In this regard, it can act as a facilitation technique.[54] FES can improve functional activities.[54,64] In a single subject study, Fulbright showed that electrical

FIG. 7-6. Electrical stimulation of the triceps in conjunction with a dropout cast.

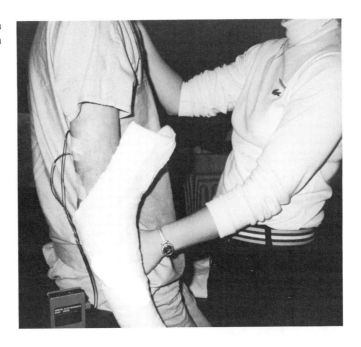

stimulation to the toe extensors successfully counteracted chronic toe flexor spasticity and improved the gait of a head-injured patient.[62] Strengthening may occur in the muscle being stimulated.[54,65-67] Using peroneal stimulation at 30 Hz for 10 minutes on 7 patients who had spasticity primarily caused by multiple sclerosis, Carnstam et al. demonstrated an increase in ankle dorsiflexion strength. Strength was measured by a force transducer. There was a simultaneous increase in the integrated EMG from the anterior tibialis muscle.[66] Although these studies give a very optimistic picture of FES, most use subjective measures and are not blind.

In using FES, the depth of the stimulus is determined in part by the distance between the electrodes. Depth increases as distance increases.[54] Because the stimulation should not penetrate to the spastic muscle, electrodes must not be placed too far apart.[54] If a contraction is not achieved, a machine may be needed with a different waveform or more output.[54]

Maximal isometric muscle contraction because of stimulation of the muscle motor endplate reportedly occurs at 2500 Hz.[67] This is classified as a medium frequency,[68] but has been called high frequency by the manufacturers and several authors.[67,69] This current has been called "Russian"[70] stimulation, when modulated at 50 bursts per second, because of the work of Kots from the USSR.[71] Recommended treatments consist of a 15-second "on" time and 50 second "off" time lasting usually for 10 maximal contractions.[69] Twelve-second "on" times and 8 second "off" times for as many as 60 contractions have also been suggested.[72]

This type of current has been primarily applied to healthy subjects[67,71] or rat muscle.[70] Reports have been made that it strengthens muscle, facilitates muscle contraction,[72] and increases blood flow.[71] Higher current intensity tolerance has been seen when a weight or cast is present to provide resistance to movement[72] (Fig. 7-7).

This current can be used in patients with spasticity. It may strengthen the weakened muscle while reciprocally inhibiting the spastic muscle. It has been used with good success at our facility on patients with spasticity secondary to head injury. It may achieve a stronger contraction than lower-frequency current in the weak muscle and thus provide more significant inhibition of the spastic muscle. This stronger contraction may be achieved because the patient is

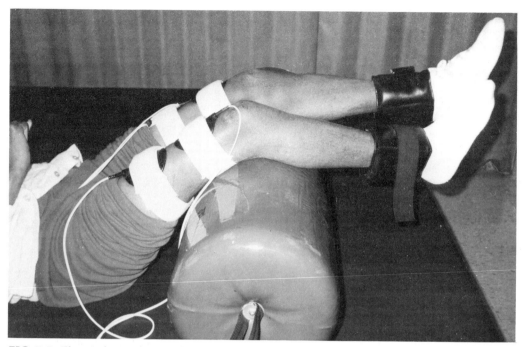

FIG. 7–7. Electrical stimulation of the quadriceps to decrease hamstring spasticity.

able to tolerate increased intensity. In a study comparing muscle force caused by electrical stimulation in healthy subjects, however, the group receiving low-frequency stimulation (25 Hz) achieved more pronounced strengthening effects than the group who received medium-frequency stimulation (2500 Hz modulated at 25 bursts per second).[67] The difference we see may be caused by the parameters we use with spastic patients. Our low frequency is generally 35 to 50 Hz to achieve a tetanic contraction. Our medium frequency is 2500 Hz modulated at 50 bursts per second. Another possibility is the difference in electrode size. Larger pads are generally used with the medium-frequency machines. Larger electrodes have been found to produce stronger contractions with less pain.[73]

At least one investigator refers to the 2500 Hz modulated at 50 bursts per second myostimulators as high voltage units.[74] In general use, however, high voltage refers to high-voltage galvanic stimulation[75,76] or so-called high-voltage pulsed galvanic stimulation.[77] High-voltage stimulation has

been shown to increase blood flow, particularly at 20 pps and under the negative pole.[75] It was not found to increase strength in healthy subjects in one study.[76] Most subjects reported discomfort during stimulation.[76] In contrast, Wong's study found that high-voltage stimulation produced a stronger muscle contraction and was less uncomfortable than that obtained from a low-frequency unit, despite the use of electrodes of equal size.[77] This indicates that high-voltage stimulation may have some advantage over low frequency in decreasing spasticity by reciprocal inhibition. Subjectively, we have found low-frequency and medium-frequency current to be tolerated better than high-voltage pulsed galvanic stimulation (twin-peaked monophasic waveform). The reason for this discrepancy is unclear. Wong used healthy subjects. Our patients generally have spasticity. Wong stimulated the plantar flexors in half of her subjects (9). We rarely find occasion to stimulate the plantar flexors. The significance of these variations may be that the technique selected should be the one that is tolerated best and is able to achieve the strongest contraction for a particular patient. With stronger contraction of the antagonist, a more significant reduction in spasticity in the agonist may occur.

STIMULATION OF THE SPASTIC AGONIST

Other authors have used stimulation of the spastic agonist. Bohannon used a low-frequency unit set at 50 cycles per second, maximum "on," minimum "off" for more than 55 seconds of every minute for 30 minutes each treatment day. In a single case report, he found that combining stimulation of the spastic quadriceps muscle with static stretching provided increased ability of the client to flex his knee.[78]

Higher-frequency stimulation can produce direct relaxation of the spastic muscle. A tetanic contraction of spastic muscle for 7 to 15 minutes is reported to cause relaxation of spastic muscle that lasts for 2 to 6 hours.[57] Lee et al. found the best results with sinusoidal current.[57] Their study was performed before the 2500 Hz machines were available. The parameters suggested for direct relaxation of the spastic muscle include a higher-frequency current.[54] The proposed theory is that relaxation is caused by fatigue at the motor end plate level, with the body unable to replace acetylcholine fast enough.[54] Jones et al. suggest that there is also decreased excitability of the muscle fiber membrane.[79]

High-voltage stimulation may also have the potential to decrease spasticity when applied directly to the spastic muscle because it is capable of achieving a tetanic contraction.[75] The machine parameters should be set to maximal "on" time and minimal "off" time. The highest frequency available from the machine should be selected. Pain and soreness are greater with this technique[74] than with longer "off" times,[80] limiting the clinical use of sustained tetanic contractions. Jones et al. found that higher frequencies cause more rapid fatigue than lower frequencies.[79] Over time, it appears logical that the spastic muscle would be strengthened, requiring increased current to produce fatigue and leading to in-creased spasticity between treatments. No studies were located that used the currently available high voltage machines on a spastic muscle.

RECIPROCAL STIMULATION

Another approach to spasticity reduction has been proposed by Vodovnik et al.[81] Ten subjects with quadriceps spasticity secondary to CVA received 30 minutes of electrical stimulation to the hamstrings followed by 30 minutes of electrical stimulation to both the quadriceps and the hamstrings. Spasticity was measured with the pendulum test. Five had a decrease in spasticity following hamstring stimulation. Three had reduced spasticity only after their spastic muscle was stimulated.[81] The reason for the variation in response is unclear.

Patterned electrical stimulation provides reciprocal stimulation. An attempt is made to produce a "normal" movement by means of surface electrical stimulation. This technique has been found to decrease spasticity.[82] The following parameters are suggested for beginning reciprocal stimulation:

Pulse rate	30–50 pps
Pulse duration	100–300 μsec
On/off	5 sec/5 sec
Treatment length	20–30 minutes[82]

STIMULATION FOR GENERALIZED RELAXATION

All the electrical stimulation techniques covered thus far are forms of transcutaneous electrical nerve stimulation (TENS). The term TENS is generally limited, however, to surface electrical stimulation for pain relief.

TENS units are manufactured with a variety of pulsatile currents, with adjustable rate and width. High-rate TENS or conventional TENS includes parameters of higher pulse rates (50 to 100 Hz) and narrower widths (40 to 75 μsec).[83] The intensity is adjusted to produce a mild tingling sensation without muscle contraction.[83] It is thought that this mode works on the "gate" theory stimulating large, myelinated Group Ia and

Group Ib fibers.[83] Group III fibers were also found to be stimulated at frequencies of 80 to 100 Hz.[5] Sjölund found that stimulation at 80 Hz resulted in a maximal suppression of a C-fiber-evoked flexion reflex in rats, indicating a temporary decrease in the nociceptive input entering the spinal cord.[5]

In a study by Bajd et al., high-rate TENS was shown to decrease spasticity. TENS was used with a rate of 100 pps on quadriceps spasticity of 6 spinal cord injury patients for 20 minutes. The electrodes were placed over the L3 and L4 dermatomes, one medially below the knee and one laterally above the knee. Significant relaxation was found immediately after stimulation in three of the six patients. Spasticity was assessed by the pendulum test.[84] This was a limited sample size study, but it appears to warrant followup.

High-rate TENS has been used with good success in our facility as a treatment for the occasional neuropathic pain which can result from a peripheral nerve phenol block. We use a rate of 85 pps and a width of 75 μsec. Electrode placement has been over the nerve involved, proximal to the painful area. This is used to provide pain relief until spontaneous resolution has occurred. The pain has generally resolved within 3 weeks. Other causes of painful peripheral nerves have been treated with conventional TENS. Sixteen of 30 patients with post-herpetic neuralgia obtained some relief from high rate TENS.[85] Mannheimer notes that pain from a peripheral nerve lesion should be treated with the electrodes placed on two points along the course of the nerve proximal to the lesion.[86] Pertovaara and Hämäläinen have suggested that high-rate TENS works by acting as a peripheral electrogenic blockade.[87] It seems reasonable, therefore, that the blockade (electrodes) should be positioned between the pain and the spinal cord.

Low-rate TENS or acupuncture-like TENS includes lower pulse rates of 1 to 4 pps and wider pulse widths of 150 to 250 μsec. Low-rate TENS is thought to stimulate small-diameter, slow-conducting afferent fibers such as Group IV fibers.[83]

The H-reflex has been shown to be decreased by low-frequency stimulation.[88] Stimulation of less than or equal to 5 Hz has been shown to diminish the flexor reflex in paraplegic patients.[89] This was attributed to habituation by Dimitrijević et al.[89] Research on skin temperature changes[90,91] and beta-endorphin levels[92,93] are contradictory. Wong and Jette found that both high-rate and low-rate TENS produced an increase in sympathetic activity as evidenced by a decrease in fingertip skin temperature.[90] Leandri et al. state that skin temperature increased significantly locally with high-rate TENS, but not with low rate TENS.[91] Hughes et al. found that the level of plasma beta-endorphins decreased in the control group but increased with treatment with high-rate TENS and low-rate TENS. The difference between the groups was not statistically significant, however.[92] O'Brien et al. state that their control group had higher levels of beta-endorphins than the groups receiving high-rate or low-rate TENS.[93] Thus, the effects of low-rate TENS remain controversial.

Electrodes can be placed on motor points, superficial areas of peripheral nerves, or acupuncture points.[86] In low-rate TENS, the intensity is set to achieve strong, rhythmic muscle contractions.[83] It has been suggested that the benefits obtained are due in part to the rhythmic contractions that act as a muscle pump to aid blood flow.[75]

Walker used subcutaneous nerve stimulation to suppress ankle clonus in pain-free patients with spasticity. She applied a 20 Hz stimulus to points 5 cm proximal to the wrist along the median and radial nerves and to two points along the saphenous nerve at the metatarsal/cuneiform junction and below the medial malleolus. Suppression of ankle clonus occurred 1 hour after stimulation and lasted for 3 hours.[94] Although this experiment used subcutaneous needle placements, there may be application to transcutaneous electrode placement.

A modified TENS device (Neurotransmitter Modulator*) has been reported to inhibit primitive motor reflexes in children with spastic cerebral palsy.[55] The electrodes are applied bilaterally in the temporal area.[86] It is applied for 10 minutes twice a

---

*Pain Suppression Labs, Inc., Elmwood Park, New Jersey.

day.[55,95] The theory proposed by these authors is that the device increases levels of serotonin and GABA.[95] It seems implausible that electrical transmission would penetrate the brain rather than be conducted peripherally along the outside fluid layer. Treatments with alternating current at 100 pps with .002 second rests between each burst, however, have been shown to improve memory.[96] Certainly further research is warranted in this area.

BIOFEEDBACK

Biofeedback has been used primarily with CVA patients,[97,98] but has also been applied to patients with poliomyelitis,[99] cerebral palsy,[100,101] and a variety of other disorders.[97,102] It has been used to obtain relaxation of a spastic muscle,[97,100,101,103,104] to facilitate the antagonist,[97,100,103–105] and for generalized relaxation.[97] Biofeedback devices are available to monitor skin temperature, brain waves, position, pressure, galvanic skin resistance, and myoelectric signals. Both EMG and positional biofeedback may be of benefit in the management of spasticity.

Electromyographic (EMG) biofeedback instruments generally process raw EMG signals obtained by means of surface electrodes to give a rising and falling voltage. This voltage then activates a variety of audiovisual devices.[97] The output devices available include oscilloscopes, meters, noisemakers, and lights. In working with head-injury clients, we have had the most success with a portable device that has a green and red LED (light emitting diode) display and a variable pitch sound. Devices with a meter or oscilloscope seem more difficult to understand.

EMG biofeedback provides immediate feedback to the patient. Immediate, quantitative feedback has been found to be more conducive to the psychomotor learning process than qualitative, delayed feedback.[99] Swaan et al. conclude from the results of their study that EMG biofeedback is more effective than a conventional rehabilitation method in suppressing the undesired activity of one particular muscle. They propose that this greater effectiveness may

be due, in part, to better retention after application of the EMG biofeedback method.[99]

Basmajian states that CVA patients who are able to inhibit spasticity using EMG biofeedback do so by using surviving pathways.[97] Shahani's research has looked at individual motor units in a spastic muscle, and found that some of the motor units behave normally (see Chapter 3). He feels that an attempt can be made with EMG biofeedback to train the normal motor units to perform better, overcome weakness, and compensate for the abnormal units. He also feels that it may be possible to modify abnormal units by increasing their firing rate.[102]

For EMG biofeedback to be successful, the patient must be motivated.[97,106] Music has been used creatively as a way to provide motivation.[101,105] The patient must be able to process and recall simple instructions.[106] The training needs to be done in a quiet area. Severe spasticity has been given as a cause for poor results.[97]

The suggestion has been made that work should begin with relaxation of the spastic muscle.[97,100,104,106] Training should progress next to facilitation of the antagonist. This method is outlined in detail for the upper extremity in the 1979 article by Kelly et al.[107] Training may be accomplished by allowing the patient to develop new movement strategies[106] or achieving increased recruitment of the weak muscle.[102] A dual-channel device allows work on relaxation of the spastic muscle to be combined with facilitation of the antagonist.

Several authors have stressed the importance of combining this training with functional activities to increase the learning response[100,107] and to maintain gains.[100] It is interesting to watch clients attempt to contract the desired muscle. They may use an associated reaction or take advantage of an asymmetric tonic neck reflex.

It has been suggested that training should proceed from proximal to distal.[104] Shahani has stated that EMG biofeedback can speed recovery of function in distal muscles of the lower extremities in some cases. He and his associates have been unable to demonstrate superiority of EMG biofeedback over conventional methods in large postural proximal muscles or in subluxed shoulders.[102] Basmajian, however, suggests that biofeedback training for the subluxed shoulder is superior to the use of a sling.[97] This discrepancy may mean only that Shahani does not consider a sling to be conventional treatment, or it may be a variation in methodology, patient selection, or time post-injury. Basmajian feels that it may not be possible to restore fine manipulative function of the hand if the function has been lost for an extended period after a middle cerebral artery lesion.[97] Leading researchers in the field have concluded that EMG biofeedback applications in appropriate patients can enhance function.[97,102,104]

EMG biofeedback can also be used for generalized relaxation.[97,108] One study by Wolf and Binder-MacLeod included a group of patients who were taught general relaxation with audio feedback proportional to the activity from the target muscles. Another group received standard EMG biofeedback training (relaxation training of the spastic muscle followed by facilitation training of the spastic muscle). There was a reduction in the mean peak EMG in three targeted spastic muscles (hip adductors, quadriceps femoris, and gastrocnemius) in response to slow or quick strength in the latter group. There was no statistical difference, however, when these two groups were compared.[108]

It has been suggested that devices that monitor position may be easier for some clients to comprehend than EMG output.[109] Such devices usually consist of a switch that completes a circuit. The switch can be set up so that a noxious auditory signal is emitted when the desired position is lost, or so that a rewarding effect is delivered when the desired position is maintained. Positioning feedback switches have been used for sitting balance[98] and head control primarily.[110] An electrogoniometer has been used to provide feedback for joint range of motion.[109] As range of motion has been used as a judge of spasticity,[29] the electrogoniometer has potential in the treatment of the patient with spasticity.

Devices are available that combine EMG biofeedback with electrical stimulation. These computerized units can be adjusted to provide electrical stimulation if a particular threshold is achieved or not achieved.

Positional feedback instruments have also been combined with electrical stimulation. The sensory feedback provided to the client by the electrical stimulation is in addition to the auditory and visual feedback provided by the EMG or positional biofeedback. This is an attractive idea, but a study by Winchester et al. found no significant change in spasticity after 4 weeks of treatment with positional biofeedback and electrical stimulation.[109] This lack of effect on spasticity may be related to the quality of the muscle contraction achieved and the muscle stimulated, the degree of spasticity present, or the lack of objective measures. Although not specified, it is assumed that the patients' spasticity was in their quadriceps muscles. The stimulation was to that same muscle, rather than to the antagonist.

VIBRATION

Vibration can either facilitate or inhibit muscle contraction according to the frequency of the stimulus. High-frequency vibration can be applied to the antagonist of the spastic muscle for reciprocal inhibition.[111,112] Low-frequency vibration can be used for its generalized relaxation effect.[111,113,114]

HIGH-FREQUENCY VIBRATION

Frequencies greater than 70 Hz are usually classified as high frequencies.[111] Most researchers use frequencies of 100 to 200 Hz for high-frequency stimulation.[115] Some devices sold for facilitation have frequencies less than 70 Hz. Close attention must be paid to the specifications of these devices to achieve the desired response.[115]

Group Ia fibers have been found to be sensitive to vibration.[112] Stimulation over the muscle or tendon produces a reflex contraction called the tonic vibration reflex (TVR).[116] The muscle contraction is stronger when the stimulation is to the tendon.[115]

When high-frequency vibration is applied to the antagonist of a spastic muscle, reciprocal inhibition of the spastic muscle occurs.[116] For best results, the antagonist of the spastic muscle should be positioned so

FIG. 7-8. Depressed H-reflex (adapted with permission from Roll, J.P., Martin, B., Gauthier, G.M., and Ivaldi, F.M.: Effects of whole-body vibration on spinal reflexes in man. Aviat. Space Environ. Med. *51*:1229). See text for explanation.

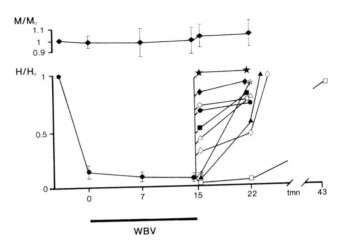

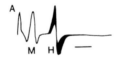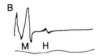

that it is on a stretch.[115] Hagbarth and Eklund hypothesize that elongation of the muscle spindles makes them more susceptible to vibration.[112] The facilitation effect is generally enhanced by active client participation.[115] Vibration has been found superior to quick strength for facilitation.[112]

Short, repeated applications produce larger contractions than sustained application.[115] The tension builds slowly. The greatest response is seen 10 to 60 seconds after the start of the vibration.[115] Subjectively, reciprocal inhibition of the spastic muscle has been noted for 20 to 30 minutes.[112] Temporary adverse reactions such as increased incoordination, rigidity, and tremors have been reported.[112]

LOW-FREQUENCY VIBRATION

A frequency less than 70 Hz is considered low frequency.[113] It is used for its generalized relaxation effect.[113,114] Much of the information available on low-frequency vibration comes from investigations of the adverse effect of vibration in helicopter flights.[117–119] Low-frequency vibration activates superficial, deep cutaneous, articular, and muscle receptors.[117] The mechanism of action is felt to be a combination of presynaptic and postsynaptic inhibition.[119] When vibration was applied to the whole body, in a study by Roll et al.,[117] the H-reflex was significantly depressed. In Figure 7–8, the decrease in H-reflex amplitude during vibration is seen (B) compared to a control condition (A). The panel above demonstrates the average time course for this decrease in a group of normal subjects. The data are plotted as a ratio of H-reflex amplitude (H) to the baseline amplitude (H_0). This ratio is markedly depressed throughout whole body vibration (WBV) and recovers at varying rates for the individual subjects whose data are plotted at the right. Note the lack of effect on the M response in the top panel. The Achilles tendon reflex was similarly depressed. Vibration of the head and trunk had a weaker effect.[117] Vestibulospinal afferents were not affected by vibration.[118] In a relaxed muscle, the tonic vibration reflex was completely abolished by low frequency vibration of the entire body.[119] Inhibition increased with increasing amplitude of the stimulus.[119]

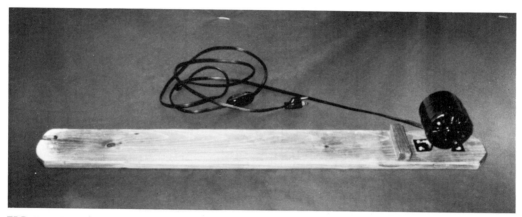

FIG. 7–9. Low-frequency vibration motor attached to board for portability.

The best response has been observed when the vibration was applied to the soles of feet,[114] the feet and back combined,[114] or the whole body.[119] Treatment time was 15 minutes in 2 of the studies reviewed.[114,117] Subjectively, we have found treatment sessions of 30 to 60 minutes to be the most effective. The duration of action seems to be from 30 minutes to several hours.

Commercially available 60 Hz vibrating motors can be purchased* and attached to a mat table or bed frame. To be portable, the motor can be secured to a board (Fig. 7–9). The board can then be slipped between the mat and the table or between the mattress and the bed frame. Massage pillows, massage action back cushions, and massage action reclining chairs are available with vibration frequency less than 70 Hz.

MAINTAINED STRETCH

Maintained stretch is used in positioning and therapeutic exercises. Figure 7–10 illustrates the use of a prone stander to obtain maintained stretch of the quadriceps. Prolonged stretch of a spastic muscle may inhibit that muscle.[115] Adaptation of the intrafusal fibers to the increased extrafusal length is thought to occur.[120] Odeen found an average increase of 255% in voluntary

range of motion following repeated maintained stretch. Passive range of motion increased an average of 48%. The 10 patients had spastic paraparesis with spasticity in the hip adductors.[121] A study by Foley used EMG recordings from the calf to document the effects of maintained stretch on a spastic muscle. Fifteen minutes of sustained stretch reduced the electrical activity considerably and diminished the tonic stretch reflex.[122] Newman et al. used maintained stretch on spinal cord injury patients with spasticity and spasms. Their patients received sustained stretch for 1 hour per day or twice a day or more plus heat to the spastic muscle. Two-thirds of the patients showed some relief subjectively for 30 minutes to 7 hours.[49]

BUCK'S TRACTION

Maintained stretch can be applied in the form of Buck's traction.[123,124] Low-force, long-duration stretching has been shown effective at producing musculotendinous elongation. The most dramatic results are obtained when the tissue is heated and stretched.[52] In addition to maintained stretch, traction of the joints may stimulate the joint mechanoreceptors to provide an inhibitory influence on some of the muscles.[125] We apply Buck's traction to the leg when there is minimal to moderate-severe spasticity in the hip or knee flexors. We generally use a 10-pound weight and wean

*Dayton brand special application vibrator electric motor #3M564, purchased from W.W. Grainger, Inc., 428 University Ave., Norwood, MA 02062

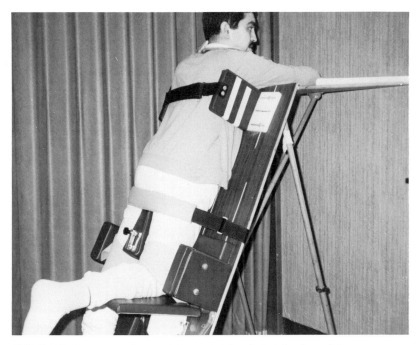

FIG. 7–10. Prone stander used for maintained stretch of quadriceps.

the client gradually until the traction is tolerated for 2 hours or more. A foam Buck's boot is applied to the lower leg. The calf is supported on a pillow, but not the heel. The pulley is adjusted so that the force is along the tibia (Fig. 7–11).

CASTING

Short leg casts have been shown to decrease the sensitivity of the plantar flexors to static and dynamic stretch.[120] This effect may be partly due to maintained stretch. The cast may block cutaneous input, thus decreasing facilitation of the underlying muscles. The application of a cast with the muscle in a lengthened position stretches the connective tissue. These changes may account for the decreased spasticity noted after the cast is removed.[126] In another study, Gossman et al. found atrophy of the casted muscle and increased connective tissue that may affect the spastic muscle's ability to produce tension.[127] Perhaps all these factors enter into the frequently dramatic reduction in spasticity that may be

observed with casting. Because of its effectiveness, casting is covered in depth in Chapter 9.

PRESSURE

Pressure may act as a counterirritant providing sensory input that closes the gate to facilitatory influences.

MANUAL PRESSURE

An immediate decrease has been shown in the amplitude of the H-reflex during tendon pressure, indicating a reduction in alpha motoneuron excitability. This depression lasts 5 to 10 seconds.[128] Umphred and McCormack state that pressure activates the Pacinian corpuscles, which then suppress other sensations in the receptor field.[24] Pressure can be applied to the tendon of a spastic muscle to inhibit the muscle, allowing ease of range of motion. An example is applying pressure to the pectoralis major tendon while performing flex-

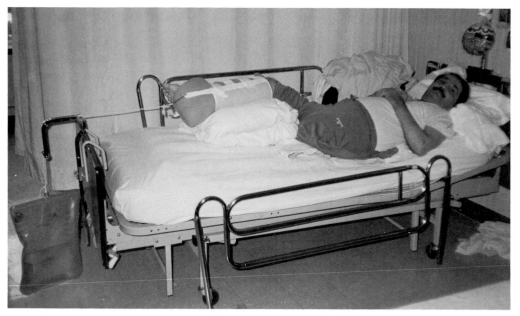

FIG. 7–11. Buck's traction.

ion/abduction of the shoulder. Pressure on either the medial or lateral calcaneus inhibits the triceps surae.[24] Maintained pressure to the abdomen, palm, sole of the foot, or above the upper lip is said to have a generalized relaxation effect,[24,35] but this has not been shown experimentally.

AIR SPLINT

An air splint may inhibit spasticity by providing maintained pressure.[129] It may also work as neutral warmth.[24,129] In addition, it incorporates maintained stretch and blocks other cutaneous input as does a cast. Johnstone recommends using an orally inflated splint, rather than a pressure pump, for spasticity.[130] This is so that the splint will not be inflated beyond the patient's diastolic blood pressure and for the warmth of the air. The air splint should be applied with the extremity stretched into an inhibiting position. With the upper extremity, the thumb should be in abduction.[130] When an air splint is used as a substitute for a cast, we wean the client into it gradually until it can be worn for several hours. An increase in blood pressure has been observed when

bilateral leg gaiters (Fig. 7–12) have been applied. The air splint can also be used as a temporary positioning device for developmental activities or functional training (Fig. 7–13). An air splint can also be used as a cold pack. One chamber of a two-chamber air splint can be filled with a mixture of two parts water and one part rubbing alcohol. The rubbing alcohol acts as an antifreeze to prevent the water from solidifying in the freezer. The other chamber is filled with air. The leg can be covered with a warm damp towel on the surface that will have the cold chamber and a dry towel or nothing on the other surface. The air splint is left on for 20 to 30 minutes, depending on the time it takes for the damp towel to cool. Edema of the foot has been seen occasionally with this treatment.

ELASTIC BANDAGES

Wrapping with elastic bandages may provide maintained pressure and neutral warmth. Twist hypothesizes that such wrapping stimulates the Group IV fibers, facilitating the autonomic nervous system to decrease muscle tone.[131] In a small study

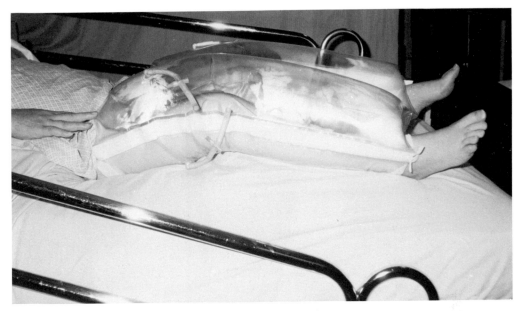

FIG. 7–12. Bilateral lower extremity air splints to decrease hamstring spasticity.

FIG. 7–13. Air splint used during gait training.

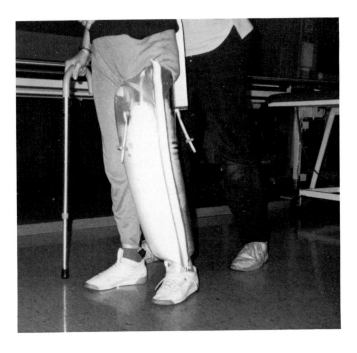

of four patients with spasticity, a significant increase in passive range of motion was found in all patients, as well as a decrease in pain. Patients received wrapping of the upper extremity with elastic bandages for 3 hours, 3 times a week for 2 to 4 weeks.[131]

ORTHOKINETIC CUFF

The orthokinetic cuff begins with an elastic bandage. A portion of the bandage is made inelastic by repeated stitching and becomes the inactive field. This section is

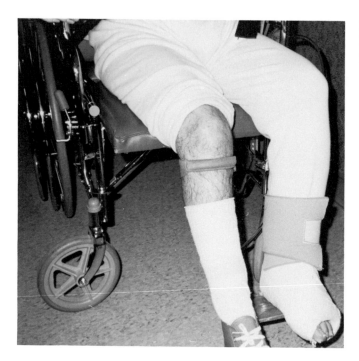

FIG. 7-14. Cho-pat® strap, Cho-Pat Inc., P.O. Box 293, Hainesport, NJ.

placed over the spastic muscle. The other side of the band is left elastic and is called the active field. In theory, the elastic section provides stimulation to the skin over the antagonist as the patient moves. The inelastic section over the spastic muscle provides pressure and decreases other sensory input for inhibition. Bands are placed serially on the extremity. Blasky and Fuchs state that the resultant orthokinetic tube decreases spasticity and, infrequently, shifts the spasticity from agonist to antagonist,[132] but no data have been presented.

CHO-PAT* STRAP

The strap applies pressure to the patellar tendon. We have found this useful when quadriceps spasticity is interfering with function. The strap may allow increased knee flexion during gait or allow the client to propel a wheelchair with the lower extremity (Fig. 7-14).

*Cho-Pat Inc., P.O. Box 293, Hainesport, NJ 08036.

INVERSION

The inverted position has been found to promote generalized relaxation.[24,35,133] Rheault et al. observed decreases in deep tendon reflexes after 8 minutes of inversion.[134] Clinically, inversion as a relaxation technique can be performed in supine, prone, or sidelying over a barrel roll, a ball, or bolster. It can be combined with slow rocking for further relaxation.[133] Facilitation techniques can be added once the client is relaxed, to work on improving control or range of motion. The patient should be monitored closely because a significant drop in blood pressure has been observed occasionally.

SLOW ROCKING

Slow rocking decreases spasticity by generalized relaxation. The movement can be in any direction or plane.[24] It provides low frequency vestibular stimulation which inhibits the reticular formation and has a calming effect.[35] Many different devices can be used such as a hammock, rocking chair, bolster, or ball. Slow rocking can be combined with inversion. Clients with spasticity in a lower extremity may begin to use that leg to rock themselves in a rocking chair once they are relaxed. The weight bearing and motion gain may carry over into an improved transfer.

WEIGHT-BEARING

Neurophysiologic investigations have established that facilitation and inhibition occur reflexively with stimulation of joint mechanoreceptors.[135] Compression of the hip that elicits a reflex from the ligamentum capitis femoris facilitates the gluteals and inhibits the other hip muscles.[135] In general, maintained joint compression may decrease spasticity in phasic muscles, i.e., the flexors in the lower extremities.[136] Static compression of the joint facilitates and inhibits different muscles according to the position of the joint. The use of the quadriped position elicits response from certain hip mechanoreceptors with resultant changes in tone. This effect is combined with maintained pressure on the patellar tendon and maintained stretch of the quadriceps.[133] The tilt table or prone stander can be used to decrease spasticity in lower extremity flexors while providing maintained stretch of the triceps surae. The inhibitory effects seen with tilt table treatments may result from the afferent inflow from joint receptors during weight load and the inhibition secondary to muscle stretch. This inhibitory effect may last up to 4 hours.[137]

JOINT MOBILIZATION

Joint mechanoreceptors show regional sensitivity to mechanical stimulation.[135] Compression, distraction, oscillation, and other joint mobilization techniques may affect spasticity through these mechanoreceptors. Stretching of a spastic muscle may stimulate Group Ia receptors, causing the central nervous system to lower the gain set. It may also stimulate Group Ib receptors, thus initiating inhibition of the spastic

muscle.[138] Cochrane notes that distraction and an inferior glide of the humerus with the arm at the side may decrease spasticity around the shoulder.[139] We have found that the technique recommended by Paris to stretch the posterior capsule of the hip[138] is often effective in temporarily decreasing extensor spasticity of the leg as well.

MASSAGE

A sedative massage performed by monotonous, repetitive stroking may cause generalized relaxation.[140,141] One study found that back range of motion in normal patients increased after massage, indicating relaxation.[142] Massage (efflurage and petrissage) has not been shown to increase levels of endogenous opiates in healthy subjects.[143] Barr and Taslitz observed an increase in most measures of sympathetic activity following a 20-minute back massage.[144] The mechanism of action is assumed to be counterirritation, but reflex effects are also suggested.[140,141] No studies were located that used general massage on spastic patients. General massage is time-consuming; the client is unable to work on functional tasks while receiving it. A less time-consuming type of massage has also been suggested. Slow stroking down the paravertebral musculature from C7 to the iliac crest for 3 to 5 minutes has been said to cause generalized relaxation.[24] Deep friction massage can be used for its reflex effects. In some clients with spasticity of the gastocnemius, deep friction massage in the arch of the foot elicits ankle dorsiflexion and may provide reciprocal inhibition of the gastrocnemius.

LASER

Low-power laser treatments have been reported to decrease pain,[145,146] increase wound healing,[147] increase skin resistance,[148] and be associated with the release of a product of serotonin metabolism.[146] A study by Snyder-Mackler et al. showed a decrease in sensory nerve conduction latency with the helium neon (HeNe) laser,[149] whereas a study by Greathouse et al. showed no change in sensory nerve conduction latency with the gallium aluminum arsenide (GaAl) laser.[150] Nissan et al. found a significant increase in action potential in the sciatic nerve with transcutaneous irradiation of rats.[151] No temperature changes in the skin have been found related to the use of low power laser.[145,150] This indicates that any effects are nonthermal in nature.[145]

HeNe and GaAl lasers are the most commonly used low-power lasers in the United States. It has been claimed that the HeNe laser is more effective in relieving pain and healing wounds than the GaAl laser.[145] The HeNe laser is a visible, monochromatic, red laser with a wavelength of 632.8 nm.[148] Therapeutic dosages are said to start at 15 to 20 seconds with a maximum intensity of 0.95 mW.[148] The GaAl laser is an infrared laser with a wavelength of 830 nm.[145]

Walker has suggested that the effects of lasers are similar to those of TENS.[146] In her study, she stimulated the same areas of superficial nerves that she had treated in her research on TENS.[94] She found laser treatment effective in decreasing pain. Pain relief was assessed by an independent interviewer. In addition, urine samples were obtained to measure excretion of a byproduct of serotonin metabolism.[146]

Although prolonged, direct exposure of the eyes is contraindicated, the low-power laser appears to be a safe modality.[145] Walker's study showed a 10% incidence of a temporary increase in pain lasting 3 to 24 hours.[146] No side effects occurred in the other studies reviewed.[145,148]

A review of the literature has revealed no claims that the low-power laser decreases spasticity. Because there have been reports of pain relief[145,146] and a decrease in nerve conduction velocity,[149] an effect on spasticity appears possible. Research in this area seems warranted.

ACUPUNCTURE

A literature search did not locate any studies showing that acupuncture decreases spasticity. Acupuncture has been shown, however, to decrease the excitability of motoneurons.[152] This implies that it may be applicable to spasticity treatment.

In a study by Homma et al., the vibration-induced finger flexion reflex was depressed 20 to 100% by acupuncture. Depression became maximal 5 to 10 minutes after the start of the stimulation. Recovery took at least 15 minutes. A similar depression of the tonic vibration reflex was found. The slow onset and long continuation suggest that inhibition is accomplished by neurochemical substances such as endogenous opiates.[152]

In addition to the suggested role of endogenous opioid substances in acupuncture, a study by Ernst and Lee found a short-term segmentally related sympathetic excitatory effect.[153] Melzack and Wall hypothesize that acupuncture, like any other intense stimulation, activates small fibers to give increased input to the reticular formation. This input closes the gate to inputs from selected body areas.[154] Winstein speculated that acupuncture could be used to inhibit abnormal motor patterns.[155]

SUMMARY

The modalities discussed in this chapter are not equally effective or objectively documented. They have been described to provide a broad selection. The technique used should be adjusted according to the response of the patient and functional goals should be kept in mind throughout the treatment. In choosing a modality, one should consider the severity and extent of the spasticity. Severe spasticity with widespread involvement eliminates many options. Those remaining include Hubbard tank, whole-body low-frequency vibration, inversion, and slow rocking.

The modality chosen should achieve the greatest number of goals simultaneously. In an unmotivated patient with lower extremity extensor spasticity, electrical stimulation to the anterior tibialis muscles bilaterally may be appropriate. Using medium-frequency electrical stimulation may strengthen the dorsiflexors while inhibiting the plantarflexors. It may also increase ankle range of motion. A flexion reflex in the entire leg may also be elicited. Seeing the leg move can often motivate the client. Thus one may be able to increase strength and range of motion, decrease spasticity, and motivate the client all at once.

The equipment available and the therapy environment are also important. For example, a noisy gym is not an appropriate setting for biofeedback. Medical stability is also relevant. In an ICU setting with an unstable patient, inversion is generally ruled out and casting may be done only as a last resort because of the need to have IV sites available and the possibility of sudden edema formation. In this case, Buck's traction or an air splint may be chosen first because they can be removed quickly.

Few modalities have been subjected to rigorous scientific research. Those that have generally have been studied in limited populations with little regard for their impact on functional goals. Some, such as heat and cold, have been used for centuries. These continue to prompt debates about efficacy. Others, like laser and medium-frequency electrical stimulation, are just beginning to be used to treat spasticity.

There is a theoretic basis for modality efficacy by means of reciprocal inhibition, direct inhibition or fatigue, and general relaxation. The link between these theoretical mechanisms and empirical observations of decreased spasticity, however, are conjectural for many modalities that lack neurophysiologic research bases.

Research is needed in all modalities. Spasticity is variable and difficult to quantify in the clinic. This has made it hard to judge the effectiveness of the various modalities and techniques. Those interested in adding to the research data base should document closely where a modality is applied, the time of application, and the parameters. Objective studies with quantifiable, clinically relevant endpoints, double-blind where possible, are of critical importance to the field. No modality is a panacea for spasticity, but many can be useful additions to a therapeutic exercise program.

REFERENCES

1. Dorland's Illustrated Medical Dictionary. 24th Ed. Philadelphia, W.B. Saunders Company, 1965.
2. Erickson, D.L., et al.: Control of spasticity by implantable continuous flow morphine pump. Neurosurgery 16:215–217, 1985.
3. Melzack, R.: Neurophysiological foundations of pain. In The Psychology of Pain. Ed. R.A. Sternback. 2nd Ed. New York, Raven Press, 1986.
4. Melzack, R., and Wall, P.D.: Pain mechanisms: A new theory. Science 150:971–978, 1965.
5. Sjölund, B.H.: Peripheral nerve stimulation suppression of C-fiber-evoked flexion reflex in rats. J. Neurosurg. 63: 612–616, 1985.
6. Ngai, S.H.: Action of general anesthetics in producing muscle relaxation: Interaction of anesthetics with relaxants. In Muscle Relaxants. Edited by R.L. Katz. The Netherlands, North Holland Publishing Co., 1975.
7. Kunesch E., et al.: Peripheral neural correlates of cutaneous anesthesia induced by skin cooling in man. Acta Physiol. Scand. 129:247–257, 1987.
8. Knutsson, E. and Mattsson, E.: Effects of local cooling on monosynaptic reflexes in man. Scand. J. Rehabil. Med. 1:126–132, 1969.
9. Bell, K.R., and Lehmann, J.F.: Effect of cooling on H- and T- reflexes in normal subjects. Arch. Phys. Med. Rehabil. 68:490–493, 1987.
10. Miglietta, O.E.: Evaluation of cold in spasticity. Am. J. Phys. Med. 41:148–151, 1962.
11. Hartviksen, K.: Ice therapy in spasticity. Acta Neurol. Scand. 38:79–84, 1962.
12. Eldred, E., Lindsley, D.F., and Buchwald, J.S.: The effect of cooling on mammalian muscle spindles. Exp. Neurol. 2:144–157, 1960.
13. Douglas, W.W., and Malcolm, J.L.: The effect of localized cooling on conduction in cat nerves. J. Physiol. 130:53–71, 1955.
14. Lee, J.M., Warren, M.P., and Mason, S.M.: Effects of ice on nerve conduction velocity. Physiotherapy 64:2–6, 1978.
15. DonTigny, R.L., and Sheldon, K.W.: Simultaneous use of heat and cold in treatment of muscle spasm. Arch. Phys. Med. Rehabil. 43:235–237, 1962.
16. Knutsson, E.: Topical cryotherapy in spas-

ticity. Scand. J. Rehabil. Med. 2:159–163, 1970.

17. Kelly, M.: Effectiveness of a cryotherapy technique on spasticity. Phys. Ther. 49:349–353, 1969.

18. Lehmann, J., and deLateur, B.: Cryotherapy. In Therapeutic Heat and Cold. Ed. J.F. Lehmann. 3rd Ed. Baltimore, Williams and Wilkins Company, 1982.

19. Newton, M.J., and Lehmkuhl, D.: Muscle spindle response to body heating and localized muscle cooling: Implications for relief of spasticity. J. Am. Phys. Ther. Assoc. 45:91–105, 1965.

20. Lorenze, E.J., Carantonis, G., and DeRosa, A.J.: Effect on coronary circulation of cold packs to hemiplegic shoulders. Arch. Phys. Med. Rehabil. 41:394–399, 1960.

21. Bassett, S.W., and Lake, B.M.: Use of cold applications in the management of spasticity. Phys. Ther. Rev. 38:333–334, 1958.

22. Boynton, B.L., Garramone, P.M., and Buca, J.T.: Observations on the effects of cool baths for patients with multiple sclerosis. Phys. Ther. Rev. 39:297–299, 1959.

23. Clendenin, M.A., and Szumski, A.J.: Influence of cutaneous ice application on single motor units in humans. Phys. Ther. 51:166–175, 1971.

24. Umphred, D.A., and McCormack, G.L.: Classification of common facilitory and inhibitory treatment techniques. In Neurological Rehabilitation. Ed. D.A. Umphred. St. Louis, C.V. Mosby Company, 1985.

25. Duncan, W.R.: Tonic reflexes of the foot. J. Bone Joint Surg. 42-A:859–868, 1960.

26. Travell, J.: Ethyl chloride spray for painful muscle spasm. Arch. Phys. Med. 33:291–298, 1952.

27. Halkovich, L., Personius, W., Clamann, H., and Newton, R.: Effect of fluorimethane spray on passive hip flexion. Phys. Ther. 61:185–189, 1981.

28. Vallentyne, S.W., and Vallentyne, J.R.: The case of the missing ozone: Are physiatrists to blame? Arch. Phys. Med. Rehabil. 69:992–993, 1988.

29. Sabbahi, M.A., DeLuca, C.J., and Powers, W.R.: Topical Anesthesia: A possible treatment method for spasticity. Arch. Phys. Med. Rehabil. 62:310–314, 1981.

30. Inacio, C., Giebler, K., Whyte, J., and Wroblewski, B.: The effects of topical anesthesia on active movement in the brain injured patient with spasticity. Poster presentation at the Braintree Hospital's 6th Annual Traumatic Head Injury Conference, November 24, 1985.

31. Lehmann, J.F., and deLateur, B.J.: Diathermy and superficial heat and cold therapy. In Krusen's Handbook of Physical Medicine and Rehabilitation. Ed. F.J. Kottke, G.K. Stillwell, and J.F. Lehmann. 3rd Ed. Philadelphia, W.B. Saunders Company, 1982.

32. Fischer, E., and Solomon, S.: Physiological responses to heat and cold. In Therapeutic Heat and Cold. Ed. S. Licht. 2nd Ed. Baltimore, Waverly Press, 1965.

33. Farber, S.D.: Neurorehabilitation: A Multisensory Approach. Philadelphia, W.B. Saunders Company, 1982.

34. Wells, H.S.: Temperature equilization for the relief of pain. Arch. Phys. Med. 28:135–139, 1947.

35. Stockmeyer, S.A.: An interpretation of the approach of Rood to the treatment of neuromuscular dysfunction. Am. J. Phys. Med. 46:900–956, 1967.

36. Farber, S.D.: Sensorimotor Evaluation and Treatment Procedures for Allied Health Personnel. 2nd Ed. Indianapolis, Indiana University Foundation, 1974.

37. Lehmann, J.F., et al.: Temperature distributions in the human thigh produced by infrared, hot pack and microwave applications. Arch. Phys. Med. Rehabil. 47:291–299, 1966.

38. Michlovitz, S.L.: Biophysical principles of heating and superficial heat agents. In Thermal Agents in Rehabilitation. Ed. S.L. Michlovitz. Philadelphia, F.A. Davis Company, 1986.

39. Kanui, T.I.: Thermal inhibition of nociceptor-driven spinal cord neurons in the cat: A possible neuronal basis for thermal analgesia. Brain Res. 402:160–163, 1987.

40. Abramson, D.I., Tuck, S., Chu, L.S.W., and Agustin, C.: Effect of paraffin bath and hot fomentations on local tissue temperatures. Arch. Phys. Med. Rehabil. 45:87–94, 1964.

41. Borrell, R.M., et al.: Comparison of in vivo temperatures produced by hydrotherapy, paraffin wax treatment, and fluidotherapy. Phys. Ther. 60:1273–1276, 1980.

42. Valenza, J., Rossi, C., Parker, R., and Henley, E.J.: A clinical study of a new heat modality. J. Am. Podiatr. Assoc. 69:440–442, 1979.

43. Knapp, M.D.: Massage. In Krusen's Handbook of Physical Medicine and Rehabilitation. Ed. F.J. Kottke, G.K. Stillwell, and J.F. Lehmann. 3rd Ed. Philadelphia, W.B. Saunders, 1982.

44. Alcorn, R., Bowser, B., Henley, E.J., and Holloway, V.: Fluidotherapy and exercise in the management of sickle cell anemia. Phys. Ther. 64:1520–1522, 1984.

45. Von Werssowitz, O.F.: Heat in neuromuscular disorders. *In* Therapeutic Heat and Cold. Ed. S. Licht. 2nd Ed. Baltimore, Waverly Press, 1965.

46. Walsh, M.: Hydrotherapy: The use of water as a therapeutic agent. *In* Thermal Agents in Rehabilitation. Ed. S.L. Michlovitz. Philadelphia, F.A. Davis Company, 1986.

47. Lehmann, J.F., and deLateur, B.J.: Therapeutic heat. *In* Therapeutic Heat and Cold. Ed. J.F. Lehmann. 3rd Ed. Baltimore, Williams and Wilkins, 1982.

48. Von Euler, C., and Soderberg, M.K.: The influence of hypothalamic thermoceptive structures on the electroencephalogram and gamma motor activity. Electroencephalogram. Clin. Neurophysiol. *9*:391–408, 1957.

49. Newman, L.B., Arieff, A.J., and Wasserman, R.R.: Present status in the management of spasticity and spasm: Preliminary report. Arch. Phys. Med. Rehabil. *35*:427–436, 1954.

50. Lehmann, J.F.: Ultrasound therapy. *In* Therapeutic Heat and Cold. Ed. S. Licht. 2nd Ed. Baltimore, Waverly Press, 1965.

51. Lehmann, J.F., et al.: Temperatures in human thighs after hot pack treatment followed by ultrasound. Arch. Phys. Med. Rehabil. *59*:472–475, 1978.

52. Warren, C.G., Lehmann, J.F., and Koblanski, J.N.: Heat and stretch procedures: An evaluation using rat tail tendon. Arch. Phys. Med. Rehabil. *57*:122–125, 1976.

53. Wessling, K.C., DeVane, D.A., and Hylton, C.R.: Effects of static stretch versus static stretch and ultrasound combined on triceps surae muscle extensibility in healthy women. Phys. Ther. *67*:674–679, 1987.

54. Benton, L.S., Baker, L.L., Bowman, B.R., and Waters, R.L.: Functional Electrical Stimulation. A Practical Clinical Guide. 2nd Ed. Downey, CA., Professional Staff Association of the Ranchos Los Amigos Hospital, 1981.

55. Malden, J.W., and Charash, L.I.: Transcranial stimulation for the inhibition of primitive reflexes in children with cerebral palsy. Neurology Report *9(2)*:33–38, spring 1985.

56. Alfieri, V.: Electrical treatment of spasticity. Scand. J. Rehabil. Med. *14*:177–182, 1982.

57. Lee, W.J., McGovern, J.P., and Duvall, E.N.: Continuous tetanizing (low voltage) currents for relief of spasm. Arch. Phys. Med. *31*:766–771, 1950.

58. Castelain, P.-Y. and Chabeau, G.: Contact dermatitis after transcutantous electric analgesia. Contact Dermatitis *15*:32–35, 1986.

59. Balmaseda, M.T., Fatehi, M.T., Koozekanani, S.H., and Sheppard, J.S.: Burns in functional electric stimulation: Two case reports. Arch. Phys. Med. Rehabil. *68*:452–453, 1987.

60. Vodovnik, L., et al.: Improvement of some abnormal motor functions by electrical stimulation. Med. Prog. Technol. *9*:141–147, 1982.

61. Baker, L.L., Yeh, C., Wilson, D., and Waters, R.L.: Electrical stimulation of wrist and fingers for hemiplegic patients. Phys. Ther. *59*:1495–1499, 1979.

62. Baker, L.L., Parker, K., and Sanderson, D.: Neuromuscular electrical stimulation for the head injured patient. Phys. Ther. *63*:1967–1974, 1983.

63. Baker, L.L., and Parker, K.: Neuromuscular electrical stimulation of the muscles surrounding the shoulder. Phys. Ther. *66*:1930–1937, 1986.

64. Fulbright, J.S.: Electrical stimulation to reduce chronic toe-flexor hypertonicity. Phys. Ther. *64*:523–525, 1984.

65. Arvidsson, I., Arvidsson, H., Eriksson, E., and Jansson, E.: Prevention of quadriceps wasting after immobilization: An evaluation of the effect of electrical stimulation. Orthopedics *9*:1519–1527, 1986.

66. Carnstam, B., Larsson, L., and Prevec, T.S.: Improvement of gait following functional electrical stimulation. Scand. J. Rehabil. Med. *9*:7–13, 1977.

67. Stefanovska, A., and Vodovnik, L.: Change in muscle force following electrical stimulation. Scand. J. Rehabil. Med. *17*:141–146, 1985.

68. Delitto, A., and Rose, S.J.: Comparative comfort of three waveforms used in electrically eliciting quadriceps femoris muscle contractions. Phys. Ther. *66*:1704–1707, 1986.

69. Owens, J., and Malone, T.: Treatment parameters of high frequency electrical stimulation as established on the Electro-Stim 180. J. Orthop. Sports Phys. Ther. *4*:162–168, 1983.

70. Greathouse, D.G., Nitz, A.J., Matulionis, D.H., and Currier, D.P.: Effects of short-term electrical stimulation on the ultrastructure of rat skeletal muscles. Phys. Ther. *66*:946–953, 1986.

71. Currier, D.P., Petrilli, C.R., and Threlkeld, A.J.: Effect of graded electrical stimulation on blood flow to healthy muscle. *Phys. Ther.* *66*:937–943, 1986.

72. Nitz, A.J., and Dobner, J.J.: High intensity

electrical stimulation effect on thigh musculature during immobilization for knee sprain. Phys. Ther. 67:219–222, 1987.

73. Alon, G.: High voltage stimulation: Effects of electrode size on basic excitatory responses. Phys. Ther. 65:890–895, 1985.

74. Balogun, J.A.: Pain complaint and muscle soreness associated with high voltage electrical stimulation: Effect of ramp time. Percept. Mot. Skill, 62:799–810, 1986.

75. Mohr, T., Akers, T.K., and Wessman, H.C.: Effect of high voltage stimulation on blood flow in the rat hind limb. Phys. Ther. 67:526–533, 1987.

76. Mohr, T., Carlson, B., Sulentic, C., and Landry, R.: Comparison of isometric exercise and high volt galvanic stimulation of quadriceps femoris muscle strength. Phys. Ther. 65:606–609, 1985.

77. Wong, R.A.: High voltage versus low voltage electrical stimulation. Phys. Ther. 66:1209–1214, 1986.

78. Bohannon, R.W.: Results of prolonged stretch and electrical stimulation on knee function in a hemiparetic stroke patient. Neurology Report 11(2):19–21, spring 1987.

79. Jones, D.A., Bigland-Ritchie, B., and Edwards, R.H.T.: Excitation frequency and muscle fatigue: Mechanical responses during voluntary and stimulated contractions. Exp. Neurol. 64:401–413, 1979.

80. Currier, D.P., and Mann, R.: Pain complaint: Comparison of electrical stimulation with conventional isometric exercise. J. Orthoped. Sports Phys. Ther. 5:318–323, 1984.

81. Vodovnik, L., Bowman, B.R., and Winchester, P.: Effect of electrical stimulation on spasticity in hemiparetic patients. Int. Rehabil. Med. 6:153–156, 1984.

82. Palermo, F.X.: Patterned electric stimulation vs. upper extremity spasticity in hemiplegia. Scientific paper presented at the AAPM&R/ACRM Conference, October 19, 1987, Orlando, Florida.

83. Mannheimer, J.S., and Lampe, G.N.: Clinical Transcutaneous Electrical Stimulation. Philadelphia, F.A. Davis Company, 1984.

84. Bajd, T., Gregoric, M., Vodovnik, L., and Benko, H.: Electrical stimulation in treating spasticity resulting from spinal cord injury. Arch. Phys. Med. Rehabil. 66:515–517, 1985.

85. Nathan, P.W., and Wall, P.D.: Treatment of post-herpetic neuralgia by prolonged electric stimulation. Br. Med. J. 3:645–647, 1974.

86. Mannheimer, J.S.: Electrode placements for transcutaneous electrical nerve stimulation. Phys. Ther. 58:1455–1462, 1978.

87. Pertovaara, A., and Hämäläinen, H.: Vibrotactile threshold elevation produced by high-frequency transcutaneous electrical stimulation. Arch. Phys. Med. Rehabil. 63:597–600, 1982.

88. Cook, W.A.: Effects of low frequency stimulation on the monosynaptic reflex (H reflex) in man. Neurology 18:47–51, 1968.

89. Dimitrijević, M.R., et al.: Habituation: Effects of regular and stochastic stimulation. J. Neurol. Neurosurg. Psychiatry 35:234–242, 1972.

90. Wong, R.A., and Jette, D.U.: Changes in sympathetic tone associated with different forms of transcutaneous electrical nerve stimulation in healthy subjects. Phys. Ther. 64:478–482, 1984.

91. Leandri, M.: Brunetti, O., and Parodi, C.I.: Telethermographic findings after transcutaneous electrical nerve stimulation. Phys. Ther. 66:210–213, 1986.

92. Hughes, G.S., Lichstein, P.R., Whitlock, D., and Harker, C.: Response of plasma beta-endorphins to transcutaneous electrical nerve stimulation in healthy subjects. Phys. Ther. 64:1062–1066, 1984.

93. O'Brien, W.J., Rutan, F.M., Sanborn, C., and Omer, G.E.: Effect of transcutaneous electrical nerve stimulation on human blood β-endorphin levels. Phys. Ther. 64:1367–1374, 1984.

94. Walker, J.B.: Modulation of spasticity: Prolonged suppression of a spinal reflex by electrical stimulation. Science 216:203–204, 1982.

95. Okoye, R., and Malden, J.W.: Use of neurotransmitter modulation to facilitate sensory integration. Neurology Report 10(4):67–72, fall 1986.

96. Childs, A., and Crismon, M.L.: The use of cranial electrotherapy stimulation in post-traumatic amnesia: A report of two cases. Brain Inj. 2:243–247, 1988.

97. Basmajian, J.V.: Biofeedback in rehabilitation: A review of principles and practices. Arch. Phys. Med. Rehabil. 62:469–475, 1981.

98. Bjork, L., and Wetzel, A.: A positional biofeedback device for sitting balance. Phys. Ther. 63:1460–1461, 1983.

99. Swaan, D., van Wieringen, P.C.W., and Fokkema, S.D.: Auditory electromyographic feedback therapy to inhibit undesired motor activity. Arch. Phys. Med. Rehabil. 55:251–254, 1974.

100. Skrotzky, K., Gallenstein, J.S., and Osternig, L.R.: Effects of electromyographic

feedback training on motor control in spastic cerebral palsy. Phys. Ther. *58*:547–552, 1978.

101. Neilson, P.D., and McCaughey, J.: Self-regulation of spasm and spasticity in cerebral palsy. J. Neurol. Neurosurg. Psychiatry *45*:320–330, 1982.

102. Shahani, B.T.: Control of voluntary activity in man and physiological principles of biofeedback. *In* Electromyography in CNS Disorders: Central EMG. Boston, Butterworth Publishers, 1984.

103. Binder, S.A., Moll, C.B., and Wolf, S.L.: Evaluation of electromyographic biofeedback as an adjunct to therapeutic exercise in treating the lower extremities of hemiplegic patients. Phys. Ther. *61*:886–893, 1981.

104. Wolf, S.L., and Binder-MacLeod, S.A.: Electromyographic biofeedback applications to the hemiplegic patient. Changes in upper extremity neuromuscular and functional status. Phys. Ther. *63*:1393–1402, 1983.

105. Asato, H., Twiggs, D.G., and Ellison, S.: EMG biofeedback training for a mentally retarded individual with cerebral palsy. Phys. Ther. *61*:1447–1451, 1981.

106. Wolf, S.L.: Electromyographic biofeedback applications to stroke patients. Phys. Ther. *63*:1448–1459, 1983.

107. Kelly, J.L., Baker, M.P., and Wolf, S.L.: Procedures for EMG biofeedback training in involved upper extremities of hemiplegic patients. Phys. Ther. *59*:1500–1507, 1979.

108. Wolf, S.L., and Binder-MacLeod, S.A.: Electromyographic biofeedback applications to the hemiplegic patient. Changes in lower extremity neuromuscular and functional status. Phys. Ther. *63*:1404–1413, 1983.

109. Winchester, P., Montgomery, J., Bowman, B., and Hislop, H.: Effects of feedback stimulation training and cyclical electrical stimulation on knee extension in hemiparetic patients. Phys. Ther. *63*:1096–1103, 1983.

110. Hallum, A.: Subject-induced reinforcement of head lifting in the prone position. Phys. Ther. *64*:1390–1392, 1984.

111. Eklund, G.: Some physical properties of muscle vibrators used to elicit tonic proprioceptive reflexes in man. Acta Soc. Med. Upsal. *76*:271–280, 1971.

112. Hagbarth, K., and Eklund, G.: The effects of muscle vibration in spasticity, rigidity, and cerebellar disorders. J. Neurol. Neurosurg. Psychiatry *31*:207–213, 1968.

113. Johnson, M.D., Hensel, C.L., and Matheson, D.W.: Vibration effects on three measures of relaxation. Percept. Mot. Skill *54*:1071–1076, 1982.

114. Matheson, D.W., et al.: Relaxation measured by EMG as a function of vibrotactile stimulation. Biofeedback Self Regul. *1*:285–292, 1976.

115. Griffin, J.W.: Use of proprioceptive stimuli in therapeutic exercise. Phys. Ther. *54*:1072–1079, 1974.

116. Bishop, B.: Spasticity: Its physiology and management. Part IV. Current and projected treatment procedures for spasticity. Phys. Ther. *57*:396–401, 1977.

117. Roll, J.P., Martin, B., Gauthier, G.M., and Ivaldi, F.M.: Effects of whole-body vibration on spinal reflexes in man. Aviat. Space Environ. Med. *51*:1227–1233, 1980.

118. Gauthier, G.M., Roll, J.P., Martin, B., and Harlay, F.: Effects of whole-body vibrations on sensory motor system performance in man. Aviat. Space Environ. Med., *52*:473–479, 1981.

119. Martin, B.J., Roll, J.P., and Gauthier, G.M.: Inhibitory effects of combined agonist and antagonist muscle vibration on H-reflex in man. Aviat. Space Environ. Med. *57*:681–687, 1986.

120. Otis, J.C., Root, L., and Kroll, M.A.: Measurement of plantar flexor spasticity during treatment with tone-reducing casts. J. Pediatr. Orthop. *5*:682–686, 1985.

121. Odéen, I.: Reduction of muscular hypertonus by long-term muscle stretch. Scand. J. Rehabil. Med. *13*:93–99, 1981.

122. Foley, J.: The stiffness of spastic muscle. J. Neurol. Neurosurg. Psychiatry *24*:125–131, 1961.

123. Becker, A.H.: Traction for knee-flexion contractures. Phys. Ther. *59*:1114, 1979.

124. Light, K.E., Nuzik, S., Personius, W., and Barstrom, A.: Low-load prolonged stretch vs. high-load brief stretch in treating knee contractures. Phys. Ther. *64*:330–333, 1984.

125. Newton, R.A.: Joint receptor contributions to reflexive and kinesthetic responses. Phys. Ther. *62*:22–29, 1982.

126. Gossman, M.R., Sahrman, S.A., and Rose, S.J.: Review of length-associated changes in muscle. Phys. Ther. *62*:1799–1808, 1982.

127. Gossman, M.R., Rose, S.J., Sahrmann, S.A., and Katholi, C.R.: Length and circumference measurements in one-joint and multijoint muscles in rabbits after immobilization. Phys. Ther. *66*:516–520, 1986.

128. Kukulka, C.G., Fellows, W.A., Oehlertz,

J.E., and Vanderwilt, S.G.: Effect of tendon pressure on alpha motoneuron excitability. Phys. Ther. *65*:595–600, 1985.

129. Goad, R.A., and Ricks, N.R.: Pressure modalities in the treatment of a hypertonic limb. Neurology Report *8(3)*:63–64, summer 1984.

130. Johnstone, M.: Restoration of Motor Function in the Stroke Patient. 2nd Ed. New York, Churchill Livingstone, 1983.

131. Twist, D.J.: Effects of a wrapping technique on passive range of motion in a spastic upper extremity. Phys. Ther. *65*:299–304, 1985.

132. Blashy, M.R.M., and Fuchs, R.L.: Orthokinetics: A new receptor facilitation method. Am. J. Occup. Ther. *13*:226–234, 1959.

133. Smith, S.S.: Traumatic head injuries. *In* Neurological Rehabilitation. Ed. D.A. Umphred. St. Louis, C.V. Mosby Company, 1985.

134. Rheault, W., et al.: Effects of an inverted position on blood pressure, pulse rate, and deep tendon reflexes of healthy young adults. Phys. Ther. *65*:1358–1362, 1985.

135. Dee, R.: Structure and function of hip joint innervation. Ann. R. Coll. Surg. Engl. *45*:357–374, 1969.

136. Wyke, B.: The neurology of joints. Ann. R. Coll. Surg. Engl. *41*:25–50, 1967.

137. Odéen, I., and Knutsson, E.: Evaluation of the effects of muscle stretch and weight load in patients with spastic paraplegia. Scand. J. Rehabil. Med. *13*:117–121, 1981.

138. Paris, S.V.: Extremity Dysfunction and Mobilization. Pre-publication Edition. Atlanta, Institute Press, 1980.

139. Cochrane, C.G.: Joint mobilization principles. Considerations for use in the child with central nervous system dysfunction. Phys. Ther. *67*:1105–1109, 1987.

140. Knapp, M.E.: Massage. *In* Krusen's Handbook of Physical Medicine and Rehabilitation. Ed. F.J. Kottke, G.K. Stillwell, and J.F. Lehmann. Philadelphia, W.B. Saunders Company, 1982.

141. Beard, G., and Wood, E.C.: Massage: Principles and Techniques. Philadelphia, W.B. Saunders Company, 1964.

142. Nordschow, M., and Bierman, W.: The influence of manual massage on muscle relaxation: Effect on trunk flexion. Phys. Ther. *42*:653–657, 1962.

143. Day, J.A., Mason, R.R., and Chesrown, S.E.: Effect of massage on serum level of β-endorphin and β-lipotropin in healthy adults. Phys. Ther. *67*:926–930, 1987.

144. Barr, J.S., and Taslitz, N.: The influence of back massage on autonomic functions. Phys. Ther. *50*:1679–1691, 1970.

145. Basford, J.R.: Low-energy laser treatment of pain and wounds: Hype, hope, or hokum? Mayo Clin. Proc. *61*:671–675, 1986.

146. Walker, J.: Relief from chronic pain by low power laser irradiation. Neurosci Lett. *43*:339–344, 1983.

147. Cummings, J.P.: The effect of low energy (HeNe) laser irradiation on healing dermal wounds in an animal model. Phys. Ther. *65*:737 (abstract), 1985.

148. Snyder-Mackler, L., Bork, C., Bourbon, B., and Trumbore, D.: Effect of helium-neon laser on musculoskeletal trigger points. Phys. Ther. *66*:1087–1090, 1986.

149. Snyder-Mackler, L., Bork, C., and Fernandez, J.: The effect of helium-neon laser on latency of sensory nerve. Phys. Ther. *65*:737 (abstract), 1985.

150. Greathouse, D.G., Currier, D.P., and Gilmore, R.L.: Effects of clinical infrared laser on superficial radial nerve conduction. Phys. Ther. *65*:1184–1187, 1985.

151. Nissan, M., Rochkind, S., Razon, N., and Bartal, A.: HeNe laser irradiation delivered transcutaneously: Its effect on the sciatic nerve of rats. Lasers Surg. Med. *6*:435–438, 1986.

152. Homma, S., Nakajima, Y., and Toma, S.: Inhibitory effect of acupuncture on the vibration-induced finger flexion reflex in man. Electroencephalogr. Clin. Neurophysiol. *61*:150–156, 1985.

153. Ernst, M., and Lee, M.H.M.: Sympathetic effects of manual and electrical acupuncture of the tsusanli knee point: Comparison with the hoku hand point sympathetic effects. Exp. Neurol. *94*:1–10, 1986.

154. Melzack, R., and Wall, P.D.: Acupuncture and transcutaneous electrical nerve stimulation. Postgrad. Med. J. *60*:893–896, 1984.

155. Winstein, C.J.: Acupuncture and its application to physical therapy. Phys. Ther. *54*:1283–1289, 1974.

8

UPPER EXTREMITY CASTING AND SPLINTING

PATRICIA A. FELDMAN

In the spastic upper extremity, hypertonicity is most commonly distributed in what is often referred to as a flexor pattern: the scapula is retracted and depressed, the shoulder exhibits adduction and internal rotation, the elbow and wrist are in flexion, and the digits are flexed and adducted. Less typically, yet not uncommonly, variations from this pattern are found: the scapula may be protracted and elevated despite flexion at the elbow, wrist, and digits. Another variation that may be seen includes scapular rotation, elbow and wrist flexion, MP hyperextension, and IP flexion. Other patterns may be found as well. At times, only certain joints are involved, but tone remains relatively normal in others. Each joint in the upper extremity can also exert influence on another joint. Each patient should be carefully evaluated so that treatment can be deliberately planned.

Early and, in some cases, aggressive management is critical in the treatment of the spastic upper extremity. Untreated, spasticity not only causes loss of motor control that results in functional disability, but can lead to contractures as well. These contractures develop primarily because of static positioning in spastic patterns as discussed. Shortening thus occurs in the muscles, tendons, ligaments, and capsules surrounding the joint. While the spastic muscle and other soft tissues are shortening, the antagonist structures are lengthening. This phenomenon sets the stage for future loss of motor control and function in the extremity because the joint and associated structures are now deprived of their delicate physiologic balance. An overstretched wrist extensor, for instance, loses its mechanical advantage and is more difficult to strengthen. In the most severe cases of spasticity, antagonist muscles and tendons can rupture or the joint can dislocate.

Another consequence of delaying the treatment of spasticity is skin breakdown caused by static positioning. The most common problems in the upper extremities are palmar maceration due to finger flexion or breakdown at the elbow caused by elbow flexion. These breakdowns result from sustained pressure, lack of air circulation, and inability to clean the skin adequately in the affected areas. Posturing secondary to spasticity can also cause discomfort to the patient and a variety of unusual problems, such as obstruction of a tracheostomy by a flexed upper extremity.

Spasticity can also lead to psychologic problems. The pain associated with posturing or ranging a spastic extremity and the frustrations resulting from the motor disability can cause the patient to become depressed. The upper extremities, and particularly the hands, have important personal and cultural associations for us, and the appearance of a spastic extremity, especially if deformity and contracture are present, can

149

cause the patient embarrassment and humiliation at the perceived threat to the body image.

As discussed throughout this book, clinicians have many techniques at their disposal to manage spasticity. Among the choices are positioning, exercise, modalities, medications, nerve blocks, and surgery. This chapter will specifically discuss the use of splinting and casting to control spasticity and its eventual consequences.

Adjunctive techniques should always be considered when choosing splinting or casting as an option. Could the extremity, for example, be better managed using positioning and electrical stimulation along with casting? Would a phenol block before the splinting program better reduce tone and lead to increased function? Should another technique be chosen and splinting or casting avoided altogether?

There are multiple frames of reference to consider in managing a spastic extremity. More conservative relaxation techniques such as those described by Rood, Bobath, and Brunnstrom should be considered. If splinting or casting is chosen as an intervention, what frame of reference is the clinician following? What complimentary or detrimental effect will this modality have, for example, on the weight-bearing techniques (Bobath) that are practiced daily in therapy?

The choice of a treatment approach can therefore be confusing and difficult. There are almost as many opinions as to management of the spastic upper extremity as there are clinicians. As will be described later, the research literature expounds conflicting theories on spasticity management with splinting or casting. Across disciplines, conflict of approach can be found. In today's health care cost containment environment, efficiency and cost of materials and labor became factors influencing the clinician's choice. Casting, especially, can be expensive and time-consuming. It can be argued, however, that its benefits are more extensive and longer-lasting than those of other modalities.

Initially, the clinicians treating the patient must decide whether or not to intervene at all, and this decision should be reconsidered periodically. Perhaps the range

of motion at a particular joint, although not normal, is functional, and the effects of the spasticity on that joint actually improve the patient's abilities. In patients without the potential for function, decisions to cast or splint to facilitate hygiene, for instance, should be weighed against the potential for skin problems that might be caused by the splinting or casting. The whole patient and his overall status should be considered. The need for range of motion at any joint may depend on the range of motion available at other joints or the functional status of the opposite extremity. Clinicians should be clear about the goals of treatment as they relate to the patient as a whole and should not automatically treat contractures and spasticity just because they are present.

In deciding to splint or cast the spastic upper extremity, the clinician should determine if he or she is doing so to decrease spasticity, reduce or manage contracture, or both. These two elements can be treated successfully with splinting or casting in selected patients.

SPLINTING

The literature reveals several controversies regarding splinting of the spastic upper extremity:

1. Whether or not splinting reduces spasticity
2. Volar versus dorsal splinting
3. Static versus dynamic splinting.

DOES SPLINTING REDUCE SPASTICITY?

In 1959, Brennan[1] provided 14 hemiplegic patients with static splints for various spastic joints of the upper extremity (elbow, wrist, and/or digits). These devices were worn for 24 hours per day, usually for a period of 3 months, and positioned the joint at maximum stretch. The results of this experiment were that spasticity was abolished in all splinted flexor groups. The extensor groups (antagonists) exhibited improved active range of motion and strength. These improvements generally remained long after splinting was discontinued.

This study was flawed in certain respects. The patients chosen had hemiplegia that had existed for 6 months or more. Although this is a relatively long time from onset, the use of a control group would have demonstrated more clearly whether the improvement was due to the splinting, and blind observations would have been appropriate. The evaluation procedures for determining presence or absence of spasticity before and after treatment appeared somewhat subjective.

Another study examined the immediate effects of various splints on spastic upper extremity muscle groups. In 1983, Mathiowetz, Bolding, and Trombly[2] compared the effects of a volar splint, hand cone, finger spreader, and no device on eight normal and five hemiplegic subjects. Electromyography (EMG) was used to determine the relative increase or decrease in spasticity in selected flexor muscles. In the hemiplegic subjects, EMG activity was not significantly reduced with any device. In fact, EMG activity was found to increase when the subject was performing work with the contralateral extremity. This study was limited by the fact that devices were worn for short periods, thus eliminating the potential for decrease in spasticity over time.

In 1984, Mills[3] compared the joint position and EMG activity of spastic muscles in eight brain damaged subjects during splinted and unsplinted conditions. The splints used (either low temperature plastic or plaster bivalves) positioned the joints studied (ankle, wrist or elbow) within five to ten degrees of full range of motion. Mills found that EMG activity did not significantly differ in the splinted and nonsplinted conditions. The effect of these splints on spasticity during activity was not evaluated.

The studies discussed below with regard to other controversies indirectly add to the above data on the effectiveness of splinting in the treatment of spasticity. In all, it seems likely that some splints reduce spasticity in some situations. The challenge that faces us is to determine the conditions in which spasticity can be successfully treated. Perhaps the most provocative feature of the three studies noted above are the varying durations of time the splints were applied.

This is certainly a factor worth further investigation.

A survey of occupational therapists was conducted in 1981 by Neuhaus et al.[4] to study rationales for and against hand splinting in hemiplegia. Ninety-three respondents were presented with a case study of a hemiplegic at three stages of recovery and asked whether or not they would recommend splinting at each stage. The results indicated that approximately one fourth would always splint, one fourth would never splint, and half would only splint given moderate to severe spasticity (at any given stage). When years of therapist experience were examined, it was noted that the less experience a therapist had, the less likely he or she was to splint spastic muscles.

It should be noted that contractures may be prevented by splinting even in the absence of an effect on spasticity. Therefore the decision to splint for contracture prevention may not be directly affected by the knowledge that spasticity is not likely to be reduced. The possibility of sustained reductions in tone once a splint is removed may, in fact, be a more important question to resolve.

VOLAR VERSUS DORSAL

Whether spasticity is increased or decreased with splinting the dorsal versus volar forearm surface has been explored by four researchers.

The first study, performed in 1962 by Kaplan,[5] looked at 10 hemiplegic subjects who wore dorsal-surface hand splints. Subjects were splinted at their maximum wrist extension and the splints were gradually modified as range of motion improved and spasticity diminished. The splints were worn an average of 8 hours per day for an average of 20 weeks. Spasticity was measured by clinical examination and EMG recording. All subjects demonstrated significantly reduced flexor spasticity. This study did not compare volar splinting effects with the same subjects, nor were the subjects followed up to assess maintenance of the reduced tone.

One study that attempted to address the

effects of both volar and dorsal splinting was performed in 1968 by Charait.[6] Ten subjects with CVA were fitted with volar surface splints and ten with dorsal surface splints. Splints were worn anywhere from 2 to 23 hours a day and from 2 months to 3 years in total. Spasticity was evaluated by clinical observation by three staff members who were not blinded. The volar splints increased spasticity in six of ten subjects. The remaining four showed no change. The dorsal splints reduced spasticity in eight of ten subjects, one showed no change, and the other had an increase in spasticity. Half of the patients with reduced spasticity also exhibited an increase in active finger and wrist extension. The main problem with this study was that it is based on unblinded, subjective observation.

Zislis, in 1962, noted that a dorsal forearm splint prescribed and worn by his hemiplegic patient was difficult to apply and caused discomfort.[7] A volar surface splint was then fabricated that fully extended and abducted the fingers and positioned the wrist at neutral. This splint subjectively reduced flexor spasticity and discomfort. To assess this reduction of spasticity more objectively, Zislis subjected his patient to EMG recordings in three conditions: unsplinted, with the dorsal splint, and finally, with the volar splint. Flexor activity was prominent in the unsplinted condition. While the patient was wearing the dorsal splint, flexor activity was significantly increased over the unsplinted condition. On application of the volar splint, flexor activity was greatly reduced and, in fact, almost matched the antagonist (extensor) activity. The limitation of this study is the lack of a large patient sample.

In a more recent study, McPherson et al.[8] examined 10 subjects who were randomly fitted with either volar or dorsal splints, both positioning the fingers and the thumb in extension and abduction. Baseline measurements of spasticity, using a spring weighted scale device, were taken for 1 week before splint application. These measurements were repeated 3 hours after splint removal for the 5 weeks the subjects wore the devices. Splints were worn for 2 hours per day. Statistical data, in the form of t-Test calculations, suggested that static volar and dorsal splints reduce spasticity.

In summary, the literature appears to be conflicting in regard to dorsal versus volar splinting. One study showed volar splinting decreased spasticity, two supported dorsal splinting for tone reduction and one study indicated that both volar and dorsal splinting reduced spasticity. The potential for other aspects of splint design, such as finger and thumb position, to affect spasticity may be an important factor in the outcome of these studies and needs further clarification.

STATIC VERSUS DYNAMIC

Another important controversy to review is the question of static versus dynamic splinting. Little formal research has been done in this area. Bunnell,[9] in 1956, advocated the use of dynamic splinting, stating that static splinting led to muscle atrophy and weakness. This led McPherson et al.[10] to study an adaptation of Bunnell's dynamic splint for tonal reduction. This splint has movable finger and thumb parts to allow positioning of the digits in varying abduction. The splint was individually fitted to four of the eight subjects who were matched as closely as possible with controls by age, sex, and time since insult. The splinted group wore the device three times per week for one hour each day. The control group wore no splints and were given only passive range of motion treatments to the affected hand. Spasticity was measured by means of a spring-weighted scale, previously studied for reliability.[11] The results indicated that the dynamic splint reduced pull of the wrist flexors by greater than three times that of passive range of motion treatment. When compared with static splinting, the dynamic splint reduced the force of the wrist flexors more than twice that of the static design. (The comparison to static splinting was made by McPherson applying previous research data to this study.)[8] Although this study had a small sample group and subjects were not followed past the 6 weeks of the experiment, it was well designed and controlled.

Although no research was done to support their rationale, Farber and Huss,[12] in 1974, advocated the use of dynamic splinting in the spastic hand. Their opinion held that static splinting led to pain because of the force required to keep the hand in the splint. Also, they felt that an increase of flexion, pronation and internal rotation was caused by static splinting. A dynamic splint, developed by Huss and adapted by Kiel, was preferred by these authors.

Clearly, not enough research has been done in the static versus dynamic controversy. One actual study demonstrated spasticity reduction with dynamic splinting.

DECISION MAKING

What is clear after this literature review is that hard and fast rules regarding splinting and spasticity cannot be formulated. Each patient should be carefully evaluated. The clinician should exercise flexibility and use his or her experience in determining the appropriate treatment approach to the spastic upper extremity. Clinicians should set treatment goals that are appropriate to the patient and reassess the treatment approach when goals are not obtained.

CASTING

It is generally well accepted that casting, as opposed to splinting, does reduce spasticity and hypertonia related to primitive motor behaviors (see Chapter 9). Although few well controlled, objective studies have been done on spasticity reduction with casting, the anecdotal evidence from the field is compelling. Most reports have studied the lower extremities.

A case report by Zachazewski et al., in 1982, cited a patient whose positive support reaction significantly interfered with gait.[13] Inhibitory casting was performed, before which the physical therapist performed an observational gait analysis. The inhibitory cast was as described by Sussman and Cusick.[14,15] In this patient, the positive support reaction was markedly reduced. On removal of the cast, before fitting in a tone-reducing AFO, the positive reaction returned. When the tone-reducing AFO was applied, the tone reduction surpassed that of the cast.

Forty-two head-injured patients were subjects in a 1983 report by Booth et al.[16]

These patients were split into groups by location of injury and types of casts applied. All casts were applied for range-of-motion loss and spasticity in the lower extremities. For patients with decreased ankle dorsiflexion, all improved in range of motion. In patients demonstrating a decrease in ankle range of motion with increased range of motion postcasting, 37% demonstrated a reduction in spasticity. Long leg-casting of the knee improved range of motion in all patients, but only 1 patient exhibited a reduction of tone.

Bernard et al.[17] described a patient who, 6 days after a head injury, demonstrated severe spasticity throughout his body. Plaster casts were applied to both ankles. Within a day after cast application, a dramatic decrease in spasticity was noted, not only at the ankles, but throughout his body. The authors acknowledged that this phenomenon could have been due to spontaneous recovery.

King[18] used plaster casting of the elbow to reduce spasticity in the elbow flexors of a 46-year-old subject. This cast, of the dropout variety, was applied at the end of comfortable elbow extension (90 degrees). During the first 12 days of treatment, the patient received six cast changes, each cast required due to increasing range of motion. On day 16, the cast was bivalved for night use only. Spasticity reduction was dramatic, allowing the patient to demonstrate and strengthen elbow extension. On removal of the bivalve for a 24-hour period, the spasticity increased significantly. When the bivalve was returned, tonal reduction then returned. The bivalve was eventually discontinued, the patient being able to extend the elbow actively to approximately −15 degrees.

INHIBITIVE CASTING THEORY

Many hypotheses have been offered to explain the phenomenon of tone reduction during casting. The rationale most commonly used for the upper extremities is that it is the effect of neutral warmth and total, constant pressure. Casting reduces the variability of the cutaneous sensory input received by the central nervous system and may cause some habituation. This may help to inhibit the level of excitability of gamma and alpha motor neurons and decrease the sensitivity of the muscle spindle to stretch. Applying neutral warmth also assists in reducing input to exteroceptors for temperature. The constant position of the joint and static length of the muscle may also contribute.[17] Excitation of the Golgi tendon organ has been thought to play a role.[18]

PRINCIPLES AND INDICATIONS FOR CASTING OR SPLINTING

The decision to cast or splint the spastic upper extremities should come after careful regard of many factors. Although the focus in this chapter is the use of casting to treat spasticity, these modalities are commonly used to reduce contractures as well, and both can occur simultaneously. Therefore, the discussion will sometimes encompass the treatment of both problems. It is imperative that clinicians carefully consider and question their reasons for using upper-extremity casts and splints, including a determination as to whether these devices are being implemented to influence spasticity, contractures or both. The following are important considerations for casting or splinting:

1. Spasticity: Patients who present with minimal, moderate, or even beginning severe spasticity can be casted successfully. If the spasticity fluctuates, it is still possible to cast or splint. In this case, however, the patient should be monitored more closely for possible splint or cast modifications or possible skin breakdown. It is important to intervene early, before spasticity becomes severe. The longer tonal influences are left to bear on the joints, the greater the risk for contractures and other complications. Patients who present with severe spasticity should not be considered for a casting/splinting program. The potential and risk for skin breakdown, edema formation and circulatory impairment are too great. These patients may be more appropriate for intervention with spasticity medication, nerve blocks, and other procedures after which splinting or casting can again be considered.

2. Position: The patient's total body pos-

ture should be evaluated. It could be that simple adjunctive positioning techniques to the head and neck (for example) will effectively reduce or eliminate spastic posturing in the upper extremities. It could also be found that simple positioning of the elbow into extension with a lap tray reduces or eliminates spastic posturing in the upper extremities. In spite of these considerations, casting or splinting may be indicated. The clinician should then observe upper-extremity positioning after application of these devices. The patient may require additional positioning interventions to prevent pressure sores and breakdown while he or she is in the device.

3. Range of Motion: Casts and splints by nature have to be as precise and close-fitting as possible. Some stretching of the soft tissues must be possible to achieve the desired goals. Therefore, adequate range of motion is necessary before proceeding. Ideally, patients considered for these devices should exhibit at least 90 degrees of elbow extension, 20 to 30 degrees of wrist movement and 20 degrees of finger motion. Even with such severe losses of range of motion, casting, more commonly than splinting, can still be successful. In some cases, casting has even been successful with less available range of motion than described, especially in the elbow. Alternately, maintenance of these deformities and prevention from worsening are the only strategy. The clinician's creativity can be greatly challenged here, especially if the patient's skin is close to breakdown. Simple devices such as gauze or towel rolls can often be used in the hand to prevent breakdown. The elbow, as mentioned before, may be successfully casted with less than 90 degrees of elbow extension. Care must be exercised, however, and quick gains should not be expected. Often a flexor hinge built into the cast may give the best results. This hinge can be extended manually with a screwdriver daily or weekly in small increments. Cast removal is not necessary.

At times it may be difficult to assess the relative contributions of contracture and spasticity to loss of joint mobility. Such a determination, however, may influence the clinician's approach. If the joint is largely under the influence of spasticity, perhaps a nerve block alone will suffice. If the joint is severely contracted, with only mild spasticity present, casting alone may resolve the problem. The difficulty with assessment arises when enough range of motion is not available to elicit the stretch reflex to assess spasticity. The most reliable way to assess what is spasticity versus contracture is to slowly extend (or flex) the affected joint, allowing the stretch reflex to abate and then continuing slow constant pressure. When, after abatement of the stretch reflex, the joint no longer moves, most likely you have discovered the beginning of the contracture. When spasticity is particularly severe, however, the clinician may be uncertain that he or she has reached the true end point. In such cases, blocks with local anesthetics may resolve the question.

4. Fractures: Careful review of the patient's history should be performed to rule out any previous fractures. In the case of a fracture history, the clinician should note if it is currently stable. If so, casting and splinting can proceed if otherwise indicated.

5. Heterotopic Ossification: Joints that present with heterotopic ossification (myositis ossificans) can be casted or splinted successfully. In the case of extensive heterotopic ossification, splints or bivalved casts are used to maintain range. When minor heterotopic ossification is present, sometimes range of motion can be gained even with serial casting or splinting. Care should be exercised during fabrication so that the joint is stretched gently. The devices should also be removed more frequently or serial casts changed more often, and the joint gently ranged to prevent solidification or fusion. In some cases, two bivalved casts or splints must be alternated, one in flexion and one in extension, to prevent loss of range in either direction.

6. Skin Condition: The patient's skin should ideally be free from breakdown in areas to be covered by splints or casts. Patients who are known to have sensitive skin can be casted or splinted but should be monitored very closely and devices should be removed more frequently for skin checks. Foam padding should be placed on either side of a susceptible area to relieve pressure within a cast. Splints that bypass an area of breakdown may assist in the healing of wounds. An example of this is an elbow extension splint that exposes an area of breakdown at the elbow crease to the air, allowing better hygiene and accessibility to the area for treatment. Patients who exhibit excessive diaphoresis can also be casted or splinted but their status must be carefully watched. Splinted patients with diaphoresis may benefit from the application of stockinette before putting the splint on. The stockinette can be changed frequently. Special splinting materials with ventilation holes may also be used.

7. Circulation: Circulation should be adequate. When the skin is pressed down and blanching occurs, color should return quickly, indicating adequate capillary refill. Patients who present with minimal to moderate edema can be casted or splinted, but these patients do require careful monitoring. The device should be checked frequently (at least daily) for slippage. Should slippage occur, this indicates resolution of the edema, and without modification of the device, rubbing and skin breakdown are imminent.

8. Rebound: In the opinion of some clinicians, splints/casts applied to the spastic upper extremity, although reducing tone while in the device, can lead to rebound after removal. Patients should be monitored for this phenomenon.

Initially, clinicians must decide whether to cast or splint the spastic upper extremity. Generally splinting is chosen when contractures and spasticity are less severe or when casting could cause limitation in the patient's functional abilities.

SPECIFIC SPLINTS

Many different splints designed to reduce spasticity in the upper extremity will be discussed and specific information on fabrication presented. With experience, each clinician will undoubtedly develop a preference for design materials and methods. A few guidelines on these decisions will be given.

MATERIAL/METHODS

This author clearly prefers the use of more rigid, less flexible, low temperature plastics when splinting spastic upper extremities. Orthoplast® and Orthoform® are ideal because of their relatively quick setting time (important in splinting spastic limbs). These materials offer acceptable conformity without the excessive stretching properties of other materials. Their strength and durability, especially when reinforced, are superior. These materials do not tend to pick up fingerprints or inadvertent marks during handling and fabrication, thereby making the finished product more cosmetically appealing. Padding of any variety is rarely used by this author. A well designed and appropriate fitting splint should not require it. If padding absolutely has to be used, Spenco® is an acceptable choice. This is a densely packed, closed-cell foam that offers more even distribution of pressure.

During actual fabrication, a few hints may help the inexperienced clinician. The splint pattern is important and the extremity must be traced as accurately as possible. Traditional relaxation techniques may prove useful in reducing spasticity to allow a drawing to be made. The use of two therapists, one to hold the extremity, the other to draw, is especially effective. Finally, the clinician can trace the opposite extremity (if unaffected) for the pattern and reverse it. The splint should, if possible, be fabricated in stages, from the forearm to the digits. It is very difficult to attempt setting wrist and digit position at the same time, especially when the influence of spasticity is fighting your efforts. The use of two therapists is helpful during fabrication as well. One therapist can position the extremity appropriately and the other can fabricate the device. Patience and fortitude are important.

SPASTICITY REDUCTION SPLINT

Designed by Julie Snook, the spasticity reduction splint is based on Bobath's principles of reflex-inhibiting postures (RIPs).[20] This posture, for the hand, includes 30 degrees of wrist extension, 45 degrees of metacarpal-phalangeal (MP) flexion, full interphalangeal (IP) extension, finger abduction, and thumb abduction. The complete splint is shown in Figure 8–1.

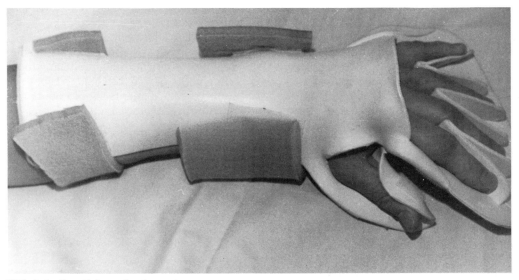

FIG. 8–1. Spasticity reduction spint.

The pattern is made by placing the patient's fully pronated hand on paper with the fingers and thumb abducted. Trace around the entire forearm, thumb and fingers. Mark the location of the MPs of the fingers and thumb. Remove the patient's hand from the paper and draw the details of splint. Using a ruler, make small marks approximately 1½ cm from the edge of the hand tracing around the whole hand. Connect these marks with a pen, and you now have the basic splint outline. Additional areas to draw in on the pattern are small circles around the MPs indicating where cutouts should be of both the thumb and fingers. Draw in a little extra material next to the MPs of the digits on either side. These are reinforcement pieces to fold over. Finally, indicate the location of the finger spreader pieces on the pattern. These are located at the base of each digit. Draw the outline of the splint onto the material (Orthoplast® is preferred), heat the material, and cut out the splint. Draw the details of the pattern on the splint and clearly mark the location of the MP cutouts and finger spreaders. Cut out the MP openings with a mat (carpet) knife. Using small strips of extra material, make the finger spreaders. These are fashioned by making three small "Vs" and are approximately 2 inches long. Heat the splint and the finger spreaders well and attach the spreaders to the splint, using the indicated location marks. Let the splint cool completely. Check the placement of the finger spreaders by placing the splint on the volar surface of the patient's hand. Make adjustments to the finger spreaders. Heat the forearm piece to the finger MP cutouts. Place the splint on the dorsal forearm surface of the patient, holding the wrist at 30 degrees of extension. Allow to cool completely. Heat the finger pan. Fabricate the 45-degree flexion angle of the finger pan independent from the patient. Cool completely. Heat the thumb piece only. Apply the entire splint to the patient, directing your attention to gaining abduction of the thumb. Cool completely. Spotheat either side of the MPs and fold over reinforcement pieces. Spot-heat and roll back MP cutouts and end of forearm. Apply the splint to the patient, checking carefully for fit. A wearing schedule should be determined individually for each patient by observing tone reduction or increase. Some patients wear this splint only at night; others wear it intermittently throughout the day (2 hours on, 2 hours off).

Initial reports by the creator of this splint indicated immediate and marked reduction of tone in the hand as well as in the entire upper extremity in all 18 patients provided with the device.[20] Follow-up study by McPherson in 1981 confirmed tone reduction with use of the splint in five subjects.[21]

FINGER ABDUCTION SPLINT

This splint, designed by Doubilet and Polkow, is also based on Bobath's principles of RIPs.[22] The splint is designed, however, only to provide for finger and thumb abduction. The completed splint is pictured in Figure 8–2.

Fabrication is easy. An 8-inch by 3-inch (approximately) square piece of splinting material is cut out. The therapist abducts the patient's fingers on the splint and marks them. The finger locations are punched out with a leather punch. The finger piece is heated separately from the thumb. The fingers are placed in the holes, and the holes widen and stretch when the material is warm. The splint should fit between the PIPs and DIPs. Next heat the thumb piece. Put patient's fingers in the splint, molding the remaining material around the thumb, positioned in abduction. Cut off excess material and round off the corners. Wearing time with this splint should also be individually determined. The creators recommend constant use throughout the day, removal occurring for therapy and meals.

Of the 15 patients originally given this device, all had a reduction of tone.[22] Mathiowetz et al., however, found no reduction of tone with this device.[2]

THE MACKINNON SPLINT

Designed by Joyce MacKinnon, this splint is easily fabricated. The belief that release of overactive finger flexors and adductor pollicis allowed balanced muscle action of the wrist was the rationale behind this

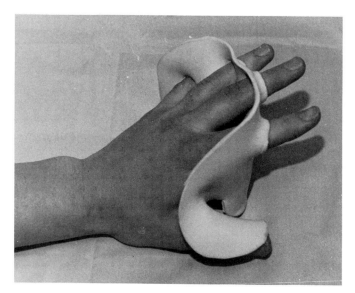

FIG. 8–2. Finger abduction splint.

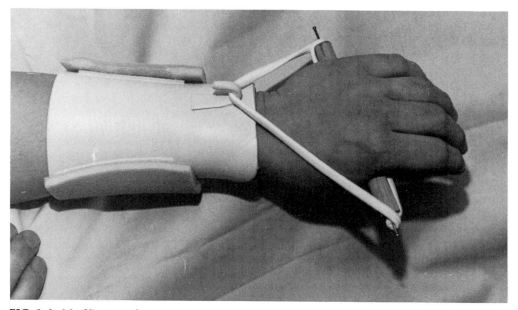

FIG. 8–3. MacKinnon splint.

splint.[23] The completed splint is seen in Figure 8–3.

The device is fabricated by attaching rubber tubing to the ends of a small circumference dowel with nails. A wrist gauntlet is fabricated by molding a strip of splinting material three quarters of the way around the wrist. A Velcro strap holds the gauntlet securely on the wrist. A small screw or piece of splint material is embedded into the dorsal portion of the gauntlet. The splint is applied by placing the dowel in the palm, maintaining contact with the metacarpal heads. The rubber tubing attaches to the screw. Clinical observation of 31 children using this device by the creator demonstrated "excellent results" in terms of hand awareness, use, acceptance, and decreased spasticity after splint removal.[23]

ORTHOKINETIC CUFF

The design of the orthokinetic cuff is said to be based on exteroceptor stimulation of the muscle spindle of the antagonist of a spastic muscle by means of an elastic band. An "active field" causes the elastic to provide small pinches to the desired muscle, thereby facilitating it. More likely, the alpha motor neuron pool is excited by exteroceptor stimulation. This cuff was designed by Farber and Chapman[12] (Fig. 8–4).

The clinician must first decide which muscle should be facilitated. Cuff fabrica-

tion will be described using an example in which the muscle to be facilitated is the extensor digitorum, to increase MP extension and reduce spasticity in the finger flexors. The therapist first determines the length of rubber-reinforced roller bandage that will be used. The circumference of the forearm is measured at the location of the extensor digitorum muscle belly (8 inches). Next the width of the extensor digitorum muscle belly ("active field") is measured (2 inches). Each cuff has a relatively "inactive field" (does not provide as much stimulation as an active field). This inactive field is determined by subtracting the muscle belly width from the forearm circumference (6 inches). Add 2 inches for the Velcro closure to be added (8 inches). Most cuffs have two layers of elastic in the active field and four

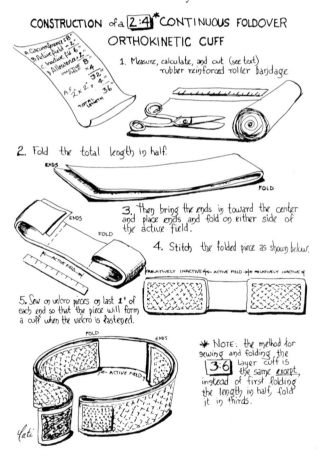

FIG. 8–4. Orthokinetic cuff (with permission from Farber, S.D., and Huss, J.A.: Sensorimotor Evaluation and Treatment Procedures for Allied Health Personnel. 2nd Ed. Indiana, Indiana University Foundation, 1974, p. 81).

layers of elastic in the inactive field. Using this formula, the active field width (2 inches) is multiplied by 2 (2 layers, which equals 4 inches). The inactive field width (8 inches) is multiplied by 4 (4 layers, equalling 32 inches). The total length of rubber-reinforced roller bandage to be cut equals 36 inches (by adding active and inactive fields). To complete the cuff, fold the bandage in half lengthwise. Fold both ends toward the center, keeping the width of the active field uncovered. Stitch the elastic closed on both sides of the inactive field. Sew Velcro hook and pile on either side of the ends of the inactive field for closure. The creators of this device do not give any information on its use and effectiveness on patients. They do, however, comment on the need to monitor the patient closely while he or she is in the device because the facilitated muscle gains in strength and girth, making the cuff too tight.

SUBMAXIMUM RANGE SPLINT

Based on the rationale described by Peterson, the submaximum range splint was designed.[19] When any muscle is splinted on full stretch or maximum range of motion, spasticity is increased. The author has also noted this to be the case in clinical observations of splints applied to the spastic hand. Incorporating this idea into splint design is simple. Ideally, this splint should position the hand with the thumb in partial opposition to the index and long fingers. The MP/PIP joint should exhibit 45 degrees of flexion with DIP extension. Pressure should occur in the palmar arch to aid in inhibition. The wrist should be positioned at 10 to 20 degrees of extension. If the patient does not have the available range of motion to position the hand ideally, each joint should be positioned in five to ten degrees less than the available range. This splint is designed and fabricated exactly like a typical resting hand splint. See Figure 8–5 for an example.

BECKER DYNAMIC SPLINT

This splint, the theory of which is based on an adaption of Bunnell's dynamic splint as described earlier in this chapter, is currently under consideration for mass marketing by Alan Becker, LPT (Mequon Care Center, Mequon, Wisconsin 53217).

The splint is made from a plexiglass type material. It has a dorsal forearm piece, attached to which are rods extending the length of the fingers and thumb. At the ends of these rods are finger loops. The

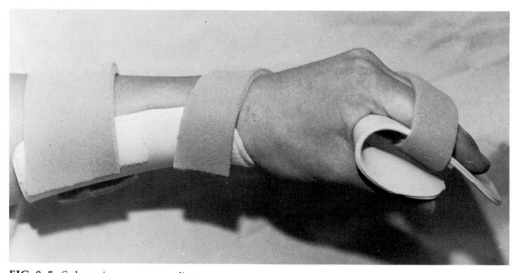

FIG. 8–5. Submaximum range splint.

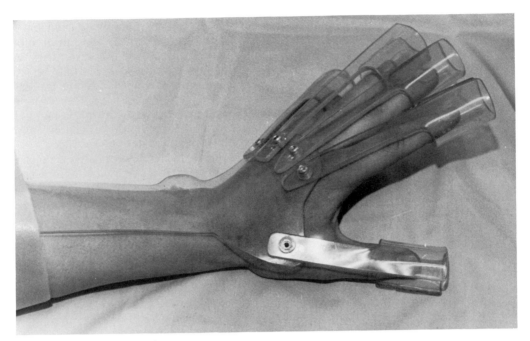

FIG. 8–6. Becker dynamic splint

rods are attached with a rivet, allowing placement of the fingers and thumb into abduction or adduction, as desired. The dorsal forearm piece is fairly flexible, allowing wrist flexion/extension. The initial reports on the effectiveness of this splint are favorable.[10] The splint is pictured in Figure 8–6.

crease, necessitating frequent cast changes. Plaster is relatively inexpensive. Fiberglass is usually the material of choice for bivalves when further range of motion gains are not expected. Fiberglass, although more expensive than plaster, is more durable, lightweight, and soil-resistant.

UPPER EXTREMITY CASTS

The two different forms of casting to be described in this section require different materials and techniques: solid casting and bivalve casting. Solid casting is usually used to improve range of motion with serial casts, and spasticity may diminish in the process. Solid casts can also be used solely to diminish spasticity on a short-term basis. Bivalve casting is used to maintain joint range of motion, decrease spasticity, or both. Occasionally serial casting is done with bivalve casts to increase range of motion when periodic removal of the casts will be necessary.

In general, plaster is used in serial casting when range of motion is expected to in-

SOLID CASTING

Spasticity management through solid casting can be quite effective. A situation in which this might be helpful is in a patient who has active hand control but whose elbow flexor tone interferes. A solid cast, applied at the point of reduction of elbow flexor tone, might help the patient to use the hand. For spasticity management, casts are applied in submaximum range of motion. Determine patient's maximum joint motion and subtract 5 to 10 degrees.

Serial casting can be an extremely effective method for reducing contractures. Gains in range of motion seen after the application of the cast are incorporated into each subsequent cast change until no further gains are seen. In patients with spasticity, serial casting is successful partly by virtue of the ability of a solid cast to reduce spasticity.

It is useful to have an organized written procedure before initiation of a serial casting program. In general, the following guidelines are recommended:

1. Good communication should occur among all team members when casting is to be initiated.
2. X-rays should be considered with significant contractures at the shoulders and elbows in patients at risk for heterotopic ossification, or where there is a question of orthopedic stability.
3. For contracture management, the initial cast is applied at the end of the easily available range of motion after allowing the stretch reflex to abate. Subsequent casts are applied at the end of available range of motion gained by minimal stretching of joint.
4. Serial casts are left on anywhere from 24 hours to 10 days. Factors influencing this decision are the degree of contracture and spasticity, the chronicity of the contracture and the goal of the casting program. More recent contractures may require shorter periods between cast changes. Some patients easily gain range of motion when casts are changed every fourth day, whereas other patients may require the constant stretch over a 10-day period to gain motion.
5. Following the application of each cast, and for the duration of the casting period, circulation, sensation and motion of the casted extremity should be closely monitored. If edema occurs, the extremity should be elevated. Should the edema not resolve, the cast should be removed. Persistent complaints of pain may warrant cast removal. Sensory loss is a relative contraindication to serial casting.
6. The patient's skin can be cleansed thoroughly with a brisk alcohol rub between cast changes. Skin should be checked closely for any redness, areas of breakdown, blisters, or other evidence of irritation. If edema is present, the extremity should be elevated. The joint should be gently taken through its available motion several times. Maximum motion gained should be measured with a goniometer and results carefully recorded. The importance of ranging the casted joint between cast changes cannot be stressed enough because it is easy to lose joint motion in the direction opposite that in which you are casting.
7. Serial casting is terminated if no gain in range of motion is noted from cast to cast.
8. Final casts (usually fiberglass) are left on for 1 to 2 weeks to ensure that range of motion gained is not lost, and are then bivalved.
9. Casting should not be initiated over, or before, weekends unless staff members are available to check the extremity daily, or the patient or a family member can be relied on to monitor the extremity.

TECHNIQUE-PLASTER CASTING

The following procedure is used for making a plaster serial cast (Table 8–1):

1. Measure and record joint range of motion.
2. The patient should be sitting or lying comfortably and be draped with sheets or towels to protect clothing and skin. Explain the procedure to the patient clearly and reassure as needed. Some brain-injured patients may become agitated during the casting procedure. Premedicating such patients with a sedative can be considered.
3. Tubular stockinette is placed over the

TABLE 8–1. GENERAL SUPPLIES REQUIRED FOR A PLASTER CASTING PROGRAM

Plaster cast bandages
Stockinette
Cotton padding (Webril*)
Bucket for water
Linens (towels, sheets, apron)
Cast spreader
Cast saw
Cast scissors

*Trademark

extremity to be casted, extending at either end 4 to 6 inches beyond where the cast will end.

4. Determine the targeted position of the extremity. Direct another person (therapist or aide) how and where to hold the extremity.

5. Strips of stick-on-foam can be placed on either side of an area that may be susceptible to skin breakdown.

6. Apply cotton padding in a taut fashion around the extremity, ending after three to four layers have been applied. Extra padding or felt may be added if needed over bony prominences. Padding is applied 1 to 2 inches above the end of the stockinette.

7. Dip the plaster roll five to six times in warm water. Squeeze excess moisture from roll.

8. Apply plaster to the extremity in a circular fashion, moving proximally to distally.

9. Direct the person assisting to stretch the joint minimally as the plaster is being applied. The casting assistant should not apply directed pressure to the plaster as it is setting (breakdown inside the cast can occur from this "point loading" effect). Rather, the assistant should stretch the joint above and below the cast or apply pressure with the whole surface of the hand to evenly distribute any pressure.

10. Four to five layers of plaster should be applied. The plaster should be smoothed with the surface of the hands in a circular fashion as it sets.

11. Before applying the last layer, turn back the ends of the stockinette onto the cast. This gives a smooth finished surface to the cast edges. Apply the last layer of plaster just below this edge.

12. Instruct the casting assistant to maintain the stretch on the joint until the plaster has set (3 to 8 minutes).

13. The plaster will be completely dry in 24 hours. Weight bearing on the casted extremity should be avoided until then.

14. Clean any dripped plaster from the patient's skin, elevate the extremity comfortably, and check either end of the cast for tightness. Check the patient's circulation.

Casting should be learned under the supervision of someone experienced in casting technique.

ELBOW DROPOUT CAST

There are two variations of this popular cast, one developed by King[18] in 1982 and one described by Booth et al.[16] in 1983. This cast, appropriate for patients exhibiting elbow flexor spasticity and contracture, begins as a long arm cylinder cast that is then trimmed from the elbow to the wrist, leaving a forearm flexion stop, or from the elbow to the axilla, leaving an upper arm flexion stop (Fig. 8–7). After the plaster is removed, the padding and stockinette beneath are trimmed to the edge, folded over, and taped. This variation allows extension but prevents flexion. Not only does this technique allow for increasing range even before a cast change, but in addition, the extensors can be exercised or stimulated electrically to further reduce spasticity in the flexors by way of inhibitory pathways.

King followed one patient who was treated with this cast, initially 24 hours a day and then at night only.[18] He noted that the "design of the cast was effective in reducing the spasticity which was probably the result of input from the Golgi tendon organs in the spastic flexors."[18] The patient did gain voluntary functional range of motion in the extremity. Booth et al.[16] report anecdotal evidence for this cast's effectiveness.

OTHER CAST VARIATIONS

Casts can be applied over two or more joints, but application is difficult and should be attempted after single joint casting experience has been gained. Because each patient presents with different range of motion and spasticity, careful determination of targeted position should be made. Generally, each cast variation should position each joint in submaximum range of motion. When incorporating the digits into the cast, attempt to position the fingers and thumb into comfortable abduction. This can be accomplished by encircling the fingers

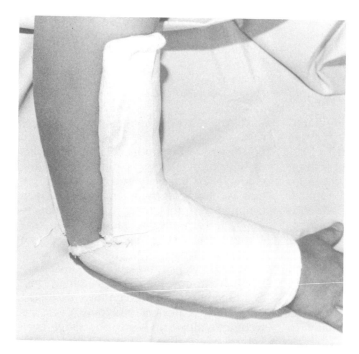

FIG. 8–7. Elbow dropout cast.

and thumb with cotton padding before application of cast material. This abduction assists in tonal reduction based on the theory described for the spasticity reduction splint.[20]

With few exceptions, casting individual fingers is extremely difficult because the plaster material is bulky when applied. If casting is attempted, however, use as little padding and plaster as possible. Fiberglass might be preferable.

Splints can be used in combination with casts. An example of this would be fabricating the forearm piece of a resting hand splint over an elbow cast to position the hand during the casting program.

With these guidelines, almost any variation can be attempted, including elbow/wrist cast; elbow, wrist and digits; short-arm wrist cock-up; and short-arm wrist, digits, and thumb.

Careful and close observation of the extremity should be made daily to determine the effects on spasticity. As with other casts, these casts can be changed approximately once a week to increase range of motion, followed by the application of a bivalve to maintain range of motion and reduce spasticity. Some individuals may require a longer time between cast changes, longer wearing time, a follow-up bivalve or more aggressive intervention, such as a phenol block.

BIVALVE CASTING

Bivalve casts are fabricated to maintain range of motion gained in a serial casting program, to prevent the development or worsening of contractures and to provide spasticity reduction by placing the extremity in reflex inhibiting postures and/or decreasing sensory input. As a result, function, comfort, or patient care may be improved. Bivalves are generally fiberglass casts consisting of anterior and posterior portions that are padded, lined with stockinette, and fastened with straps or elastic wrap.

As with any splint or positioning device, the patient should be weaned into the bivalve to ensure proper skin tolerance. Although fiberglass is preferable for reasons stated previously, plaster casts can also be bivalved.

TECHNIQUE-FIBERGLASS CAST MATERIAL

Fiberglass casts (Table 8–2) are made in generally the same fashion as plaster casts, with the following exceptions.

1. Plastic gloves should be worn by anyone touching the fiberglass material during fabrication. The plastic gloves should be coated with petroleum jelly initially and throughout the procedure. Fiberglass adheres to the skin or unlubricated gloves and is difficult to remove.
2. The fiberglass roll is submerged in *cool* water and gently squeezed six to eight times, then removed from the water and applied dripping wet to the extremity to facilitate handling of the material.
3. Fiberglass roll packages should be opened one at a time and applied within a minute. Fiberglass hardens and does not bond to itself when left exposed to the air.
4. Fiberglass must overlap itself by half a tape width.
5. Firmly blot the exterior of the cast with open palms in a circular fashion after all layers have been applied. This is to facilitate maximum bonding of all layers. Rubbing in a longitudinal fashion disrupts the bond.
6. If one layer of the cast is allowed to cure (harden), subsequent layers do not bond well. All three to four layers should be applied in efficient succession.
7. The fiberglass can be molded by maintaining the extremity in the desired position for 30 seconds during the last few minutes of the 5 to 7 minutes of setting time.
8. The cast will be completely set in 7 to 10 minutes. It can be removed after that

with a cast saw. Weight bearing can occur in 20 minutes.

The fiberglass cast can be made into a working bivalve cast in the following manner:

1. Using the cast saw, cut the cast into anterior and posterior portions. Remove the cast with the cast spreader.
2. Remove the padding and stockinette from the extremity with the cast scissors and discard them.
3. Inspect both fiberglass shells for protrusions and rough edges. Trim the ends of each shell and file until smooth.
4. Using cotton padding, reline the shells, taking care to rip padding edges off to provide a smooth inner surface with no ripples. Reline with same amount of padding used to fabricate the original cast. Extend the padding over all edges and sides of the shells.
5. Fold the padding over the edges of the shells and secure with adhesive tape.
6. Cut a length of stockinette approximately 4 to 6 inches longer than the length of each shell. Line each shell with stockinette. Secure both ends with adhesive tape.
7. Fashion straps using 1 to 3 inch wide webbing and buckles. These can be taped or sewn onto stockinette covering the shell. Bivalves can also be secured with ace wraps.
8. Carefully wean the patient into the bivalve, modifying and adjusting as needed.

SUMMARY

Making a decision to either splint or cast the spastic upper extremity requires a thorough knowledge of anatomic, physiologic, and neurologic principles and the effects on each individual patient. Splinting is generally chosen when spasticity is more localized and less severe. Casting is a better approach when spasticity is more generalized and/or severe.

Spasticity can be managed by the rehabilitation team in many different ways. Described in this chapter have been tech-

TABLE 8–2. ADDITIONAL SUPPLIES REQUIRED FOR A FIBERGLASS CASTING PROGRAM

Fiberglass cast bandages
Petroleum jelly
Gloves
Metal file
Elastic wrap or webbing and buckles
Adhesive tape

niques involving splinting and casting of the upper extremities. Whichever approach is used, it is very important that collabora-tion and communication occur between team members to ensure a consistent ap-proach to each individual case.

REFERENCES

1. Brennan, B.J.: Response to stretch of hyper-tonic muscle groups in hemiplegia. Br. Med. J. 1:1504–1507, 1959.
2. Mathiowetz, V., Bolding, D., and Trombly, C.: Immediate effects of positioning devices on the normal and spastic hand measured by electromyography. Am. J. Occup. Ther. 37:247–254, 1983.
3. Mills, V.: Electromyographic results of in-hibitory splinting. Phys. Ther. 64:190–193, 1984.
4. Neuhaus, B., et al.: A survey of rationales for and against hand splinting in hemiple-gia. Am. J. Occup. Ther. 35:83–90, 1981.
5. Kaplan, N.: Effect of splinting on reflex in-hibition and sensorimotor stimulation treat-ment of spasticity. Arch. Phys. Med. Reha-bil. 43:565–569, 1962.
6. Charait, S.: A comparison of volar and dor-sal splinting of the hemiplegic hand. Am. J. Occup. Ther. 22:319–321, 1968.
7. Zislis, J.: Splinting of the hand in a spastic hemiplegic patient. Arch. Phys. Med. Rehab. 45:41–43, 1964.
8. McPherson, J., Kreimeyer, D., Aalderks, M., and Gallagher, T.: A comparison of dorsal and volar resting hand splints in the reduc-tion of hypertonus. Am. J. Occup. Ther. 36:664–670, 1987.
9. Bunnell, S.: Surgery of the Hand. Ed. 3. Philadelphia, J.B. Lippincott, 1956.
10. McPherson, J., and Becker, A.: Dynamic splint to reduce the passive component of hypertonicity. Arch. Phys. Med. Rehab. 66:249–252, 1985.
11. McPherson, J.J., Kreimeyer, D., Gallagher, T., and Aalderks, M.: Reliability of spring weighted scales in assessing hypertonicity. Occup. Ther. J. Res. 2:118–119, 1982.
12. Farber, S.D., and Huss, J.A.: Sensorimotor Evaluation and Treatment Procedures for Allied Health Personnel, 2nd Ed. Indiana, Indiana University Foundation, 1974.
13. Zachazewski, J.E., Eberle, E.D., and Feffer-ies, M.: Effect of tone inhibiting casts and or-thoses on gait. Phys. Ther. 62:453–455, 1982.
14. Sussman, M.D.: Use of casts as adjunct to physical therapy management of cerebral palsy patients. Read at Orthopedic Aspects of Developmental Disabilities, Division of Physical Therapy, University of North Ca-rolina at Chapel Hill, 1978.
15. Sussman, M.D., and Cusick, B.: Preliminary report: The role of short leg tone reducing casts as an adjunct to physical therapy of pa-tients with cerebral palsy. John Hopkins Med. J. 45:112–114, 1979.
16. Booth, B.J., Doyle, M., and Montgomery, J.: Serial casting for the management of spas-ticity in the head injured adult. Phys. Ther. 63:1960–1966, 1983.
17. Bernard, P., et al.: Reduction of hypertonic-ity by early casting in a comatose head in-jured individual. A case report. Phys. Ther. 64:1540–1542, 1984.
18. King, T.: Plaster splinting as a means of re-ducing elbow flexor spasticity. Am. J. Occup. Ther. 36:671–673, 1982.
19. Peterson, L.T.: Neurological considerations in splinting spastic extremities. Unpublished paper.
20. Snook, J.: Spasticity reduction splint. Am. J. Occup. Ther. 33:648–651, 1979.
21. McPherson, J.: Objective evaluation of a splint designed to reduce hypertonicity. Am. J. Occup. Ther. 35:189–194, 1981.
22. Doubilet, L., and Polkow, L.: Theory and design of a finger abduction splint for the spastic hand. Am. J. Occup. Ther. 31:320–322, 1977.
23. MacKinnon, J., Sanderson, E., and Buch-anan, J.: The MacKinnon Splint—A func-tional hand splint. Can. J. Occup. Ther. 42:157–158, 1975.

9 DYNAMIC CASTING AND ORTHOTICS

NANCY HYLTON

HISTORY OF DYNAMIC CASTING

Serial casting has been used for many years as a part of the orthopedic treatment of cerebral palsy to allow prolonged stretching of contractures. Equinus deformities, both dynamic and fixed, have been of particular interest. In many children with cerebral palsy, especially those who are upright and walking or running, equinus tends to be progressive and difficult to control without immobilization of some kind. Serial casting is short-term immobilization directed at providing greater working mobility in these individuals.

In 1971, while I was participating in a refresher course taught in Seattle by Dr. and Mrs. Bobath, the topic of selective use of serial casting in conjunction with treatment was addressed. Dr. Bobath, like other orthopedic physicians, had been using casting to reduce dynamic and fixed deformities, especially in the foot and ankle. The Bobaths described in some detail the positioning and technique they used to get the best results. I stored this, like much information that comes through a course, for future reference and gave it little thought at the time. Although I had learned in physical therapy school some basic information about plaster and how to make posterior resting splints, I had little reason to believe that I would ever use this information in pediatrics.

Within two months, a fellow therapist,

Nancy Kahn, asked if anyone would consider helping her do serial casting with a young patient. I thought this an interesting challenge and agreed to help her.

It was October 1971. The patient, Shelley, age 4, was a moderate spastic diplegic with greater involvement on the right, who had been treated at our clinic for 2 years. When treatment began, she was crawling reciprocally, "W" sitting independently, pulling to standing, and standing holding on with abnormal extensor and flexor hypertonus (hip adduction, internal rotation, some knee and hip flexion, and steep plantarflexion with supination).

During therapy, it was possible to inhibit the hypertonus in her legs and hips and to achieve supported standing with knee and hip extension and abduction and heels on the floor. She was, however, unable to maintain the control on her own. The equinovarus foot deformity (greater on the right) was increasing and becoming more fixed with time. Even a trial with a long-leg brace on the right failed to help her achieve stable weight bearing. Surgery, involving heel cord lengthening and posterior tibialis transfer, was one of the few alternatives remaining.

Because of the patient's lack of progress and the imminent surgery, we decided to try serial casting as described by Dr. and Mrs. Bobath, with the thought of maintaining a more normal foot and ankle position. The casts were applied with the patient standing because this was the best way to control her foot and ankle position and maintain adequate control of hypertonus. The casts were standard short leg casts with a plaster extension under the toes to prevent clawing. Shelley's mother noticed an immediate dramatic reduction in hip adductor hypertonus, which was totally unexpected. We were both puzzled and pleased, and the casts were left on for 2½ weeks. During this time, Shelley made more progress in developing trunk and hip control in the upright position than we had seen in the previous 2 years of intensive therapy. The following changes were observed both in therapy and at home:

1. Pulling to standing with weight over both legs and with abduction and external rotation at the hips.
2. Improved hip and trunk control grading and balance. She began to stand without arm support resting her back against furniture.
3. High patient motivation. Before casting, Shelley, though a bright little girl, had become totally disinterested and frustrated with working on standing and balance. When the casts were on, we could not keep her off her feet.
4. Independent walking around furniture.
5. Greater freedom to move quickly, with more variety and better quality of movement throughout her body.
6. Sustained dramatic reduction of hypertonus in arms, trunk, hips, and legs.

Immediately after the casts were removed, Shelley was able to stand, cruise, and even push a small chair forward while actively maintaining hip abduction and external rotation and near neutral foot/ankle control and balance. Although these actions were obviously more difficult for her without the casts, the equinovarus pattern was not seen in association with the effort. We were excited, but within two to three days after cast removal, the old pattern of hypertonus reappeared and began increasing again. Frustrated, we decided that the best alternative was to make new casts and prevent continued regression.

The second set of casts was left on for 4 weeks, then bivalved for use during the daytime in connection with Shelley's therapy program. She recovered the previous gains and continued to progress toward independent standing and walking balance.

A third set of casts was made to accommodate growth and, by May 1972, Shelley was taking slow, controlled independent steps in the bivalved casts. At this time she was fitted with bilateral double Becker short-leg braces to provide needed ankle stability, and she became fully ambulatory in July of that year.[1] When she was 7 years old, an open heelcord lengthening was done to improve a "rockerbottom" foot position, and she remained involved in an active therapy program throughout her school years. Shelley has now graduated from high school. She has remained active, busy, and independently ambulatory without aid.

After this initial casting experience, we remained cautious and puzzled about the results, and tried casting several other children in our therapy clinic population whose tone had been difficult to manage with therapy alone. During this period, the support of Lynn Stahlie, M.D., the head of orthopedics at Children's Orthopedic Hospital and Medical Center in Seattle and the orthopedic consultant at Children's Clinic and Preschool, was very helpful. His primary interest was in the rapid improvement in dynamic foot and ankle deformities seen with the casting. Our primary interest and motivation were in the global tone changes and the greater possibilities to work actively in therapy, less impeded by moderate or severe hypertonus.

Results in successive subjects were strikingly similar. When hypertonus was controlled before and during application of casts, sustained global inhibition of hypertonus continued while the casts were on. When the casts were bivalved, usually after 4 to 5 weeks, a certain percentage of tone control was lost. This loss of control varied from child to child, but inhibition of tone was maintained with 75 to 95% effectiveness in the bivalved casts. We speculated that the decrease in effectiveness of the bivalves was related to looser fit, or perhaps to something in the fabrication process.

In addition to global tone reduction, more rapid motor gains in therapy, and better carryover of newly developing balance and skills outside of therapy, another typical result of casting became apparent. Many children with a history of very slow foot growth before casting showed rapid foot growth initially in the casts (as much as ½ to ¾ of an inch in 3 to 6 months). The growth rate tapered off with successive casting, but the feet continued to grow at a fairly typical rate for the children's ages. We speculated that this phenomenon could be related to improved circulation and nutrition along with improved muscle tonus, more normal muscle activity, and improved weight-bearing position. Although we have continued to observe this phenomenon, it does not yet have a full explanation.

We were excited about developing casting further as a useful therapy technique because we observed the following changes in all of the children we casted:

1. Marked reduction in associated reactions in both the feet and other parts of the body, both while the casts were on and for varying lengths of time with casts removed.
2. A progressive reduction in hypertonus while the casts were being applied.
3. Inhibition of hypertonus throughout the legs and hips, also affecting the trunk and arms while the casts were on; varying degrees of carry-over of tone control when the casts were removed.
4. Increased freedom of the children to move in all situations, especially in the upright position. Increased variety and quality of movements seen; more normal movement and postural control (i.e., balancing, weight-shifting) when the children were moving on their own, uncontrolled.
5. A decrease in fear and an increase in confidence.

During this period, we gained confidence that we had stumbled onto a general phenomenon, rather than an effect that was isolated to only a few children with cerebral palsy. We continued to try the casting cautiously with different types of cerebral palsy. We had some very frustrating and unpredictable results with athetoid and mixed-athetoid involvement and avoided casting those children for several years. We cautiously shared the information with the

Washington State group of pediatric therapists in the fall of 1973 and wrote an article, "Casting Used as an Adjunct to NDT," which was published in the Bobath Alumni Newsletter that same year.[1] With this information, others began to explore. Someone coined the term "inhibitive casting" which I used although I never really liked it.

Continual problems with plaster breakdown, especially at the toes, led to development of a plywood footboard system by a group of therapists at Good Samaritan Hospital in Puyallup, south of Seattle. Contoured support and inhibition could be designed into the footboard at a time separate from the time of casting. The actual casting time was shortened because of less need for reinforcement around the toes and base. It was hoped that this system would also provide more exact control of the foot. Therapists at the Children's Therapy Unit at Good Samaritan, with the support and supervision of Donald Mott, M.D., orthopedist, began to do a great deal of inhibitive casting as a part of their therapy program.

Donald Mott, M.D., Linda Yates, O.T.R., and John T. Chapman, M.D. made a special presentation to the American Academy of Cerebral Palsy and Developmental Medicine in Boston in 1980 detailing inhibitive casting as a part of an active neurodevelopmental treatment (NDT)-oriented therapy program.[2] Pretesting measurement was done with Dr. Bleck's *Locomotor Prognosis in Cerebral Palsy* scale, and the outcome was measured in functional motor skills. The study noted dramatic improvement in functional motor skills, and attainment of independent free ambulation in a number of children who had a very poor prognosis for ambulation precasting. In their article, "Foot Reflexes and the Use of the 'Inhibitive Cast'," Drs. William Duncan and Donald Mott outline a possible neurophysiologic explanation for the inhibitory effect and describe the results in 111 children with cerebral palsy who had inhibitive casting as a part of their therapy protocol between 1975 and 1978. Of 86 children who were considered to have poor prognosis for ambulation, 60% became independent free ambulators within the time frame of the study. Thirty-three percent of spastic quadriplegic children became independent free

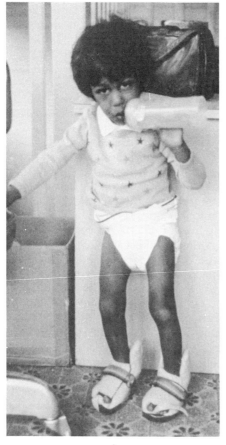

A

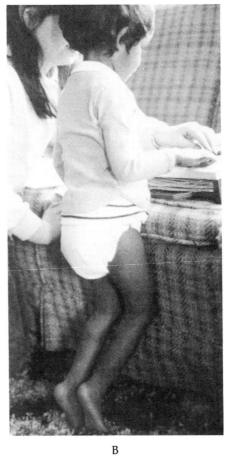

B

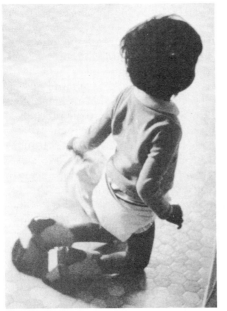

C

FIG. 9–1. Boy with severe spastic diplegia. A, Standing. B, Standing without casts. C, Kneeling with casts.

ambulators.[3] Other investigators in different parts of the country were beginning to report improved therapeutic results from inhibitive casting techniques.[4]

While, in most other parts of the country, short-leg, fixed 90-degree ankle casts were the typical style for "inhibitive" casts, the beginning development of ankle height inhibitive casts was occurring in the mid to late 70s in the Seattle area. Supramalleolar inhibitive casts allowed ankle movement in either dorsi or plantar flexion or both while providing secure medial-lateral support to the foot and ankle in a neutral position. In the beginning, these were used to provide some continued tone control in ambulatory children with milder hypertonus, but they have gradually become the standard style of cast in this area, even for children with very severe hypertonus (Fig. 9–1A and C).

The key to maintaining good tone control while allowing more freedom of ankle movement has been in the refinement of the footboard contouring. Initially, there were slightly recessed areas under the metatarsal heads and the calcaneus with buildup to support under the medial-longitudinal arch and under the toes. For a severely pronating foot, there was buildup under the 1st metatarsal head to inhibit the downward pressure. For the supinating foot, there was buildup under the 5th metatarsal head and under the entire lateral border to counteract increased downward pressure.

The routed recessed areas became larger to allow the entire metatarsal head pad area and calcaneus pad to rest in a recessed "nest." Some significant tone reduction came from simply placing the foot on the routed footboard. The drive to make it better and more exact fueled intuitive curiosity, as did the real feedback from patients' bodies. The puzzle and questions continued and so did delightful contributions and accidents from unlikely sources. The importance of the metatarsal arch was learned from an unnamed shoe repairman, who stopped for a few minutes to share some of his wisdom with a curious therapist. Curiosity won out over skepticism, and I discovered that a little "bump," supporting just behind the metatarsal heads in the center of the forefoot, made a tremendous difference in tone control and forefoot alignment for some children. With this support, the toes did not need to be dorsiflexed above horizontal to gain tone control. Toes could become more active in balancing. The need for buildup under the first or fifth metatarsal for varus and valgus control could be greatly reduced or eliminated with even better tone control!

While casting a little boy in 1984, I decided to try buildup under the peroneal notch (under the lateral border between the base of the fifth metatarsal and calcaneus) to see if his severely pronated foot would relax even more. To my surprise it did, but I was sure that this was a fluke. Curiosity made me mention this to a group of therapists in a casting workshop practicum in the spring of 1984. The room was full of patients whose feet were very similar to those of the little boy whom I had casted. I suggested that therapists try the same plaster buildup under the peroneal notch and observe for any change in tone. Until this point, upward pressure under the peroneal notch was considered an inhibitive force that worked well to control forceful supination. To our perplexity and surprise, with support under the peroneal notch, each of the stiffly pronated feet of the patients in the room settled more softly into the support of the footboard. We had expected increased eversion because of the "foot reflexes"; what happened was just the opposite. Later I was to learn about the importance of midline control of the subtalar joint, and it would make more sense.

A name change occurred that same spring when, on the way to the Austin Airport, a therapist from the casting course just completed said to me, "This is DYNAMIC CASTING!" The term "inhibitive casting" was replaced by "dynamic casting and orthotics" from that day.

The most recent developments and refinements in this technique have been in the area of orthotics. Early inhibitive orthotics were used and developed at the Children's Therapy Unit at Good Samaritan Medical Center in Puyallup and at Children's Therapy Center in Kent in the late 1970s. At first they were short-leg AFOs with inhibition contouring built into the soleplate. Later the idea of allowing some ankle movement, which had proved successful with casts, was transferred to inhibitive orthotics. The first ankle-height AFOs had fixed 90-degree posterior stops that extended 2 to 3 inches above the malleoli, allowing ankle movement into dorsiflexion. The specific anatomic locations of the top and edges of the AFOs, or trimlines, became lower and more circumferential. Fairly soon it became common to trim the back down to allow some plantarflexion. Soleplate control had made equinus much less of a problem. AFOs were pulled thinner and thinner, with increasing success.

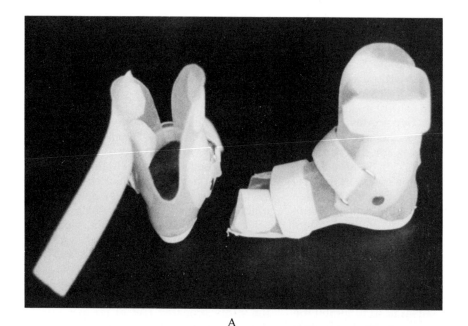

A

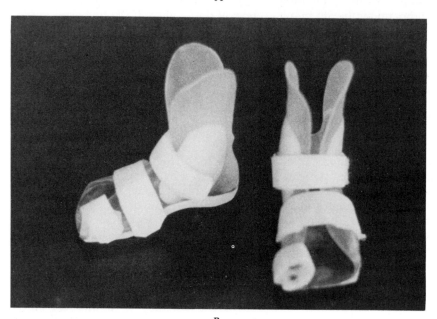

B

FIG. 9–2. A and B. Dynamic AFOs showing placement of straps.

The thinner and more circumferential they were, the more easily they were tolerated by children with severe tone problems. Placement of straps to hold the heel securely down and in the splint was critical, as was placement of straps at the forefoot to stabilize the hallicus (Fig. 9–2A and B). By the early 1980s, dynamic AFOs were so thin and flexible that they could be easily twisted in one's hands. They proved easy for patients or their parents to put on. Children and adult patients adjusted to them quickly, and many times children did not want to take them off. Growth accommodation for children was 6 months to a year. The need for new orthotics was made clear by statements of discomfort or of decreasing tone control.

In the mid-1980s we began experimenting with even lower trimlines in children who had gained sufficient balance and voluntary control to no longer need support across the ankle joint. The new dynamic foot orthoses (FOs) (Fig. 9–3D and E) gained popularity quickly at our center because they allowed a smoother transition toward no orthotic support at all.

At the present time, trimlines for dynamic AFOs (DAFOs) or casts vary considerably, based on the specific needs of the individual (Fig. 9–3A through E). Most commonly used trimlines are (A), standard supramalleolar AFO allowing plantarflexion and dorsiflexion while providing secure medial-lateral ankle/forefoot control, and (D), standard dynamic FO, which typically has a flexible pelite extension under the toes and plastic extended forward to the metatarsalphalangeal joints. Though we rarely use standard short-leg trimlines, except in braces specifically designed for a floor reaction lever arm for knee extension, (B) with a plantarflexion stop can be used in patients with constant moderate to severe equinus. In adults post-CVA or head injury with difficult-to-control equinus, the posterior shell is often extended up to mid-calf height, and can be gradually trimmed down as equinus becomes more controlled. In children, a posterior shell extended 2 to 3 inches above the malleoli is effective in controlling moderate to severe equinus. Low-profile floor-reaction options, (e.g., C), have proven useful in individuals needing

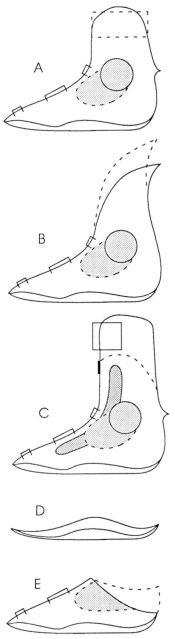

FIG. 9–3. A through E. Dynamic orthoses. See text for discussion.

a slight knee-extension assist, in patients with over-lengthened heelcords, or in low level (L-5, S-1) spina bifida where plantarflexion is weak or nonfunctional. Free plantarflexion is allowed to facilitate more movement options at the knee and hip. When significant floor-reaction forces are required, thicker plastic and/or carbon fiber reinforcement across the ankle is used to prevent buckling of the AFO across the forefoot. A maximum control dynamic FO (E) can be used where more secure forefoot stabilization and control are required. The polypropylene is pulled extremely thin and is flexible in most cases. DAFOs are volume-critical orthotics (exact volume of the patient's foot/ankle plus a thin sock is the exact volume of the inside of the DAFO) that require precise molding and fitting to

work well. There can be no extra room for movement of the foot and no extra relief, especially at the heel, or malleolus, within the brace. A D-ring, 45-degree Velcro ankle strap is fastened snugly to maintain exact heel position within the brace. A comparison of AFOs in standard use (Table 9–1) provides a composite view of various factors of AFO support and control.

Standard short-leg AFOs of ⅛ to ¼″ thick polypropylene are used commonly in an attempt to control equinus in the adult and

TABLE 9–1. COMPARISON OF AFOS IN STANDARD USE

Standard AFO	TRAFO	Dynamic AFO	Neurophysiologic AFO (See Reference 15)
ARCHES:			
Some minimal support, medial-longitudinal arch often present.	Subtalar neutral produces natural arch contours.	Support of natural arch systems provides control at and around subtalar neutral and neutral forefoot.	Metatarsal arch
ANKLE:			
Position: Fixed at 90 degrees or some dorsiflexion or plantar flexion. Could have jointed ankle, but not commonly.	Fixed at 90 degrees or jointed, allowing dorsiflexion.	Midline medial-lateral ankle support; movement available plantar and dorsiflexion and inversion/eversion along ankle axis. Possible to limit plantar and/or dorsiflexion with velcro strap.	Three-point pressure system to control calcaneovarus. Lateral ankle stabilization. Free dorsiflexion and plantarflexion along ankle axis. Dorsiflexion can be graded by widening plantar surface.
TOES:			
Often not supported at all. Trimline to metatarsal heads (usually).	Supported: sometimes hyperextension is used to inhibit tone– moderate extension of proximal phalanx, slight flexion of middle phalanx is preferred.	Supported horizontal from MP joint to allow active balancing (MP flexion and extension.)	Use of metatarsal arch to unweight the heads and thereby inhibit toe grasp.
BIOMECHANICS:			
Three-point pressure system controls movement. Neutral alignment; heel and toe lever arms produce abnormal knee/hip forces.	Subtalar neutral with fixed ankle lever arms or jointed ankle for some movement.	Subtalar neutral with active plantarflexion/ dorsiflexion possible movement around normal ankle axis; stabilizing inversion/ eversion provides grading for plantar/ dorsiflexion (triplane joint effect).	Subtalar, midfoot, and forefoot neutral. Medial trimlines distal and posterior to malleolus to counterbalance and prevent excessive pronation and rotation of orthosis in shoe. Lateral trimline as far anterior as possible to facilitate eversion and recruit more proximal control.
BALANCE POSSIBILITIES:			
Blocks plantar/ dorsiflexion unless free ankle.	Jointed ankle allows some balance in plantarflexion and dorsiflexion. Fixed ankle does not.	Allows balance reactions at ankle and in foot. Toe strap stabilizes hallux. 45-degree ankle strap holds heel down and in neutral.	Free ankle allows balance in plantarflexion and dorsiflexion. Eversion facilitation attempts to override inversion.

child neurologic patient. These usually have an anterior tibial band at the top and are designed to be held to the foot by the patient's shoe. TRAFOs, or tone-reducing AFOs, are a short-leg inhibitive type of orthotic commonly fabricated of fiberglass casting tape or rigid polypropylene, and are used to control extensor tone, most often in children with spastic CP. The foot and lower leg are strapped securely into the orthosis, which may or may not require a shoe for street wear. The neurophysiologic AFO is a relative "newcomer" developed to help control the strong inversion tone in many adult neurologic patients. It can be fabricated relatively easily, directly on the patient, of low temperature plastics (e.g., aquaplast or orthoplast) and is a spiral stirrup designed to provide neutral calcaneal support and upward pressure under the metatarsal arch and lateral border of the foot. The flexibility of fabrication materials permits movement into plantarflexion and dorsiflexion while providing a measure of inversion and equinus control. The dynamic AFOs described above are circumferential supramalleolar orthotics constructed of thin polypropylene.

THERAPEUTIC ASSESSMENT FOR DYNAMIC CASTING

Because most of my 20 years of clinical experience have been with pediatric cerebral palsy (CP) patients, the information and focus in this section will reflect and draw upon that experience. I have had considerable contact with other pediatric and adult disabilities through my teaching, treatment, and consultation experiences. My close professional association with therapists treating primarily adult neurologic patients is also drawn upon when more general therapeutic comments are needed. Although there are specific differences within the realm of varying neurologic disabilities, there is also much common ground in therapeutic assessment, especially in the area of tone management.

To understand the rationale and development of the use of dynamic casting and orthotics, it is important to look at the significance of midline control (secure graded control of the body or any of its parts in and around neutral range) and stability (or lack of it) in cerebral palsy or other neurologically impaired individuals. Whether the motor control problem is mild or severe, the basic underlying similarity is a difficulty with stable and graded postural control. This lack of normal postural stabilization, which is a critical component of balance and all volitional movements, causes abnormal adaptive responses within the CNS, including hypertonus and tone fluctuations. Hypotonia, which is often seen, especially in the trunk, is an example of the primary instability within the postural control system. Individuals with cerebral palsy or head injury share the problem of lack of control of movement and posture. The maintenance or appearance of primitive or abnormal reflexes is directly related to this lack of postural control and stabilization.

"Biomechanical neutral" is a term I learned in November of 1982 while attending a fascinating course on normal and abnormal foot biomechanics. The course title was "When the Foot Hits the Ground, Everything Changes,"[5] (Fig. 9–4), and I had certainly found this to be true in my experience with neurologically impaired children and adults. Biomechanical neutral, the point from which maximum functional movement can occur in all directions relative to any joint or part of the body, seemed connected to the NDT concept of "midline." I puzzled over the information presented in that course and how it correlated with our experiences with the dynamic casting and orthotics and with therapy itself.

The dramatic importance of subtalar joint stability in and around its neutral position made sense as the weight-bearing chain reaction effect was seen on the forefoot, calcaneus, tibia, and knee in subtalar pronation and supination (Fig. 9–4). As you can see in A, with subtalar pronation the forefoot pronates and everts, becoming more mobile and less stable, the calcaneus everts, the talus adducts and plantarflexes, and internal rotation of the tibia causes a mandatory knee flexion in the last few degrees of knee extension. With subtalar supination in B, the forefoot supinates and inverts, becoming less mobile and more stable to pro-

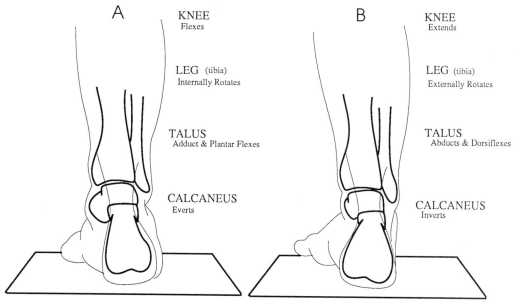

FIG. 9-4. A, Subtalar pronation. B, Subtalar supination. See text for discussion.

vide greater efficiency and stability for propulsion. At the same time, the calcaneus inverts, the talus abducts and dorsiflexes, and the tibia externally rotates, facilitating knee extension. The way in which the foot functions normally as a "mobile adapter" and "shock absorber" in subtalar pronation at heel strike and the way in which it functions as a "rigid lever" in push-off in subtalar neutral and supination began to take some of the mystique out of so-called "abnormal patterns of movement" and weight bearing in CP. In normal walking during a 0.6 second weight-bearing cycle, the subtalar joint moves smoothly through 7 degrees of movement, from supination at heel strike to pronation (shock absorption) at foot flat to resupination at push-off. The normal range for the subtalar joint is 20 to 25 degrees of movement, with the movement needed for normal gait being about 7 degrees of combined pronation and supination close around the subtalar joint biomechanical neutral or "midline" position. Subtalar joint neutral can be palpated in adults as the "midline" or balanced position of the talus just underneath the ankle joint. Being able to smoothly grade, stabilize, and control movement of this joint appears critical for any hope of normal up-

right balance and gait function. It requires a degree of refinement of movement and postural control similar to a fine pincer grasp of a pen while writing.

The problem of "midline" stability or control around biomechanical neutral and the impact on efficiency of balance and postural control in upright with even slight neurologic impairments becomes obvious. Add to this the indication that movement, postural control, and even joint organization favor the greatest efficiency of movement around "biomechanical neutral" or in "midline" ranges, and the problem for neurologically impaired individuals compounds itself. Find a way to externally provide stability and control to the subtalar joint around neutral, and to give "neutral" support to the dynamic arching systems of the foot without immobilizing the ankle, and you help the entire system to regain tremendous biomechanical and postural stability and control.

The terms and understandings presented gave words and explanations to some of the unexplainable clinical phenomena we had experienced. Through our exacting plaster footboard contouring, we had discovered "subtalar neutral" without knowing what it was. Now it appeared that the exact point at which tone became most "normal" in the CP foot was "subtalar neutral," the point at which the talus "slipped into place" and one felt a slight give of soft tissue when palpating the medial aspect of the foot. So biomechanical neutral, at least in the foot, appears to be connected to tone control and stability in our experience.

This wonderful introduction to biomechanics helped us to look critically at the placement of inhibitive and controlling "bumps" of plaster that formed the contour of our footboards. Out of that information has come the most recent explanation of why the footboard contouring is so important and how it works. Dynamic arches of the foot are seen most prominently when extra stability and balance are needed for difficult upright skills, but they are probably functioning continuously as a part of our postural control system in the upright position. They are the areas of the undersurface and sides of the foot that "lift up" through soft tissue and joint mechanisms to provide dynamic stability and improved postural feedback from the supporting surface. The person who invented Birkenstock sandals discovered this while staring at human footprints in the sand. Years ago, a good friend had mentioned the footboards' similarity to Birkenstock contouring, but it was much later that the connection was understood.

Walking in sand is difficult. We must accentuate postural control to do it well, thus dynamic arch systems are more active and apparent. Why do people experience such an attachment to Birkenstock sandals? Why do they comment without exception that their feet are more comfortable, even after hours of standing and walking all day? Dynamic arches of the foot affect our dynamic foot and ankle control and the ease and efficiency with which we are able to balance and move on our feet. When we need them, a combination of long and intrinsic foot muscles and other soft tissue and bony structures work together to simultaneously lift certain areas on the sole of the foot in weight bearing. These areas, which include the medial-longitudinal arch, the metatarsal arch, the peroneal notch area, and the space under the toes directly distal to the metatarsal heads, in CP are typically either completely flattened to the ground or tightly held up away from the ground and non-functional. Examples are the classic "rockerbottom" or equinovarus foot deformity (Figs. 9–5A and B and 9–6A and B). Even in mild neuromotor impairment, there is no graded and smooth simultaneous control of these systems. Without these systems functioning to provide a stable and balanced base, all more proximal motor control is affected negatively.

Inhibition, it seems, is a secondary rather than a primary phenomenon. It occurs because of balanced secure support under the dynamic arch systems and stable midline forefoot, subtalar, and ankle control. When dynamic arches are securely supported, the biomechanics of foot position and function change dramatically. Abnormal neurologic control can cause abnormal biomechanics, which then cause abnormal wear and tear on joints and soft tissue structures. In my experience, it is common for adults with CP to have early onset of joint problems and osteoarthritic symptoms. Our hope is that, by providing for more normal biomechanics and foot/ankle function, we can minimize future problems.

CHILDREN

The effect of global tone change and improved variety and control of movement proved to be the motivating factor in the continued development and refinement of dynamic casting and orthotics. We can still only speculate as to why this occurs, even though it is clearly a repeatable and long-standing clinical phenomenon. Drs. Duncan and Mott refer to the control of "superficial foot reflexes," reflex support, and righting reactions that are normal to infants, and "recruitment which can be seen at the knees and hips" as an explanation. "In many cerebral palsy children, one or more of these reflexes may persist as an increasing active hypertonic movement in response to superficial stimulation. Habitual reflex-induced deformities of the foot may become fixed, and proximal cocontracting musculature may become hypertonic, creating balance problems."[3] Although this

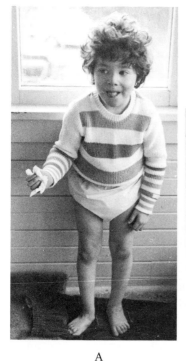
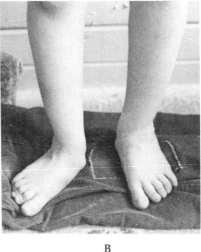
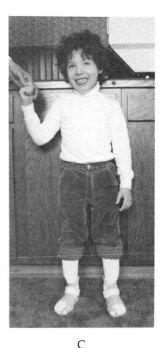

A   B   C

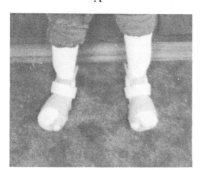

FIG. 9–5. Boy with spastic diplegia. A and B, Equinovarus foot deformity without dynamic AFOs. C and D, Patient wearing AFOs.

D

may be a partial explanation, it would predict that pressure under the peroneal notch should increase a tonic eversion response. Instead, in our experience, it has caused a decrease in tonic eversion when used with other contouring.

In ambulatory or preambulatory patients, an abnormal positive support response frequently is seen leading to increased extensor hypertonus throughout the lower extremities (Fig. 9–6A and B). As these children are more upright, often the extensor tone becomes much stronger and less controlled. A pattern of increasing dynamic deformity that is more and more resistant to change is commonly seen, leading to fixed

deformity. The abnormal posturing out of a midline control position and the related ankle and forefoot instability affect balance and movement control throughout the body. The use of dynamic casting and orthotics as a part of therapy management in these children has helped to bring the flexor and extensor hypertonus under control, greatly reducing the problem of increasing foot/ankle deformity and allowing more rapid acquisition of controlled balance and upright skills (see Fig. 9–6). Children with primary hypotonia and resultant foot/ankle instability also show improved therapeutic results with this system.

In assessing the potential usefulness of

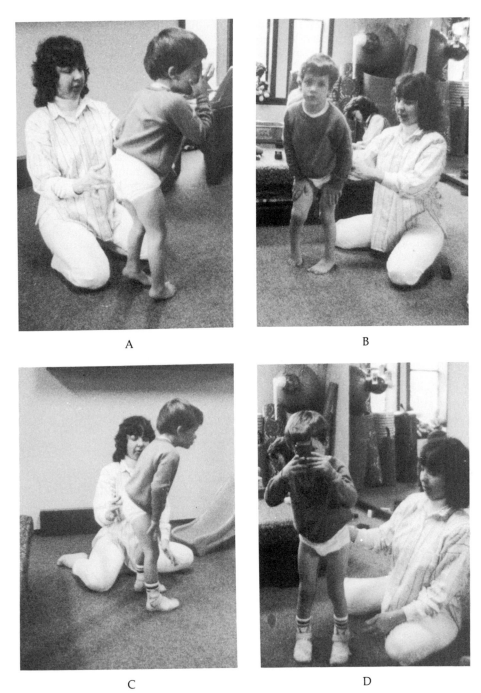

FIG. 9–6. Boy with spastic diplegia. A, Side view and B, Anterior view without dynamic casting. C, Side view and D, Anterior view with dynamic casting.

this technique with any given individual, numerous other factors must be taken into account. In a therapy situation, it is often possible to assess the impact of stabilization or pressure to certain areas of the foot on tone in the knees, hips, and trunk. Tone changes seen consistently in this situation predict a good result from more prolonged control. Sensory tolerance to tactile and deep pressure input must also be carefully assessed. Hypersensitivity in these areas often accompanies motor control problems and can accentuate the hypertonic response to weight bearing. In some cases, patients are unable to tolerate the footboard process. A period focused on desensitizing, molding with another individual's close-fitting footboard, or making the cast or mold without a footboard are all possible options. We

have found that the use of these casts or orthotics tends to decrease hypersensitivity to deep pressure stimulation. Also, a few individuals have required a longer initial adjustment phase because of hypersensitivity. We have yet to see a child or adult able to tolerate the process of casting or molding who was unable to adjust comfortably to extended wear within 1 to 2 weeks.

Dynamic casts and orthotics can cause dramatic changes in tone and therefore affect the proprioceptive feedback systems in children. If children have been moving primarily using hypertonus, they may be unable to figure out how to move with casts on (see Chapter 4). This posed much more of a problem with fixed ankle casts, which were not bivalved for several weeks. Immediate bivalving and allowance of some

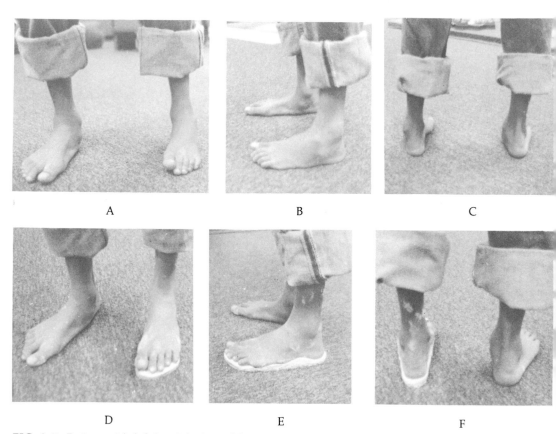

A   B   C

D   E   F

FIG. 9–7. Patient with left hemiplegia and biomechanical forefoot valgus/plantarflexed 1st ray. A, Anterior view before casting. B, Side view before casting. C, Posterior view before casting. D, Anterior view with footboard. E, Side view with footboard. F, Posterior view with footboard.

ankle movement permits a more gradual adjustment period and less fear in these children. The reactions to casting must be carefully assessed and caring support given when dramatic tone and sensory changes are experienced.

Finally, an assessment must look carefully at the ability of the dynamic arch systems and balancing to work together in a smoothly controlled way. Sometimes, even in very mildly affected individuals, dynamic arches and balance are not smoothly controlled, making more complex balancing skills difficult or impossible. Even the tendency to curl the toes whenever balance is challenged can block the normal weight-shifting and trunk adjustments necessary to maintain control. We have found that use of dynamic FOs in these cases allows greater ease with balance and control, and development of one-leg standing, hopping, skipping and balance beam skills (see Fig. 9–3D).

Biomechanical misalignments, which may be familial or developmental, can also affect the severity of a foot deformity seen in individuals with neuromuscular problems. Most of us have seen patients whose feet looked much worse than the rest of their bodies. They generally have a combination of tone control and biomechanical problems. Forefoot varus can accentuate an already existing pronation problem. Forefoot valgus can accentuate an equinovarus foot deformity. The boy in Figure 9–7 demonstrates continued difficulties with supination and lateral foot/ankle instability even after corrective tibialis posterior transfer surgery to improve equinus. Increased calcaneo/varum and tibio/varum are commonly seen developmental alignment problems that must be compensated for in the casting process. The bottom of the footboard is made perpendicular to a neutral weight-bearing line taken from midpoint between femoral condyles to midpoint between malleoli (Fig. 9–8). This essentially builds an intrinsic biomechanical rearfoot varus post into the orthotic and allows the calcaneus to remain vertical to the ground. Many hypotonic children have an increased posterior pitch to the ankle axis, which makes the joint mechanically much less stable.

A four-year-old girl with cerebral palsy, specifically a mild to moderate right hemiplegia, demonstrates the combination of these factors well. When referred for a consultation, she had a persistent problem with equinus and varus on the right, even though hand use had shown good improvement. She could even stand and balance momentarily over her right leg, but lost control when she started to walk or run. Passively ankle dorsiflexion was limited to 5 degrees above neutral, and her forefoot was stiff. When tone was reduced through slow stretch and deep pressure, instability and forefoot hypermobility were present. She also had a 10-degree forefoot valgus with a plantarflexed first ray bilaterally. When she was molded for a DAFO, an additional ⅛-inch depth was routed under the first metatarsal head to partially

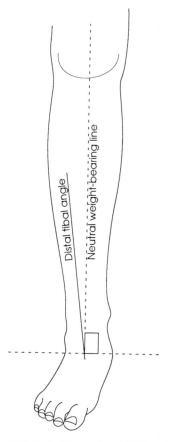

FIG. 9–8. Neutral weight-bearing line. See text for discussion.

accommodate for the biomechanical forefoot valgus/plantarflexed first ray problem.
External posting (an external build-up
under 2 through 5) on the bottom of the
DAFO was used to adjust for forefoot valgus. In the new orthotic, she was immediately more stable, her tendency to equinus
and varus corrected completely when she
was weight-bearing on the right, and she
was able to stand and balance for several
seconds over that leg.

The 9-year-old boy with left spastic
hemiparesis in Figure 9–7A, B, and C demonstrates a similar biomechanical forefoot
valgus/plantarflexed first ray problem
which persists in causing lateral foot/ankle
instability and increased tone problems with
supination even 1 year after a posterior tibialis transfer surgery to correct his equinovarus foot deformity. His right foot demonstrates a compensatory pronation pattern
which has developed through hypermobility in the midfoot to gain added stability in
weight bearing. Biomechanical forefoot valgus posting, as well as support to dynamic
arches, changes weight-bearing alignment
and stability dramatically (see Fig. 9–7 D
through F, standing on footboard). In this
situation, the use of a dynamic FO with biomechanical posting provided good tone
control and stable weight bearing over the
left leg in walking, running, and other upright activities.

In our experience, the use of dynamic
casts and orthotics is not limited to individuals who are potentially ambulatory. Improved tone control, symmetry, head/
shoulder/trunk/hip control in supported
sitting, standing and other positions has
been noted in each case with their use in
the very severely involved. Typically, we
use ankle height trimlines and allow ankle
movement to occur even with severe
equinus. The use of a removable posterior
Velcro strap to provide some plantarflexion
control is common (see Fig. 9–2A) and tolerance, even in some children who have
been unable to tolerate shoes of any kind,
has been good.

The tendency for dynamic tone patterns
to lead to dynamic deformities and later to
fixed deformities is usually more prominent
in severely affected individuals. This pro-

gression can lead to extreme difficulties
with positioning in sitting or supported
standing and later to difficulties even with
basic hygiene. Because global tone reduction from dynamic casting and orthotics is
seen even in non-weight-bearing positions,
their use can minimize these problems. Associated foot deformities can be prevented
and sometimes corrected with this technique, allowing supported standing and assisted transfers.

In situations where there is marked hypersensitivity to touch and pressure on the
feet, the use of adapted inhibitive shoes
(Fig. 9–9) is much less restrictive and more
easily tolerated as an initial step toward dynamic orthotics. These adapted shoes rely
on the same soleplate contouring for control and stabilization, but soft padding material such as aliplast or pelite are used instead of plaster. The toe of the shoe is cut
out and the tongue cut on one side to allow
easy application and removal. D-ring Velcro straps hold the heel and forefoot securely down in the shoe. A stabilizing strap
for the hallicus usually improves tone control. Such a pair of adapted tennis shoes
was fabricated for a 13-year-old girl with
severe dystonic athetoid quadriplegia. Before the use of these shoes, she had been
unable to tolerate shoes of any kind. To the
surprise of her mother and all therapists involved, she was able to adjust to wearing
the shoes all day within a few days, with
improved tone control and stability seen
throughout her body. Within six months,
she was ready for fabrication of standard
DAFOs with a full ⅛″ aliplast liner.

This kind of adapted shoe is also a useful
inexpensive problem-solving tool in determining the potential effectiveness of dynamic AFOs. Sensory difficulties and
changes in proprioception, mentioned before, can be even more dramatic in individuals with severe motor and tone disturbances. They should be carefully assessed
and acknowledged in all cases. In our experience, global tone changes produced by
adapted shoes, casting, or orthotics have
improved symmetry and the ease of symmetric positioning, arm function, and oral
motor and feeding possibilities, as well as
decreased abnormal tone, i.e., adduction,

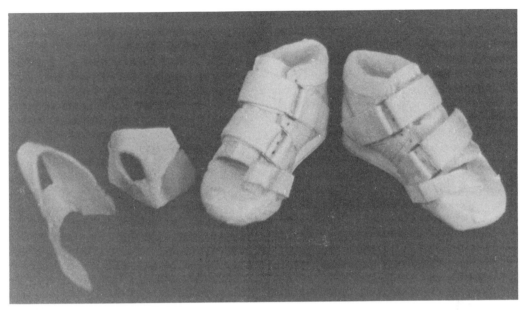

FIG. 9-9. Adapted inhibitive shoes.

knee flexion, and plantarflexion, even in individuals with moderate to severe hypertonus and very limited independent function.

An example of a fairly typical child in whom the use of dynamic AFOs has been very helpful is a 9-year-old with severe mixed athetoid-spastic quadriplegia. When first seen at age 5 years, he was unable to control any movement in his body and even to lie comfortably on the floor without total flexor spasm or flying into total rigid extension. He brought with him a pair of fixed ankle "inhibitive" casts, which were very difficult to put on and were to be worn only in sitting and standing. My first chore was to cut the casts down so that his ankles could move into plantarflexion and dorsiflexion. He immediately tolerated them better, and still got improved tone control from them. I could work with bouncing him on my lap and stimulating improved trunk co-contraction and stability, and his opisthotonic posturing started to decrease. These casts were replaced with standard ankle-high dynamic AFOs within a month, with no plantar or dorsiflexion control. Those have now been replaced for growth several times, with the following functional improvements seen:

1. He now enjoys lying softly on the floor and can independently roll from back to stomach and stomach to back.
2. The wheelchair headrest and arm retraction supports are no longer needed and have been permanently removed.
3. He is beginning to develop independent long-sitting when tone is prepared.
4. He is able to work actively, sitting on a therapy ball, with shoulder/trunk/hip control, supported only at the knees.
5. He is actively involved in a therapeutic pony-riding program.
6. He can stand softly with slight support at the shoulders, and is learning control in going slowly up to standing and down to sitting with support at shoulders or arms.
7. He has achieved facilitated walking with control at the shoulders.

Progress has been slow and steady with excellent therapy follow-through at home, and he is continuing to learn greater control over his tone and movements.

ADULTS

Although I have much less experience with casting adults with cerebral palsy, CVA, or closed head injury, the effects on improved tone control and movement appear to be quite similar, with the following specific differences. In a post-CVA case with a marked sensory deficit (i.e., total anesthesia from the knee down), global tone reduction into the trunk and arm was not seen as clearly, even though excellent control of moderate to severe extensor tone and a severely supinated foot position was obtained. Before use of the dynamic AFO (with a posterior shell, extended to mid-calf height), partial foot/ankle control had been obtained by a double metal upright with a lateral T-strap. AFO molding was done 10 years post-stroke, and the patient began to take three-mile walks with maintained neutral foot/ankle position and extensor tone control. Usually, when there is a strong equinus component to tone and significantly decreased sensation, a fixed plantarflexion stop extended several inches above the malleoli is necessary to achieve tone control. This was the case with this particular individual, who needed to be able to go into a few degrees of knee hyperextension to securely stabilize his knee.

There is typically a much stronger toe curling and forefoot component in hypertonus in adults after stroke. With careful attention to placement of support under the metatarsal arch and the toes, I have watched a foot "grow" in length ¼ to ½ inch and heard comments about sensory and blood flow changes as this was happening. This, of course, was not true growth, but rather a release of forefoot spasticity, which had caused the relative shortening in the first place. When sensation has been more intact, spontaneous tone changes and movement in the affected upper extremity have also been observed.

An unusual adult example is a man whom I first met 7 years after his stroke. He was middle-aged and active, the husband of a local pediatric therapist. He had fairly intact sensation, moderate to severe spasticity, and limited volitional motor control on the right side. He walked with a cane

and informed me that his "midline" was halfway between his cane and left leg. By this he meant that, because of marked instability over the right side, his functional center of gravity was somewhere between his cane and his left leg. During the footboardmaking process, he enjoyed the sensation of tone reduction, especially in his toes, and showed spontaneous active right forearm supination during the casting for the AFO mold.

When I saw him several months later, he shared with me a diary account of his experience with tone and other changes after he began to wear the dynamic AFO. His AFO provided medial-lateral control to just above the malleoli and allowed free movement in plantarflexion and dorsiflexion. The following are his experiences.

"Week 1:   Decrease in pain and tone; increase in stability (lower extremity)
Week 2:   Same as week 1
Week 3:   Same as week 1
Week 4:   Decrease in pain and tone; nausea; midline shift (shift in functional center of gravity)
Week 5:   Same as week 4
Week 6:   Decrease in pain and tone; decrease in stability (lower extremity); marked decrease in upper extremity tone.
Week 7:   Same as week 6
Week 8:   Increase in fine motor ability because of decreased tone; better range of motion (upper extremity)"

10/29/86 "At the present time I feel the need of therapy to regain musculature (motor control) and regain or increase stability of lower extremity and gain usage of right arm."

Functional gains also noted:

Week 2:   Raise hand above head
2nd month: Hold coffee cup in right hand and drink coffee without spilling
10/15/86:   Trim nails using right hand
10/25/86:   Active right wrist supination

General: Decreased need for spinal manipulation; increased ability to walk on uneven surfaces.[6]

He had stopped using a cane indoors, and was beginning to venture outside without his cane as well. He was delighted with the orthotic changes and those in motor function. Though he is not typical, his history is helpful in showing the possibility for functional change long after a stroke.

EXPECTATIONS FOR PROGRESS

The use of dynamic casts and AFOs has dramatically altered our expectations of therapy progress. In many cases, this has happened as a part of an ongoing assessment of each person's response without our being especially conscious of the process. Among *immediate anticipated outcomes* are decrease in hypertonus and improved stability and control of movement through the body. *Long-term anticipated outcomes* would include more rapid development of balance and control in all positions, especially upright; increased foot/ankle mobility; improved volitional control of isolated leg movements, e.g., knee extension, hip abduction, hip extension (see Fig. 9–5A through D and 9–6A through D); gradually less need for orthotic control as volitional control and balance improve.

The process of weaning individuals into and out of orthotic control is a complex one. Dramatic sensory and "body image" proprioceptive changes are fairly common and require considerable care and sensitivity (see Chapter 4). Though children are usually unable to verbalize what is happening to them, behavioral changes can help us understand what they are dealing with. A 2½-year-old girl with a mixed spastic/athetoid quadriplegia fussed as her new DAFOs were first put on. They obviously felt strange and made her body "feel strange." Within 2 days, her mother reported that she didn't want to take them off at bedtime. An adult with moderate spastic diplegia commented during the molding process, "It feels very strange. It feels kind of good but very strange. I doubt that I could stand up!" Later, after wearing the DAFOs for several months, she commented that they made her feet and ankles "very secure and stable," like a pair of "custom boots" or rather more like a pair of "support pantyhose." A young adult with severe athetoid CP had involuntary movements and posturing in his feet that were causing painful recurring tendonitis. Custom soft leather DAFOs with polypropylene soleplates provided "very comfortable" stability and control of forefoot, toe, and ankle positioning without causing him any sensation of being controlled too rigidly.

With a reduction in tone, individuals must work harder, even though the quality of movement has improved. A child who has been walking around on tone all day with no complaints is suddenly exhausted after short distances, and wants to be carried. *There must be active emphasis in therapy on teaching individuals how to use new movement available to them efficiently.* Using a modified "bear position" with hands forward on a chair or table, the individual can be taught to actively extend the knees isolated from hip extension and prepare tone and proprioceptive feedback for more stable walking with decreased spasticity. Though increased fatigue is common, children usually like the "feeling" of wearing their DAFOs. In adults, increased fatigue with DAFO wear is much less common for some reason. As active control over knee extension or plantarflexion is seen, trimlines offering extra control are lowered to allow the development of greater volitional control. Equinus is seen as "plantarflexion out of control,"[7] with the need to bring it under control, not do away with it. More complex upright skills, e.g., hopping, jumping, require forceful but controlled plantarflexion.

As medial-lateral ankle control emerges, weaning to dynamic FOs is considered. In most cases, weaning patients out of dynamic FOs has not been successful. Increased falling and balance difficulties or foot and leg pain have been most often seen over time after discontinued use. Children, if old enough, have requested a new pair of orthotics or parents have noted regression in motor skills. This regression is corrected when FO wear is resumed. We have seen several children with moderate spastic or athetoid involvement move from DAFOs to FOs, sometimes on one side and not the other.

If motor impairment is severe enough, attempts to wean the patient from DAFOs will be unsuccessful. We have had several families who have seen dramatic improvements in their child's function and decided there was no further need for orthotic control. Usually the loss in function on discontinuation is not immediately noticed, but occurs gradually over several months until it becomes noticeable. Several of these children have required serial inhibitive casting for 1 to 2 weeks before DAFO molding, and functional regression begins to reverse almost immediately. In more severely involved children, a gradual increase in tone with mild regression is seen as the child outgrows the orthotic. We are usually most aware that this has happened when we see a rapid improvement in tone control and function with a new pair of orthotics.

GOAL SETTING FOR DYNAMIC CASTING

It is important to remember in any goal-setting process that dynamic casts or orthotics are a therapy tool. To achieve their maximum benefit, they must be used in conjunction with an active intensive therapy program. As therapists, if we do not expect change and actively work for it, it is unlikely to occur. We must have "dreams" for each of our patients. By the same token, we know and work for the small increments that will build into functional changes. Early in their development, these casts were described as "a window for therapy" by a local physiatrist, Dr. Morris Horning. In ambulatory or preambulatory patients, therapy focus should be on active development of shoulder/trunk/hip control in sitting, "bear position," and standing with emphasis on increased leg separation, control of isolated knee and hip extension without overflow into plantarflexion, graded plantar and dorsiflexion in weight bearing, reciprocal leg movements, balance, and rotation. (Bear position is symmetric

weight bearing on hands and feet with trunk in the air, commonly seen before independent walking or as a transition to coming to stand without arm support in young toddlers.) In preambulatory patients, specific emphasis is on sidestepping along furniture for abductor hip control, and working toward independent standing balance and safe falling in preparation for independent walking. We deliberately avoid placing these children in any assistive walking device during this period, to have the greatest control over developing ambulation patterns of movement. In a study that compared the development of independent standing balance in a 4½ year old moderate spastic quadriplegic boy both in and out of inhibitive AFOs, a rapid increase in duration of independent standing balance was seen with orthotic wear compared with no change without the orthotics.[8] The child became independently ambulatory without aides after the study was completed.

Global tone changes affecting upper extremity function might suggest the value of goals directed at improved fine motor function. A recent study of fine motor performance in an ambulatory boy with spastic diplegia both in and out of inhibitive AFOs rather dramatically points out the improvement of fine motor function in sitting while wearing AFOs.[9] Active work in weight bearing over extended arms, especially in "bear position" or "bear walking," ties shoulder/trunk/hip control, reciprocation, and balance together to prepare for more graded use of these functions in upright. Compensatory flexion in arms because of poor trunk and shoulder stability needs continued active work in therapy to improve the protective extension response in falling.

To get maximum benefit from tone reduction to improve joint range of motion, *active stretching* needs to be a part of the therapy program. Goals for improved hip abduction, hamstring length, and dorsiflexion can be worked on actively in functional situations in sitting on a ball or in a number of weight-bearing positions. DAFOs are often left on in therapy to maximize tone control. An example of the rapid increase in range of motion sometimes seen with the initial use of dynamic orthotics is a 14-year-old girl with spastic diplegia who, after a number of years of persistent heelcord tightness, gained 20 degrees of passive range into dorsiflexion within 1 month after receiving bilateral dynamic FOs.[10]

In nonambulatory patients a similar emphasis on therapy and developing balance and control is necessary for benefit from dynamic casts or orthotics. Improved head control, shoulder/trunk/hip control and stability in supported sitting and supported standing, improved symmetry, especially in trunk and hip positioning, and improved arm and hand use are all reasonable goals even for severely involved children with spastic or athetoid involvement. Preventing or minimizing contractures and deformities also becomes an attainable goal with active therapy and a specifically designed positioning program. Actively being able to control their own tone can be a very important and achievable goal, even in very severely involved individuals, especially if intervention is begun at a young age.

In adults, there is a similar pattern of goal setting with emphasis on tone control, weight shifting, trunk balance, active weight bearing and balance with neutral ankle and foot positioning, and active control of the hip and knee in weight bearing. A daily program of physical activity including active stretching in functional positions and antigravity movements will optimize maintenance of functional movement control. Recently, a 31-year-old woman with moderate spastic diplegia shared with me some interesting side benefits to acquiring a lightweight sports wheelchair for her longer distance mobility needs. She had come to consult me about the potential benefit of using DAFOs. Being a functional cane and crutch walker from age 6, she had never considered a wheelchair. Supramalleolar DAFOs fabricated to replace her standard short-leg AFOs provided much improved stability, ease of active knee extension, and improved leg separation. In addition, she weighed very seriously the issues of long-term mobility, wear and tear on her joints, and her fatigue level at the end of the day. In addition to offering mobility choices that she had never had before, she found that crutch walking had developed considerable shoulder and upper body flexor tightness that was actively lengthened as she used her wheelchair. I noticed that her hand and arm function was considerably smoother, and was surprised at how easily and quickly she manipulated the lightweight chair up and down inclines and over long distances. She noted that, for the first time in her life, she is experiencing and enjoying speed, she has a way to exercise forcefully, and she has a way to "burn off" the effects of a particularly stressful day.

Adults must be actively involved in goal setting. Although I could not foresee all of the potential physiologic and psychologic benefits of the lightweight chair, I was ethically bound to present my serious concerns about her long-term mobility needs, as painful as this information was to her initially. Sooner or later, individuals with high-energy ambulation requirements find the energy cost too high to continue functional ambulation. Offering low- to moderate-energy mobility alternatives early may help to preserve their functional ambulation much longer.

Goals must be reassessed constantly during the course of treatment. Therapy must be active with functional objectives understood, gradually demanding more control of the patient as new movements and skills emerge.

Ankle movement into plantarflexion and dorsiflexion is an important factor in the development of secure shoulder/trunk/hip control and rotation, and graded righting and balance reactions. In prone or rolling, it is unnatural to move with an ankle fixed at 90 degrees. Subtle movements into inversion and eversion, dorsiflexion and plantarflexion are very connected to pelvic and trunk activation in the intact postural control system. Certain refinements of balance are prevented if the ankle is kept immobilized, even if it is in a very good position. The same is true on hands and knees, getting into and out of sitting with rotation, half-kneeling, pulling to standing, and balance in standing and walking. If the therapy emphasis is to be on developing the maximum graded control of movement, balance, posture and position, the ankle must remain free to move.

With the use of dynamic casts or AFOs, the ankle is free to move, but is prevented from extremes of movement and tone. Casts and orthotics can be worn in therapy sessions because they promote tone control and improve movement possibilities while allowing relatively free movement in most positions (see Figs. 9–1 and 9–6.) Tone and stability building techniques, such as rhythmic stabilization and intermittent joint compression, can be used much more freely with less worry of "uncontrolled hypertonus." Patients can actively learn to control hypertonus and associated reactions during therapy by developing control of active movements out of spastic synergies (i.e., in "bear standing") to hold and then move into active knee extension and external rotation with feet flat on the floor. This helps the individual gain active control over hamstring spasticity, which converts to better control in ambulation. Hamstrings are also actively stretched in a functional situation. Therapy is active, first focusing on maintaining control in normal balancing positions, then on losing and regaining control with balance, and finally to smoothly graded transitions into and out of different functional positions. These are all vitally important components of normal postural control that are most often impaired in individuals with neuromotor deficits. In this way individuals can learn to actively control and inhibit associated reactions that might otherwise dominate many of their movements, such as active weight bearing with arm extension forward in a hemiplegic child who typically displays flexor spasticity in the arm with any effort. Therapy is both hard work and fun because it is a successful exploration of new movement possibilities.

The use of dynamic casting and orthotics has made a tremendous impact on what we are able to expect and achieve in therapy. It promotes carryover of newly emerging skills and motor control into daily activities because of the tone control, stability, and more normal proprioceptive feedback provided when individuals are not in therapy. Good functional gains can be expected with an intensive therapy program consisting of one or possibly two hours of therapy a week with an active daily home program.

INTEGRATING DYNAMIC CASTING WITH TOTAL PROGRAM

CHILDREN

Because dynamic casts promote more normal functional skills in children with cerebral palsy, the wearing of these casts has been accepted fairly easily by families and children. In a 2½-year-old boy with severe spastic diplegia, mixed flexor and extensor spasticity compromises balance and active leg movement (see Fig. 9–1B) and he can bear weight only in steep equinus. Dynamic casts with medial-lateral support 3 to 4 inches above the malleoli and free plantar/dorsiflexion provide tone control, foot flat weight bearing, and improved active hip abduction and hip and knee extension (Fig. 9–1A and C). In our center, casts are painted with water-base Latex enamel to protect the plaster. This has an added benefit because children or their parents are allowed to choose the color and design for the casts. We have had casts designed as hiking boots, soccer shoes, Nike tennis shoes, or in pink with "Strawberry Shortcake" trim. This adds a sense of ownership to the casts, as well as making them more fun and a conversation piece. We have found that investment in using them is higher in the children and their parents when this is done. Dynamic casts integrate easily into the daily life of a child, except outdoors in the wintertime in our area. Sometimes, with extremely active children, wear needs to be restricted to indoors to maintain durability. In these situations, we have moved quickly to dynamic AFOs which are much more durable and are worn with shoes to protect them in the out-of-doors.

Casts tend to improve general mobility and function and facilitate improvements in other areas. The speech therapists at our center have noticed repeatedly that oral-motor function and feeding improve and oral-motor pathology decreases when some sort of dynamic footwear is used. Ease for parent carry-over of therapeutic handling and feeding at home seems to improve also. Improvements in fine motor control and hand function have positive implications for improved ADLs and school needs.[9]

Teachers have often commented that children are falling less, drawing and writing better, and are generally more able to pay attention in class. I am sure that improved stability and balance play an important role in these observations.

In young children, we often use inhibitive adapted shoes as a relatively simple, inexpensive, and less restrictive way to achieve tone control and improved stability. These are accepted easily by the children and families as they improve tone and positioning. They are an excellent problem-solving medium before a decision is made on the potential value of any other inhibitive or dynamic footwear. In older, severely involved children or adults, in whom shoe wear has become difficult to impossible, inhibitive adapted shoes have proven an excellent means of gaining control of tone and foot/ankle positioning. Adjustment to tone control can be very gradual, and these adapted shoes are usually tolerated very quickly for fulltime wear. Families, therapists, and school and caregiving personnel all appreciate the improved ease of handling that accompanies improved global tone control. Inhibitive adapted shoes are also a useful transition to dynamic AFOs in individuals with severe foot and tone problems, combined usually with marked hypersensitivity to touch and pressure on the bottom of their feet. After a period of several months' wear, sensitivity and general adjustment to global tone control can significantly improve, allowing the possibility of orthotic molding in a neutral position with inhibitive control.

Dynamic AFOs provide a cosmetically unobtrusive and effective bracing system (see Fig. 9–5C and D and 9–6C and D). Although the orthotics are constructed of thin and flexible polypropylene, they have proven durable even with hard wear. As with the casts, they tend to facilitate other aspects of a child's total day and program, rather than interfere in any way. With the increasing variety of trimlines developed to suit individual needs for tone control and stabilizing forces, effective functional bracing can now be achieved with minimum weight, the lowest possible trimline, and least restriction of movement (see Fig. 9–3). Similarly, orthotics initially require some

extra time and effort from parents to make sure that they are on properly. Tone must be reduced and foot position held in neutral while the brace is being put on, and the heel held securely down into the heelcup until the ankle strap is securely fastened. Parents usually become more proficient at this process than therapists. The children often let their tone decrease in anticipation of putting on the braces or casts, after a short period of intensive wear.

ADULTS

The general tolerance and level of acceptance among adults has been similar to that described above. Orthotics are almost always used for durability and cosmetic reasons, except in the case of some hospitalized patients in the early stages of recovery when casting is generally the more accepted procedure and allows for problem solving of ultimate orthotic needs.

I have had lengthy discussions on numerous occasions with adult neurotherapists about the feasibility of using standard supramalleolar DAFOs fabricated immediately on intake for tone control, positioning, and stability through all phases of recovery and rehabilitation following severe head injury. Other than the fact that it simply has not been done, it has intrigued them all. The system initially proposed by a therapist from Spokane, Washington, would fit a patient immediately during the flaccid phase to help provide tone control before sudden changes in tone occur. A posterior strapping system or, if needed, an external posterior cast shell could be used to control extreme extensor tonus. DAFOs could later be used during the rehabilitation process and could be trimmed down to FOs if the recovery process warrants this. Inhibitive adapted shoes have also been used in this way with considerable success. Integration of DAFO or dynamic FO wear into daily life and function seems natural and unimpeded. They are especially liked by patients because they allow ankle movement to occur. Numerous adult patients have shared their dislike and frustration with standard short-leg AFOs because of jarring and hip or knee discomfort, and not being able to smoothly move over their affected leg. In some cases, specific trimline variations have been made to DAFOs to allow ease of application with one hand.

With one exception, dynamic AFOs have resulted in good fit and tone control in my experience. The exception brings up some important issues and limitations of dynamic AFOs. A 24-year-old patient was seen for consultation approximately 1 year after a severe closed head injury, and was experiencing increasing extensor spasticity which was becoming more and more difficult to control in the leg and foot as she worked on functional activities in the upright position. With difficulty, her right foot could be positioned in slight eversion with the knee and hip flexed. When she attempted to stand, it was impossible to maintain control of the foot and ankle position because of severe equinus and varus posturing.

An AFO mold was made using the maximum everted foot position to control hypertonus. When it was fitted, she could wear the orthotic for up to 2 hours without discomfort several times a day, and she was able to stand and take weight over that leg with equinus and supination completely controlled. The orthotic required a high posterior extension two thirds of the way up the calf to control extensor spasticity. When she returned home with a new ability to take weight over her right leg, she was determined to become upright. During consultation, she was warned that she needed a great deal of preparation work on balancing in sitting and standing, weight shifting, and graded weight bearing over her right side before tone would remain under control with aided walking. With the increased effort to walk instead of focusing on balance and graded weight bearing, the brace for a time masked the associated reactions causing increasing spasticity. She began having discomfort under the base and head of the fifth metatarsal. With antispasticity medication, the inhibitive brace, and valiant therapy efforts, the hypertonus was barely manageable. We decided to have an orthotist in her area look at the brace and relieve slightly the area under the fifth metatarsal.

The brace again became tolerable. The plan had been to remold the AFO in 3 to 4 months in a more neutral position using a footboard. The molding failed; the patient's spasticity was extremely difficult to control; she was supinating inside the orthotic because of the extra room from relieving the area under the 5th metatarsal. The relieved areas, which I had agreed upon over the phone, were a big mistake. The problem would have been much better solved by increasing support under the peroneal notch inside the base, had I fully understood what was happening.

A new orthotic was made from the original mold. Extra support and contouring under the peroneal notch and metatarsal arch were made to affect tone, position, and stability more in the new AFO. She has tolerated this well, but I fear that her tone will again get out of control if upright position or posture is pursued prematurely with increased vigor.

Dynamic AFOs have limitations like any other brace. They are a working tool, within the limits of the improved tone control and stability which they provide. This young woman, by pushing the limits to be upright, was taxing a small piece of plastic beyond its limit of control and risked losing the tool completely. Had her energy been directed at gaining balance and control over her right hip and knee in weight bearing, the result might have been different

TECHNICAL ASPECTS OF DYNAMIC CASTING

Because this technique can produce dramatic changes in body tonus, it is very important that a period of time in therapy be allowed for experiences with tonus change and proprioceptive adjustments in working on balance and postural control under the hands of a therapist before inhibitive casting. It can be a very frightening and negative experience to suddenly have spasticity, grown accustomed to and used for function for years, gone with no idea of how to move or what to do with this "new body" (see Chapter 4). Preparation time before casting not only allows a better chance of acceptance of the new proprioception as positive, it also allows better baseline data for measuring changes seen with the casting.

The second important consideration is having adequate passive mobility in the foot and ankle to allow neutral positioning for the casting. If fixed contractures prevent the ankle from coming to at least 90 degrees and neutral medial-lateral alignment, a period of inhibitive or standard serial casting is indicated to achieve the necessary passive mobility. In addition, we have used inhibitive taping (using athletic taping methods to produce stabilizing and inhibitive corrective forces) as an alternative way to gain needed mobility before orthotic molding.

A third factor to consider when planning to use dynamic casting or orthotics is tactile or proprioceptive hypersensitivity. Parents or adult patients can be given suggestions for foot rubbing with a towel, deep rubbing as in massage, or numerous games to play to improve tolerance to touch and pressure. It is important to remember that individuals who are hypersensitive to deep pressure will also probably be hypersensitive to cast removal with the vibrator. In extremely hypersensitive individuals, it is usually more successful to start with inhibitive adapted shoes and allow a more gradual adjustment period to proprioceptive and tactual input as well as tonus changes. In some cases, modified shoes have been tried and used successfully. Following this and significant work to desensitize, hypersensitivity can still be so marked that AFO molding must be done without a footboard. When this is the case, additional contouring under the medial-longitudinal, metatarsal, and peroneal arch areas, as well as under the toes, is carved into the plaster positive mold for improved orthotic control. If there is significant concern about tolerance of pressure directly against the plastic, the entire orthotic can be lined with ⅛-inch aliplast.

With the use of a custom-contoured footboard, we seek to achieve neutral foot/ankle positioning, exact support under all of the dynamic arch systems of the foot for improved stability, and refined inhibitory control of tone (Fig. 9–10C).

Dynamic arching in the foot occurs as a result of a complex interplay between bony configuration, balanced intrinsic and long muscle pull, ligament and other connective tissue tension, and graded neuromotor control in response to dynamic balancing situations.[11] Dynamic arching functions to allow dynamic stability in weight bearing, graded adjustments and adaptability to surface changes, and stable control in weight bearing in and around midline or biomechanical neutral.

For years our casting method affected these systems without our understanding them, simply adjusting to tone changes that occurred with pressure or stabilization to a certain area of the foot. As we have begun to understand the interplay between graded stabilization, tone control, and normal biomechanics, we have discovered that exact mirror image support of the natural arch systems of the foot with stabilization of primary weight-bearing areas (metatarsal

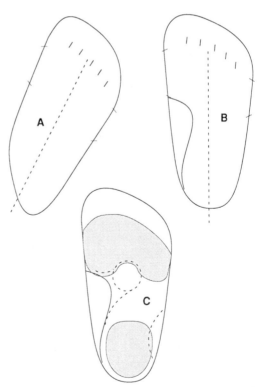

FIG. 9–10. A, Pronated foot. B and C, Neutral alignment. See text for discussion.

heads region and calcaneus) creates ideal tone control and offers maximum opportunity for devleopment of graded balance and postural control.

More specifically, the combined support under the medial-longitudinal arch and peroneal notch provides stability and graded control around subtalar neutral, which affects stability of the calcaneus and the rest of the foot and the leg through biomechanical and postural relationships. The metatarsal arch, a bony indentation immediately proximal to the metatarsal heads, is traversed by numerous vital soft tissue structures and plays an important role in midline forefoot stability and control of the toes. Finally, immediately distal to the MP joints is a natural arch space under the toes, as well as slight natural spacing between the toes, which allows the toes to function in normal balancing with proximal and distal IP extension and MP flexion and extension. The

correspondence of these anatomic features to the design of the footboard is shown in Figure 9–11.

Support under the toes, which must vary according to the thickness of the fatpads and the contour of the transverse arch (requiring often greater elevation under the second and third toes), is built up only to horizontal, allowing the toes the possibility of active dorsiflexion and plantarflexion in dynamic casts and AFOs. With exact support and control around midline and/or biomechanical neutral, more active balancing in the foot is made possible, with better advantage taken of residual motor function and recovery.

There is another interesting hydraulic effect as well. Raised areas provide upward pressure into soft tissue spaces and increased hydraulic pressure into those tissues supports bones in those areas. In midline or biomechanical neutral, the pressure

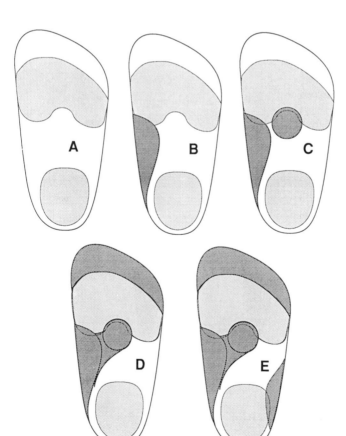

FIG. 9–11. A through E. Steps in the fabrication of a foot board. See text for discussion.

is distributed evenly below and around the foot and ankle. As a person begins to shift weight (or lose balance) either laterally or medially, the upward stabilizing and correctional pressure into the soft tissue increases proportionally. The brace, therefore, creates its greatest correctional forces in the situation of greatest postural and mechanical instability. Upward pressure also gives a clear and consistent proprioceptive feedback that parallels the mechanical effects.

A local orthopedist was surprised by comparison weight-bearing x rays of a young boy with moderate spastic diplegia in and out of DAFOs (Fig. 9–12). In Figures 9–5B and 9–10A, normal arch structures are flattened because of body weight, spasticity, and instability. In Figures 9–5D and 9–12B, ankle/foot alignment is supported in a neutral position and natural arches and more normal bony inclination angles have emerged in the x ray. It is not surprising that this child's total posture and sense of security in the upright position changed when he was wearing the DAFOs (see Fig. 9–5A and C).

Because the base of support is more stable and secure, improved control possibilities in the knees, hip, and trunk are fostered. It is intriguing that, in our experience, children with meningomyelocele (poor or

FIG. 9–12. Weight-bearing X rays of 3½-year-old boy with spastic diplegia. A, Without DAFO. B, With DAFO.

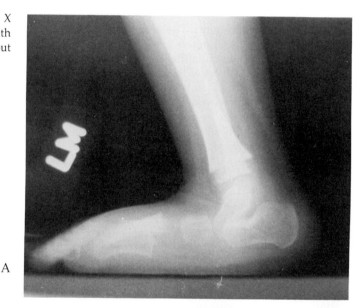

A

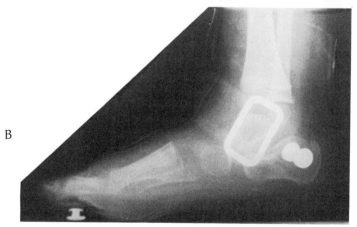

B

no sensation in the lower legs and feet) show improved balance, stability, and hip function when a dynamic soleplate is put in their braces. This is perhaps because of a more consistent foot/ankle positioning, allowing interpretation of proprioceptive information higher in the leg/hip or trunk.

NEUTRAL FOOT DRAWING AND FOOTBOARD

It is often difficult or impossible to hold a foot with significant spasticity in neutral in weight bearing. Neutral drawings (rearfoot aligned neutral to the forefoot) are done in non-weight-bearing, usually in sitting, with some loading through the knee. In Figure 9–10A, the outline of a pronated foot is shown. In Figure 9–10B and C, this is corrected to neutral alignment. The completed drawing includes designated areas to be routed under the metatarsal head pad area and the calcaneus pad area. Footboards are usually constructed of ⅜ inch plywood, routed, then cut out with a jigsaw. Routed areas provide a "nest" effect for support and stability to major weight-bearing areas.

Recently, a composite system constructed of a bottom layer of ⅛ inch masonite rubber cemented to a top layer of pelite (usually 5 mm) has simplified the process somewhat. For the routed areas, the pelite layer can be cut out completely with a utility knife. Plaster built up areas are applied in a specific sequence which facilitates problem solving (see Fig. 9–11). First the foot is held on the routed footboard (A) with heel and forefoot centered on the board. Size and precise location of routed areas for calcaneus and metatarsal areas can be evaluated at this time, as well as any tone changes. The medial longitudinal arch should begin to emerge and plaster is packed gently under this arch area (B). In a severely pronated foot, it may also be necessary to gently lift the navicular and medial talus and hold while placing the plaster to get a more accurate arch contour. In a foot with a strong supination tone pattern and a tight plantar fascia, it is helpful to apply firm pressure downward over the midfoot to lengthen and lower the arch and apply plaster under the arch area very lightly. This avoids an unnaturally high arch contour in the footboard, allowing gentle support so that tight structures can lengthen in weight bearing. A small mound of wet plaster is then applied to the area of the metatarsal arch (C). While the plaster is still soft, it is molded to the exact height and contour of the patient's foot by placing the forefoot down over the plaster with toes in maximum dorsiflexion. This support is the ideal height if the metatarsal heads rest gently down into the routed area with the toes dorsiflexed. If the toes are not held in dorsiflexion, it is much easier to make this support too high, causing discomfort for the patient in wearing. Exact support under the toes (D), usually more under the second and third to accommodate the influence of the transverse arch and less under the first to accommodate a larger bone and fat pad, is now applied to bring the toes softly to horizontal. If the toes persist with excess pressure on the distal fat pads, slightly more support under the proximal phalanx usually improves the tone. At the same time, a small amount of plaster is applied to join and smooth the transition between the metatarsal and medial longitudinal arches. Stabilizing support under the peroneal notch (E) is now applied and shaped with a similar contour to the medial longitudinal arch. The apex of this support should be ⅔ as high as the apex of the medial longitudinal arch in a pronated foot. Soft tissue compression and wrinkling above the apex of this support are normal and desirable to provide needed stability. Care should be taken to center the apex of support directly in the center of the soft tissue notch area, avoiding elevation of the base of the fifth metatarsal.

Further specific inhibitive refinement is done next, if needed, e.g., additional support under the medial side to provide more exact support for a talus and navicular either falling or pressing medially. In addition, it is possible at this point to post under the first metatarsal head for a biomechanical forefoot varus. In the case of a forefoot valgus and plantarflexed first ray, additional routing of ⅟₁₆ to ⅛ inch under the first head is done prior to plaster build-up to improve alignment. When the contouring is complete, a heelcup can be added in cases of significant instability, and the entire footboard is covered with two layers of plaster for unity and smoothness.

CAST FABRICATION

The foot is held at 90 degrees in neutral position while two layers of cotton stockinette are applied from toes to midcalf. The first layer is taped to the shin and at the toes with all wrinkling stretched and smoothed out. The second layer is left untaped, but is also smoothed. After a thin layer of non-compressible foam or felt is taped to the footboard, the board is taped securely to the foot across the forefoot with a single 1½ inch piece of athletic tape (Fig. 9–13A). Because of a cross-inhibition effect, the less involved side is often done first, allowing easier tone control for the more difficult foot.

Because exact neutral positioning and stability are required for maximum usefulness, minimal compressible padding is used in the fabrication of dynamic casts. Thin, noncompressible pads (double thickness directly over the bony prominence) are applied over the malleolar areas and surrounding soft tissue. A thin rectangular pad is applied over the entire forefoot to just past the MP joint, and just above the heel to cushion the Achilles tendon (Fig. 9–13B). A single layer of cast padding is wrapped over the forefoot and heel, with two to four extra layers wrapped above the malleoli (Fig. 9–13C). It is critical that, while all this is happening, a holding therapist or parent is maintaining the foot securely on the footboard at the heel and the forefoot, while managing general body tone and movement. Children must be either cooperative or distracted, to keep movement and tone to a minimum. They are usually fascinated with the process, but it does require them to be still for a long time (between a half hour and an hour per cast).

The position of the footboard is checked a final time, and an adjustment made if the child's foot has slipped back on the footboard. Plaster is circularly wrapped snugly around the forefoot to secure the footboard, then around the heel and ankle with mod-

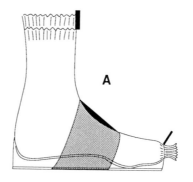

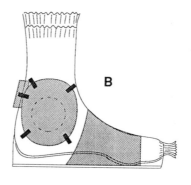

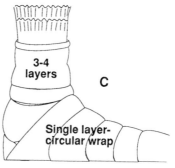

FIG. 9–13. Steps in cast fabrication. A, foot in two layers of stockinette is taped to footboard. B, Rectangular pad is applied. C, Foot is wrapped. See text for detailed discussion.

erate tension to ensure close contouring. Reinforcing strips of plaster are usually applied behind and in a stirrup under the heel, and up the sides of the cast, for additional strength with the least bulk. Close attention is given to secure midline heel molding and holding the forefoot securely down on the foot board while the initial layer of plaster sets. To compensate for increased tibiovarum angle, the footboard is eyed perpendicular to a line bisecting the femoral condyles and ankle (see Fig. 9–8). During the initial setting process, light loading from the knee helps to stabilize the heel down on the footboard. Reinforcement plaster pieces at the toe serve a dual function of securely attaching the front of the cast to the footboard and providing a medial and lateral nesting effect for the toes. If the toes are allowed to abduct or adduct around the front edge of the cast, it will be much more difficult to maintain forefoot and rearfoot control in neutral.

Casts are bivalved immediately after both are completed with a cast cutter (always referred to as a "tickle machine" or a "vibrator" to reduce anxiety and resultant hypertonus when working with children). Bandage scissors used to cut the padding at the bivalve line are referred to as "snippers" for the same reason. "Snippers" are slipped between the two layers of stockinette, and children are occupied by listening for the "snip, snip, snip." The inside stockinette is the last thing to be cut, and both layers remain a part of the finished cast.

BIVALVING AND FINISHING

Bivalve lines are kept as anterior as possible, barely allowing enough room to remove the foot in corrected alignment (Fig. 9–14). This allows maximum medial/lateral support to the foot and ankle from the posterior portion of the cast, and usually requires that the foot be positioned in neutral or slight supination to exit or enter the cast. Exact trimlines (rounding supramalleolar extensions, cutting "V" in the back to allow plantarflexion, trimming anterior piece to allow dorsiflexion) are done after the casts have been removed. Casts must dry completely and the edges are finished with athletic tape to hold the stockinette in place and to make a hinge opening for the top. Cotton or nylon webbing with a D-ring Velcro closure is used for the ankle strap. Naugahyde or thin leather sole, toe, and heel protection, and latex enamel paint protect the plaster and allow a less clinical ap-

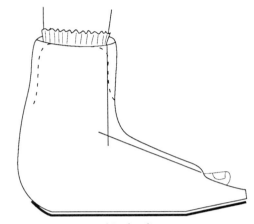

FIG. 9–14. Anterior bivalve lines on cast.

pearance. We have the patients or their parents choose the color and design of the casts, as mentioned previously.

ORTHOTIC FABRICATION

Because the dynamic AFO is a critical volume brace, molding must be very exact around the entire circumference and the footboard is incorporated into the molding process. Instead of the standard piece of rubber tubing, we have found that a piece of cotton webbing ½ to ¾ inch wide works well for the anterior cutting strip, referred to as a "zipper" in front of children. Other than the details of the footboard and very close molding, the dynamic orthotic molding process is the same as the molding of any other orthosis. One layer of cotton stockinette and a layer of tube gauze are used, and the footboard is taped in place across the forefoot and held securely at the heel and forefoot throughout the molding process. Markings for malleolar pads, trimlines, and any unusual bony prominences are made with indelible pencil. Plaster wrapping starts at the forefoot and proceeds in a manner similar to the initial wrap with the cast. Again, as the heel is securely cupped to the board and the forefoot held firmly in place, the tibiovarum angle is compensated for, and light loading from the knee is used to stabilize the foot on the board.

Making the plaster positive mold is typical except for specific artifacts resulting from the use of a footboard. Ridging around the edge of the board, which always occurs to some extent, must be trimmed off and smoothed for best results. Relieving at the malleoli or heel is contraindicated because it allows room for movement inside the brace and reduces tolerance. The exact contouring from the footboard should remain on the bottom of the mold and be transferred to the AFO. Malleolar pads can be enlarged to include the navicular or lateral head of the talus when necessary, and are usually constructed of ⅛-inch aliplast or PPT, thicker for adults. Other troublesome bony prominences can be relieved in this way as well. To distribute pressure, a slight flair is added at the top of the splint and at the back cutout. AFOs are vacuum-formed of ³⁄₃₂ inch polypropylene with greater thinning on the anterior surface. It is important that the D-ring ankle strap be set at a 45-degree angle across the anterior ankle to hold the heel securely into the heelcup. Dynamic AFOs usually include a wide forefoot strap, a hallucis-stabilizing strap, and frequently an adjustable posterior Velcro strap attached above the malleoli for some degree of plantarflexion control. If needed, a similar strap can be placed anteriorly to give dorsiflexion control, or completely around the top of the brace to limit ankle movement at 90 degrees for certain activities. Pelite is glued to the undersurface of the brace to provide protection and a non-slip surface if the brace is worn in therapy without shoes.

A dynamic FO mold is fabricated in the same fashion using the custom footboard and a circular plaster wrap of the foot and around the heel. Alignment considerations and tibiovarum compensation are the same. Recently, we have developed a new type of dynamic FO which is very easy and can be fabricated quickly. It has also become a useful problem-solving tool. The FO is fabricated of pelite using the same principles as used in footboard fabrication to recess the metatarsal pads and calcaneus pad areas and build up under dynamic arches (see Fig. 9–11). The base is 3 mm pelite with cut-outs for the metatarsal and calcaneus pads. Build up is done with 5 mm pelite except for the metatarsal arch and under the toes. The entire pelite FO can be covered with thin leather or naugahyde, or simply taped together with athletic tape and painted. The dynamic FO replaces the insole removed from the shoe. We use this system extensively with young children with milder motor involvement, or after head injury in children to problem-solve orthotic needs. It has also proven useful in adult treatment settings, providing significant tone control and improved stability after CVA or head injury, in MS, or in partial spinal cord lesions.

FITTING

In applying casts or dynamic AFOs, hypertonus must always be inhibited and foot/ankle alignment must be at neutral before the foot is put into the device, to ensure that the fit is proper and that the heel is well situated back and down in the heelcup. The patient or parents must be taught how to keep the heel in place while the straps are being securely fastened. If this does not happen, rubbing, irritation, and poor tolerance will occur. A tight fit with some soft tissue compression is crucial with both casts and AFOs, especially in patients with small, pudgy, hypermobile feet. Initially, it may appear that the cast is too small (top will not close completely) or that the heel will not go completely down in the brace, but if the brace or cast is fastened for a few minutes, additional tone reduction will allow the foot to go completely down into the device. As patients adjust to wearing these devices, this is less and less of a problem, but they must clearly understand this process if they are to use the devices effectively.

Typically, as children grow, casts begin to gap at the anterior closure and toes grow over the end of the casts. Four to six months is the typical growth expectancy of a pair of dynamic casts. Of course, there are always active children who mutilate them in short order, and others who are able to wear them for a year or more without the need for change. Dynamic AFOs typically begin to wing out above the malleoli as tarsal bone growth occurs, allowing movement and increased spot pressure within the brace. If the plastic is adequately thin, the anterior trimlines can be trimmed back ⅛ to ¼ inch on either side with bandage scissors, accommodating tarsal growth. The supra-malleolar extensions will again conform closely around the ankle and pressure will be evenly distributed. Typically, children can grow ¼ to ½ inch over the end of the splint without any complaints or signs of decreased tone control. It is usually very clear when the splints no longer fit, but even then they can often be worn for 1- to 2-hour periods during the day while new AFOs are being fabricated. Nine months to one year is a typical growth cycle for a pair of dynamic AFOs. Dynamic FOs are typically outgrown in 1 to 1½ years.

This time frame, while children are outgrowing splints, has proven to be helpful for solving the problem of a change in trimlines, i.e., moving from a fixed plantarflexion stop to free plantarflexion with an adjustable strap, or moving from AFO to FO control. A period of 1 to 2 months can be used to assess the change before the new orthotic is needed, or the FO can continue to be worn if it works well.

Adults present us with unique problem-solving needs. Often, there is a need for a fixed plantarflexion stop and a posterior extension up the calf, to distribute the force of the tone over a larger area. Unless there is a need for ground reaction forces to assist with knee extension, no anterior strap is required, thus allowing dorsiflexion. The plastic needs to be slightly thicker, pulled from ⅛" polypropylene, to be more durable. Trimlines can be creatively modified to allow one-handed application, while still providing secure three-point stabilization, especially of a strong tendency to supinate or pronate.

A previously discussed patient, with right hemiplegia and no right arm function, required such creative modification. He was molded for a DAFO with a high posterior extension to assist with knee stability and distribute plantarflexion force along a broader area. Modification (extra flaring) was made to the posterior shell to allow

slight knee hyperextension, necessary for secure ambulation. The AFO was trimmed more posteriorly at the medial malleolus and ankle to allow extra room for entry. Trimlines remained anterior over the lateral head of the talus and along the medial aspect of the forefoot and hallicus to prevent supination and forefoot adduction. This allowed one-handed ease of entry, comfort, and secure inhibitory control. Inserting an anterior ankle pad under his sock provided protection from pinching when he fastened the ankle strap forcefully.

As mentioned previously, option "A" of the trimlines is most typical for children and "B" is often used with severe equinus, especially in adults (see Figure 9–3), but each individual should be carefully assessed as to specific needs. Trimlines can be creatively designed to meet individual tone and control problems while allowing maximum movement possibilities.

DOCUMENTATION AND RESEARCH

As is typical in applied medical fields, clinical practice techniques are often years ahead of an exact understanding and a quantifiable documentation of their effects. This does not make these techniques any less useful as tools, or of any less interest to those in primary clinical practice. It does tend to cause raised eyebrows and skepticism among academicians in our field, and those in other related fields. Some are curious enough to want to see and reproduce the effects themselves, and then set about studying them. Others remain skeptical until significant research proof of clinical changes is available.

Most of the published studies done to date have been done on short-leg, inhibitive casting systems, which we do not use anymore. Some specific clinical research studies, most of them "single-case" format, are being done now, to look at the various aspects of control and changes that come about with dynamic casting and orthotics. One such study, involving an adult with CVA, comparing numerous gait parameters barefoot, in a standard polypropylene AFO, and in a dynamic AFO, has been completed in Milwaukee, Wisconsin, but the report is not yet published.[12] Significant improvement over barefoot and standard AFO measures in stance time, weight shifting, and other balance and stability-related parameters over the involved side was seen while the patient was wearing the dynamic AFO. A pilot study done in Seattle with two children with cerebral palsy compares traditional orthopedic casting and inhibitive casting using, among other measures, assessment of movement quality and balance in standing and walking on videotape by physicians and therapists blinded to whether the children wore casts A, B, or standard tennis shoes.[13] Spearheaded by a local pediatric orthopedist, the study found some of the chosen parameters difficult to measure, but enough trends were seen in the data to warrent future research. In both cases, the children, one with athetoid ataxic involvement and the other with a mild to moderate spastic diplegia, performed best in the inhibitive casts and worst in the standard orthopedic casts, with tennis shoes in between. I am currently involved in fabricating dynamic AFOs for four children with cerebral palsy, more specifically two with hemiplegia, one with diplegia, and one with asymmetric quadriplegia, for a comparison study recently funded here in Seattle.[14]

It is gratifying that the trend toward careful study of different aspects of this treatment approach is growing, sparked by positive clinical results. We are hopeful that this will continue with increasing interest among therapists, physicians, and orthotists in these systems. Sometimes in studies, inadequate measures are chosen and documentation of clearly valuable subjective changes and improvement eludes our measurement tools. There is no question in my mind that adequate measures are available and will be found to quantify the changes that are found in therapy. Nor is there any question in my mind that further research is needed using measures as objective as possible to compare the relative effectiveness of different bracing systems on different patient populations, both children and adults. In the meantime, clinical practice, as always, will forge ahead and continue to develop and refine useful techniques out of the specific needs and responses of our patients.

In the final analysis, our patients teach us what works or does not work for them. They are the ultimate critics of our success of failure. It is for them and because of them that dynamic casting and orthotics have developed, and will continue to develop as a vital therapeutic system.

REFERENCES

1. Hylton, N., and Kahn, N.: Casting Used as an Adjunct to N.D.T. Bobath Alumni Newsletter, 1973.
2. Yates, L., Mott, D., and Chapman, J.: An Appraisal of Inhibitive Casting as an Adjunct to the Total Management of the Child with C.P. Presentation to the American Academy of Cerebral Palsy and Developmental Medicine, Boston, MA, 1980.
3. Duncan, W., and Mott, D.: Foot reflexes and the use of the inhibitive cast. Foot Ankle 4:145–148, 1983.
4. Sussman, M., and Cusick, B.: Preliminary report: The role of short-leg tone-reducing casts as an adjunct to physical therapy of patients with cerebral palsy. Johns Hopkins Med. J. 145:112–114, 1979.
5. Gray, G.: Course: When the Foot Hits the Ground, Everything Changes, Denver, CO, November 1984.
6. Houck, L.: personal diary, May 1986–October 1986.
7. Quinton, M.: NDT Course, Seattle, WA, 1978.
8. Harris, S.R., and Riffle, K.: Effects of inhibitive ankle-foot orthoses on standing balance in a child with cerebral palsy. Phys. Ther. 66(5):663–667, May 1986.
9. Harris, S.R., and Taylor, C.L.: Effects of ankle-foot orthoses on functional motor performance in a child with spastic diplegia. Am. J. Occup. Ther. 40(7):492–494, July, 1986.
10. Brandon, M.: Case Record, Chehalis, WA, 1985.
11. Bojsen-Moller, F., and Lamoreux, L.: The

significance of free dorsiflexion of the toes in walking." Scand. J. Orthop. *50:*471–479, 1979.

12. Diamond, M.: The Effect of Tone Inhibiting Dynamic Ankle-Foot Orthosis on Adult Hemiplegic Gait. Master's Thesis for the University of Wisconsin, Madison, 1987.

13. Hinderer, K., Harris, S., Purdy, A., et al.: Effects of tone reducing vs. standard plaster casts on gait improvement of children with cerebral palsy. Dev. Med. Child Neurol. *30:*370–377, June 1988.

14. Haigh, K.: Effects of Dynamic Ankle-Foot Orthoses on Gait in Children with Hypertonia. Master's Thesis Research for the University of Washington, 1988.

15. Ford, C., Grotz, R.C., Shamp, J.K.: Neurophysiological AFO. J. Clin. Prosth: Orthot. *10(1):*15–23, 1986.

10 PHARMACOLOGIC MANAGEMENT

JOHN WHYTE
KEITH M. ROBINSON

Pharmacologic treatment is a major component in the management of spasticity. Over the last several decades, numerous medications have been studied for their physiologic and clinical effects on animals and humans with upper motor neuron syndromes. Several of these drugs have been abandoned because of lack of efficacy or unacceptable adverse effects. Others are in common clinical usage. Many more are in various stages of investigation.

In preparation for the writing of this chapter, a computer search of the English language literature on pharmacologic treatment of spasticity from 1970 to 1989 was conducted. These articles were supplemented with selected references on diazepam from earlier dates. References were grouped according to whether they were double-blind placebo-controlled studies of individual medications, double-blind comparisons of two or more drugs, or open studies. For the purposes of this chapter, conclusions will be drawn mainly from double-blind studies to minimize subjective bias. The results of these studies will be reviewed with an attempt to answer the following questions:

1. What are the limitations in the research to date in this area and how might they be overcome in future investigations?
2. What is the effectiveness of particular medications against various target symptoms seen in the upper motor neuron syndrome?
3. What is the effectiveness of particular medications in various diagnostic groups?
4. What is the optimal approach to selecting an antispasticity medication for the individual patient and evaluating the response?

METHODS OF STUDYING THE PHARMACOLOGIC TREATMENT OF SPASTICITY

Although drug treatment of spasticity has been under investigation for many years, it is still difficult to come to firm conclusions in answer to these questions because of the way in which previous research has been designed. A consideration of some of these research limitations will not only assist in a critical evaluation of existing data, but also may assist future investigators in furthering such research. Moreover, to the extent that clinical decision making is analogous to single case research, awareness of these limitations should also improve patient care.

Spasticity is a set of clinical symptoms that may appear grossly similar regardless of etiology. Because different drugs have different mechanisms of action, however, they may act differently on spasticity of varying neurophysiologic origins.

201

If selection of the ideal medication is to be grounded in the underlying neurophysiology, problems may be encountered in generalizing from one diagnostic group to another, e.g., from adults to children (because of developmental changes in neurophysiologic organization) or from acquired lesions to congenital. This issue sometimes arises even within a single diagnostic group. For example, patients with multiple sclerosis may have spinal, cerebral, or mixed pathology.[1] Patients with traumatic brain injuries may have multifocal and highly variable neuropathology.[2]

Most pharmacologic studies in the literature are of a heterogeneous patient population. Even studies confined to "spinal spasticity" often include a mixture of traumatic spinal cord injury (SCI), multiple sclerosis (MS), and hereditary spastic paraparesis. In general, the patients in such studies are too few to allow assessment of diagnostic subgroups within them. Clearly, more research is needed on the efficacy of specific medications in etiologically and neurophysiologically defined patient groups.

Once the appropriate patient population has been identified, a decision must be made about how changes in spasticity are to be measured. The upper motor neuron syndrome may display both positive and negative symptoms. Positive symptoms include both those of spasticity (e.g., resistance to passive stretch, hyperreflexia, clonus) and those due to other aspects of the UMN syndrome (e.g., flexor spasms induced by nociceptive stimuli, unmasked primitive reflexes). Negative symptoms include such things as weakness and incoordination. It is generally agreed that the stretch-related positive symptoms are more direct reflections of spasticity than the negative symptoms.[3] Therefore measures of amelioration of positive symptoms (e.g., decreased clonus) are more likely to detect drug effects than are measures of improvement in negative symptoms (e.g., increased strength). Furthermore, functional assessments, such as activities of daily living (ADL) scales, are likely to detect benefits of medications only to the extent that *positive* symptoms are the cause of the ADL deficit. Thus, a patient who has difficulty ambulating because of clonus may experience improvement with drug treatment, whereas a patient whose difficulty is primarily caused by weakness may not, even though both patients have clinically detectable spasticity. Although in this chapter we will be primarily concerned with the treatment of spasticity, some of the drugs that decrease spasticity also decrease other positive symptoms such as flexor spasms. Therefore, drug effects on all types of positive symptoms will be reported, rather than just those related specifically to spasticity.

Measures of spasticity can be thought of as existing on a hierarchy from the most molecular to the most global (Table 10–1). In general, measures at the molecular end of the continuum are most sensitive to drug effects, but will be of uncertain clinical relevance, whereas changes at the global end of the continuum are less sensitive to drug effects (because they reflect the interaction of many factors) but, if effects are seen, they are of clear clinical relevance.[4]

Research at the molecular level reveals likely sites of drug action and suggests appropriate dosage protocols but does not, in

TABLE 10–1. LEVELS OF ASSESSMENT OF SPASTICITY AND OTHER POSITIVE SYMPTOMS

Molecular	Neurophysiologic	Clinical	Functional	Global
Receptor binding	H/M ratio	Resistance to	ADL ability	Discharge outcome
Pharmacokinetics	Tonic vibration	passive	Gait pattern	Employment
Pharmacodynamics	reflex	stretch	Pain	status
	Vibratory inhibition	Manual muscle	Amount of	Patient preference
	of DTRs	testing	nursing	Clinician
		DTRs	care	preference
		Spasms		
		Range of motion		

itself, determine whether such drugs have clinical utility. Neurophysiologic measures may help clarify sites and mechanisms of drug action (e.g., a drug that affects the DTR differently from the H-reflex, may act on the spindle) but will not document clinical response unless validated by prior research. Clinical examination is, in general, only semi-quantitative (e.g., manual muscle testing) and is still not directly relevant to functional changes. Functional effects of medication can be assessed through a variety of scales and are of great clinical relevance. Expectations of functional improvement, however, must be based on a clear understanding of the individual patient's symptom pattern. Global measures of outcome such as discharge status or employment are usually too insensitive to serve as helpful markers of medication effects. Global patient or clinician preference for a particular drug is relevant, but may be misleading, especially during initial research. A patient may show no preference for a specific drug, suggesting that it is of no benefit. Quantitative data, however, might reveal that the drug has subtle beneficial effects that could be increased with a larger dose.

Within each level of the measurement hierarchy, it is possible to design clinic- or laboratory-based measures. For example, the reflex examination in the clinic can be equated with the integrated EMG activity evoked by a standardized hammer tap in the laboratory. Similarly, the angle or speed of stretch at which muscle contraction occurs can be assessed clinically or in the laboratory. Clonus and flexor spasms can be recorded in a patient diary, elicited by a clinical examiner, or evoked by a standardized stimulus. The laboratory measurement of these phenomena is more reliable and quantitative but no more removed from "real life" than the clinical examination.

Ultimately, it is important to understand the site and mechanism of drug action as well as its effect on clinical and functional parameters. Therefore, ideal research must involve the measurement of outcome at various levels. This allows greater understanding of the relationship between the neurophysiologic changes and corresponding functional changes. Furthermore, it may

at some point allow the measurement of relatively simple physiologic changes that could reliably predict more complex behavioral outcomes.

Aspects of study design may affect the ability to draw accurate conclusions about drug effects regardless of the level of the hierarchy at which effects are measured. Many studies are conducted in an open fashion, encouraging clinician and patient bias. Within the domain of double-blind studies, crossover designs (where each patient receives both drug and placebo) are superior to group designs (where some patients receive drug and others placebo) because they control for individual differences in drug response. Studies that look at a variety of doses or allow individualized dosing more definitively assess the benefits of drugs for clinical use. Finally, studies that compare two or more medications in individual patients are particularly useful in addressing *choice* of medication rather than simply efficacy or lack thereof.

Criterion measures are measures of the *achievement of a particular goal* rather than *movement in the direction of a goal*. Criterion measures of drug effects were almost never used in the reviewed studies despite the fact that these would be expected to most closely parallel the factors used by patients and clinicians to assess medication efficacy. A drug might, for example, produce a 50% reduction of clonus (a change measure). A patient attempting to transfer, however, might be as disabled by 10 beats of clonus as by 20. In this instance, "number of patients experiencing abolition of clonus" (a criterion measure) might be more relevant.

CLINICAL CLASSIFICATION OF SPASTICITY

Spasticity, as previously defined (see Chapter 1), is only one component of the upper motor neuron (UMN) syndrome. Clinical examination may reveal a variety of both positive and negative symptoms. Some of these may document only the presence of the UMN syndrome and others may be of profound clinical significance (Table 10–2), depending on the pattern of

TABLE 10–2. UNDESIRABLE ASPECTS OF THE UPPER MOTOR NEURON SYNDROME

	Positive Symptoms				Negative Symptoms	
	Spasticity	Other Positive Symptoms				
	Spasticity	Clonus	Spasms (nociceptive)	Unmasked primitive reflexes	Weakness	Decreased coordination
SYMPTOM:	Increased resistance to passive stretch					
CLINICAL/ FUNCTIONAL RESULT:	Contractures Poor bed and wheelchair position	Unsafe transfers Unsafe ambulation Impaired grasp and hand use	Pain Sleep disruption Impaired transfers Impaired ambulation Impaired wheelchair positioning	Impaired bed and wheelchair positioning	Decreased voluntary activity Decreased mobility	Decreased fine motor function Decreased mobility

symptoms and the functional level of the patient. There is little evidence that abnormal motor signs "hide" underlying patterns of skilled performance. Rather, they may be the remaining movement strategies after more skilled systems have been damaged.

CHARACTERIZATION OF THE CLINICAL PROBLEM

When considering pharmacologic, or indeed any, treatment of a patient with the UMN syndrome, it is useful to begin with an identification of the variety of positive and negative symptoms present. Thus, a patient may have increased resistance to passive stretch, clonus, and flexor spasms (positive symptoms) and weakness and poor coordination (negative symptoms). Subsequently, the patient's functional deficits can be identified. For example, difficulty in performing a stand pivot transfer, in remaining in an upright position in the wheelchair, or in performing skilled manual movements may be encountered.

The challenging task for those evaluating the patient is then to attempt to relate the first list to the second. That is, which of the positive and negative symptoms seem to be most responsible for the functional deficits encountered? Is the patient having difficulty in stand pivot transfers primarily because of clonus or primarily because of weakness of the knee extensors? Are skilled manual movements limited principally because of spasticity in the finger flexors or because of incoordination of the relevant muscle groups? To make matters even more complicated, other deficits in cognition, sensation, etc., may also be partly responsible for the functional deficits seen.

To the extent that functional deficits seem to be related to positive symptoms of the UMN syndrome, antispasticity treatment may offer considerable benefit. Negative symptoms are less likely to respond. Thus, this initial classification may help determine whether antispasticity treatment of any kind is likely to be beneficial.

If antispasticity treatment is undertaken, the initial evaluation should assist in the development of operational treatment goals. In the case of a patient with ankle clonus interfering with independent ambulation, reasonable treatment goals might be elimination of ankle clonus and decreased frequency of loss of balance during ambulation. Improved ambulation as measured by speed of walking may not be a reasonable goal, because slow ambulation is less likely to be a direct result of clonus. Clear formulation of operational treatment goals in advance can help the patient to understand what benefits to realistically expect from treatment, and can reduce the pursuit of treatments that result only in improvements of functionally irrelevant symptoms.

When evaluating treatment outcome for either clinical or research purposes, a few caveats are in order. Repeated or prolonged assessments within one evaluation session should be avoided because spasticity may fluctuate as a result of the testing itself (fatigue or muscle stretching effects). Furthermore, day-to-day fluctuations in spasticity are common, and are magnified by differences in general health, bladder fullness, pain, and many other factors. Therefore, it is unlikely that a brief assessment on one occasion will provide an accurate picture of the average effects of any treatment. Finally, it is important to consider the potential positive role for spasticity in certain functional settings. Thus extensor tone may facilitate standing, transfers, and ambulation, and treatment may lead to deterioration of these functions.

NEUROPHARMACOLOGY AND SITES OF DRUG ACTION

A neuroanatomic classification of antispasticity medications can be generated, based on multiple potential neuroanatomic sites of action, from the motor cortex to the sarcolemma. At each of these sites, there is a system of neurotransmitters and/or ions in operation. Anatomically, these drugs can be viewed as either centrally acting or peripherally acting. Centrally acting drugs act at various sites from the cerebral cortex to the spinal cord. Peripherally acting drugs act potentially at various sites from anterior horn cells to subcellular structures in muscle. All drugs, either directly or indirectly, influence activity of the stretch reflex arc as the ultimate end organ in the system.

Burke[5] delineates several sites where it is postulated that certain drugs act to modify stretch reflex activity (Figure 10–1). At each of these sites are receptors whose systems of neurotransmitters and transmembrane ionic flow can be identified. These systems are postulated to be modified by the presence of specific drugs. Davidoff[6] and Young and Delwaide[3] discuss these systems for each of the major antispasticity drug categories:

1. Benzodiazepines enhance inhibitory neurons in the spinal cord and at the supraspinal level by means of the inhibitory neurotransmitter gamma amino butyric acid (GABA). There is evidence to suggest that these drugs act at postsynaptic sites at various supraspinal levels, and at both pre- and postsynaptic sites in the spinal cord. It appears that benzodiazepines do not act directly on the GABA receptor, but bind to a site near the GABA receptor. This modifies either the affinity of the receptor for GABA, or the coupling between the GABA receptor and the flow of chloride ions.
2. Baclofen, although a GABA derivative, does not seem to inhibit the stretch reflex arc through the GABA system. It appears to act both pre- and postsynaptically. Presynaptically, it has been postulated to inhibit the release of excitatory neurotransmitters such as glutamate, aspartate, and substance P. Davidoff[7] in earlier discussion has suggested that baclofen acts by way of the glycine system postsynaptically.
3. Phenothiazines appear to have alpha-adrenergic blocking properties, probably in the descending bulbospinal pathways which influence alpha and gamma motor neurons.
4. Dantrolene sodium* acts directly on skeletal muscle by suppressing the release of calcium ions from the sarcoplasmic reticulum. Calcium ions are needed to activate the contractile apparatus. Whether this suppression is direct or indirect is unknown.

Several strategies have been used to identify the anatomic sites of drug action and the associated neurotransmitter/ionic flow systems. These include *in vivo* animal studies, *in vitro* nerve tissue culture studies, and *in vivo* human studies. Animal and tissue culture studies have the expected construct validity problems when attempts are made to generalize for clinical use in humans, but these methods are very specific in elucidating mechanisms of action. Human studies have used both clinical and neurophysiologic indicators to identify mechanisms of drug action. Generally, clinical indicators are not as helpful as neurophysiologic indicators in identifying a specific anatomic site of action, but, considered together, they point to gaps in the neuroanatomic knowledge base.[6,8] For example, diazepam is described to be more effective in incomplete than in complete spinal cord injury in neurophysiologic studies,[9] but is described as equally effective in incomplete and complete spinal cord injury in clinical studies.[10]

Neurophysiologic indicators may be useful in identifying an anatomic site of action of a drug because they differentiate among specific mechanisms of spasticity. Many neurophysiologic indicators are used concurrently in human studies, and there has been some attempt to quantify these.[8,11] (See Table 10–3).

The neurophysiologic indicators really are an extension of the different clinical indicators of the UMN syndrome, but perhaps with more precise application of stimuli by means of various standardized mechanical devices, and more sensitive measurement of response by means of EMG recording over specific muscle groups. Again, there is an issue of construct validity when these indicators are used to direct clinical decision making, because either alone or in combination, they do not relate to functional performance.

From this discussion, then, it becomes clear that spasticity is not an entity that is easily measured by one or a few tests. The indicators used to measure spasticity in drug studies represent the conceptual uncertainty that exists in defining spasticity. Thus, many kinds of measurement in different kinds of experimental contexts (animal versus tissue culture versus human) have been developed to seek out different kinds of information regarding mechanisms of drug action.

---

*Manufacturer's recommended dosage not to exceed 400 mg/day.

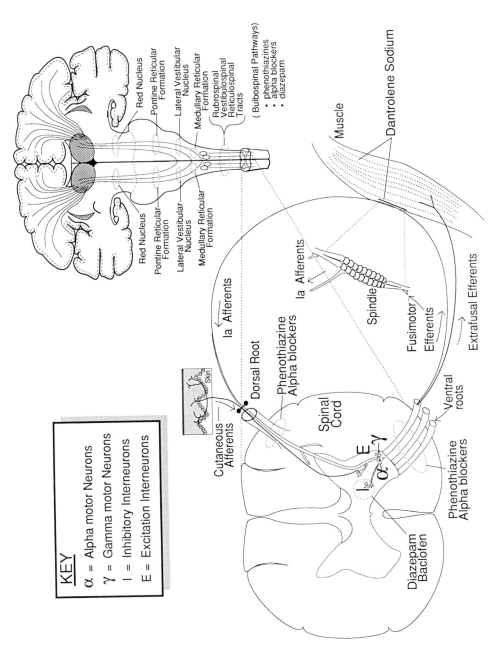

KEY

α = Alpha motor Neurons

γ = Gamma motor Neurons

I = Inhibitory Interneurons

E = Excitation Interneurons

Red Nucleus
Pontine Reticular Formation
Lateral Vestibular Nucleus
Medullary Reticular Formation

Rubrospinal
Vestibulospinal
Reticulospinal
Tracts

(Bulbospinal Pathways)
• phenothiazines
• alpha blockers
• diazepam

Red Nucleus
Pontine Reticular Formation
Lateral Vestibular Nucleus
Medullary Reticular Formation

Muscle

Dantrolene Sodium

Ia Afferents

Ia Afferents

Spindle

Fusimotor Efferents

Extrafusal Efferents

Dorsal Root

Phenothiazine
Alpha blockers

Spinal Cord

Cutaneous Afferents

Skin

Ventral roots

E
γ
α
I

Phenothiazine
Alpha blockers

Diazepam
Baclofen

FIG. 10–1. Proposed Sites of Drug Actions (adapted from Young, R.R., and Delwaide, P.J.: Spasticity. N. Engl. J. Med. 304:28–33,96–99, 1981).

TABLE 10–3. NEUROPHYSIOLOGIC
INDICATORS OF SPASTICITY

Deep tendon reflexes
H-reflex
H/M ratio
TVR (tonic vibration reflex)
Mechanomyographic methods
Pendulum test
Cryotest (effect of local cooling on resistance to pas-
sive stretch)

The site(s) of action of a particular drug
may have clinical relevance in relation to
the pathophysiology of different disease
states and their resulting spasticity. Thus,
one would predict that drugs acting on descending brainstem influences would be
relatively ineffective in complete spinal
cord injury. Furthermore, the site of drug
action may be relevant to prediction of side
effects. For example, many of these drugs'
affinity for higher centers in the CNS may
account for their adverse effects on mental
status and cognitive function.

REVIEW OF SPECIFIC MEDICATIONS

DANTROLENE SODIUM

Dantrolene sodium is unique among antispasticity medications in clinical use in acting peripherally at the level of the muscle
fiber. It uncouples the electrical excitation
from the contraction mechanism by inhibiting the release of calcium ions from the
sarcoplasmic reticulum.[12,13] This inhibition
of contraction occurs in both intrafusal and
extrafusal fibers,[14] raising the possibility
that part of its efficacy may be related to alterations in spindle sensitivity. Dantrolene,
however, produces equivalent decrements
in muscle force evoked by tendon tap and
H reflex, despite the fact that the latter by-
passes the spindle.[15]
The effects of dantrolene on force of contraction are most evident in fast twitch fibers, at low frequencies of neural stimulation, and at shorter muscle lengths.[16]
Dantrolene does reduce maximal voluntary
power, but only modestly (to 93% of baseline).[15] Evoked electromyographic activity

in response to either tendon tap or nerve
stimulation is not reduced.[15]
The above findings are all consistent with
the proposed mechanism of action of dantrolene. Because it interferes with the release of calcium, but incompletely, its effects are most noticeable when a single
nerve impulse must produce contraction
(e.g., at low-frequency stimulation). At
higher rates of stimulation or in slow twitch
fibers, the amount of available calcium can
build up and result in greater force. Similarly, in voluntary contraction, the patient
can sense the decrement in force and compensate through greater recruitment. Because neurally mediated electrical activity is
unaffected, electrophysiologic assessments
of muscle activity are misleading, and effects must be measured with reference to
the force generated.
Excessive muscular contraction is the
final pathway in spasticity of all causes.
Consequently, dantrolene is potentially of
use in all diagnostic groups. This lack of se-
lectivity, however, is also at the root of
some of the drug's adverse effects. Furthermore, different symptom patterns may respond differently to dantrolene. Therefore,
with this particular medication, etiologic diagnosis may not be as relevant in patient
selection as symptom type, severity of functional impairment, and goals of treatment.
Several studies in patients with spinal
cord pathology have demonstrated the efficacy of dantrolene in reducing deep tendon reflexes, resistance to passive motion,
muscle spasms, and clonus, assessed
through clinical examination.[17–19] In one
study, clinical examination and neurophysiologic studies were able to correctly identify the active drug condition versus the
placebo in 15 of 19 patients.[20]
No changes were seen in ADL function
in one study,[17] but another study did identify ADL improvement in 43% of patients.
The authors appeared to select ADL measures which were highly related to spasticity
(e.g., "clonus when applying braces").[18]
Even in this study, the proportion of patients who improved in ADL function was
much smaller than the proportion who had
reduced clonus or improved "overall clinical response," consistent with the multifac-

torial nature of ADL deficits discussed earlier.

Dantrolene is the antispasticity medication most commonly recommended in spasticity of cerebral origin. The data on which this is based, however, are limited. Chyatte et al.[21] studied nine patients with cerebrovascular accident (CVA) in terms of physical examination changes, timed ambulation, and quantitative measures of ADL function and upper extremity performance. During the dantrolene phase, patients had reduction of deep tendon reflexes and resistance to passive range of motion. Some aspects of upper extremity performance were improved on active drug, but ambulation and ADL function were unaffected. Loss of strength and difficulty in stair climbing were more prominent during dantrolene treatment.

Ketel[22] studied 18 CVA patients in an open trial of dantrolene. Those who responded in the open trial entered a double blind phase in which they either remained on dantrolene or were switched to placebo. Clinical deterioration was seen only in patients switched to placebo. Deterioration, however, was defined in global and subjective terms, so it is difficult to assess the effects of the medication on specific symptoms and aspects of function.

Children with cerebral palsy (CP) have also been treated with dantrolene.[23] The medication was found to decrease deep tendon reflexes and scissoring, and to improve the scores on an occupational therapy assessment. Passive and active range of motion and tone were improved, but not to a statistically significant degree, and no change in clonus was observed.

Two studies of treatment of multiple sclerosis suggest that dantrolene is generally a poor treatment option for these individuals. Gelenberg and Poskanzer[24] studied 20 MS patients, of whom 14 were ambulatory. Resistance to passive motion, clonus, reflexes, and strength were serially assessed. Although spasticity decreased in most patients, in 13 of the 20, drug-induced weakness or other adverse effects outweighed clinical benefits. In another study, mild reductions were also noted in resistance to passive motion, but once again,

clinical weakness was seen in 50% of patients.[25]

Dosages of dantrolene* vary in the cited studies, ranging from 50 to 800 mg/day in adults and up to 12 mg/kg/day in children. Doses as high as 800 mg/day were used in the MS studies, raising the question whether the high incidence of clinical weakness may have been partly dose-related. In a group of patients with mixed spinal diagnoses, the optimal dose was 100 to 200 mg/day.[19]

A variety of adverse effects are found with dantrolene sodium treatment. Weakness is a prominent complication, especially in patient groups with marginal strength, and is probably related to the therapeutic action of the drug. Drowsiness, lethargy, dizziness, paresthesias, nausea, and diarrhea are the symptoms most consistently reported in the literature reviewed. In addition, hepatic injury can occur especially in long-term, high-dose treatment, repeated courses of treatment, patients over 30, and women.[3] As many as 1.8% of patients treated for at least 60 days may suffer from hepatic injury, but most cases are reversible on prompt discontinuation.[26]

In summary, dantrolene sodium seems to consistently improve measures of resistance to passive movement, decrease deep tendon reflexes, and control clonus and muscle spasms. No consistent changes are seen in ADL function or ambulation, but the studies reviewed were not designed to assess patients whose ADL or ambulation deficits were specifically related to spasticity. Because weakness is a common adverse effect of treatment, this drug is likely to be of most use in patients with good strength, limited by their spasticity, or those with complete paralysis in whom additional weakness is not of concern.

Treatment with dantrolene sodium should be initiated after a baseline assessment of liver function. Treatment is generally begun with a dosage of 25 mg b.i.d. with small dosage increments at 5- to 7-day intervals. Liver enzymes should be reassessed frequently during dantrolene treatment and the medication discontinued if abnormalities develop. An upper limit in dosage is generally 400 mg/day, although

---

*Manufacturer's recommended dosage not to exceed 400 mg/day.

doses as high as 800 mg/day are not uncommon. Patients who show no benefit from moderate doses, however, rarely show dramatic benefit from high-dose treatment.

BENZODIAZEPINES

The vast majority of research on benzodiazepines in spasticity concerns diazepam. This is the oldest antispasticity medication still in widespread clinical use. Most of this section addresses diazepam, but studies on other benzodiazepines will be discussed as appropriate. Diazepam, unlike dantrolene, exerts its antispasticity action within the central nervous system. Although diazepam appears to bind in both the brainstem reticular formation and spinal polysynaptic pathways, the former seems to be more sensitive to the drug's effects.[27] Diazepam is believed to potentiate the presynaptic inhibitory effects of gamma amino butyric acid (GABA), an inhibitory neurotransmitter.[28] Because diazepam acts selectively within the CNS, it might be predicted that its effects would differ among different diagnostic groups or patients with lesions in different parts of the CNS. This issue will be addressed below.

Diazepam has been used most extensively in patients with spasticity of spinal cord origin. In one double-blind study of 22 patients with traumatic spinal cord injury given gradually increasing doses of diazepam, amytal (to control for general sedation), or placebo, diazepam was superior in decreasing global spasticity scores assessed clinically.[29] Although patients with complete and incomplete lesions were included in this trial, there is no comment regarding any differences in response. On the basis of studies showing drug binding in the brainstem, however, one might predict little drug response in those with complete spinal cord lesions. In another study of 21 patients with chronic MS or spinal cord injuries, resistance to passive motion and spasms were decreased more by diazepam than placebo and the trend for improvement was greater at a dose of 16 mg/day than at 8 mg/day.[30]

An open trial designed specifically to compare responses in complete and incomplete spinal lesions did find greater inhibition of reflex activity in MS patients and those with incomplete traumatic injuries than in those with complete injuries, supporting the hypothesis that diazepam augments brainstem reflex inhibition when the relevant pathways are intact.[9] This trial, however, assessed only neurophysiologic measures of spasticity, so it is not clear whether the clinical effects of diazepam in these patient groups also differ markedly. Another open trial using clinical measures showed no differences in the effectiveness of diazepam in incomplete and complete spinal cord injury.[10] Thus this question remains controversial.

A small study of hemiplegic patients showed some reduction of resistance to passive movement of the lower extremities with diazpam. A nonsignificant trend toward similar improvement was also seen in the upper extremities. A test of hand function showed no difference between diazepam and placebo, and ambulation speed actually deteriorated slightly on diazepam.[31] Sedation was a mild problem for 2 and a severe problem for 1 patient out of 12. It should be noted that the dosage was only 6 mg/day, which may account for the modest therapeutic effect, but may also mean that adverse effects were underestimated.

Cocchiarella et al.[32] studied diazepam, phenobarbital, and placebo in 24 patients with mixed diagnoses. However, 16 of the 19 patients who finished the study were hemiplegics. Diazepam dosages in this study ranged from 6 to 15 mg/day. No therapeutic effects of diazepam on spasticity were seen, although the methodology focused more on functional changes than on direct measurement of changes in spasticity. In contrast, sedation was a significant problem, and grip strength and walking speed were adversely affected by the drug.

The effects of diazepam in children with cerebral palsy have also been studied. A double blind cross-over study of diazepam and placebo in doses of 3.75 to 20 mg/day revealed greater improvement on diazepam in 12 of 16 children, assessed through subjective clinical evaluation.[33] Many of the children, however, improved primarily behaviorally rather than in specific indicators of spasticity. Despite the positive outcome, improvement was not dramatic. This study involved a number of athetoid children who apparently benefited as well. A methodologically weaker study also found improvement in CP with diazepam which was greater in athetoid than spastic children.[34] Here again, however, much of the improvement was attributed to general relaxation.

Clorazepate, which is metabolized to the same active metabolite as diazepam (desmethyl diazepam), was studied in a small double-blind study of MS and CVA patients.[35] Clorazepate decreased the intensity of the ankle reflex in response to quick stretch in all patients, and increased the sensory threshold for elicitation of the ankle reflex. Rigidity (defined as the resistance to slow passive stretch induced by a hanging weight) was unchanged. In this study, there was a suggestion that CVA patients benefited. If clorazepate is confirmed to be an effective antispasticity drug in this and other populations, it may offer some specific therapeutic advantages, especially in those with cognitive impairments. Clorazepate is not reported to impair learning and memory, in contrast to diazepam.[36,37] Ketazolam, a benzodiazepine not yet licensed in the United States, is reported to produce benefits comparable to those of diazepam.[38,39] The use of mixed diagnostic groups and the reduction of data to simple rank order preferences, however, preclude the drawing of more analytic conclusions.

It is more difficult to draw firm conclusions about the effects of diazepam than those of other medications because the research that led to widespread use of this drug was done in an era when methodology was less sophisticated, and little basic research has continued in recent times. Nevertheless, it appears that diazepam is effective in decreasing resistance to passive movement, deep tendon reflexes, and painful muscle spasms. It appears to be ineffective in reducing muscle rigidity (nonrate-dependent tone). There is some suggestion that diazepam is more useful in incomplete spinal cord lesions and MS than in complete lesions, but this has been incompletely studied. Similarly, the effects of diazepam on hemiplegic spasticity appear to

be less dramatic or at least more often overshadowed by adverse effects, but here, too, definitive data are lacking. Effects on cerebral palsy appear to be primarily due to nonspecific tranquilization because athetoid patients benefit as much or more than spastic patients, and benefits are seen in areas unrelated to spasticity.

The studies reviewed used doses of diazepam ranging from 3.75 mg/day (in children) to 30 mg/day. Treatment is generally initiated at a dose of 2 mg b.i.d. and gradually titrated upwards in 2 mg increments to a maximal dose of 40 to 60 mg/day. Rapid dosage increases are more likely to lead to sedation and other adverse effects. Other side effects include weakness, depression, ataxia, memory disturbances, and drug dependence.

BACLOFEN

Baclofen is the other centrally acting antispasticity medication in common clinical use. It was developed as an analog of the inhibitory neurotransmitter GABA, but subsequent research has suggested that its therapeutic effects are not caused by direct action on GABA receptors.[6] Baclofen appears to act primarily in the spinal cord on polysynaptic inhibitory pathways.

The bulk of research on baclofen concerns patients with spinal cord pathology or MS.[40-49] The majority of MS patients (60 to 70%) treated with baclofen show reduction in resistance to passive movement and in sudden and painful flexor and extensor spasms and clonus.[44,49] Similar patterns of symptom relief are seen in traumatic spinal cord injury, confirmed by reductions in elicited EMG activity.[46] Mixed studies of patients with a variety of forms of spinal cord pathology and MS generally reveal similar patterns, with relief of spasms, clonus, and resistance to stretch.[40,43,45,47,48]

Improvement in resistance to passive stretch is sometimes of interest in its own right, as in paralyzed patients who must be passively exercised, appropriately positioned in chairs or braces, etc. Improvement in active movement is often inferred, however, because that movement would be able to take place against less spastic resistance.

Along these lines, baclofen may decrease the resistance to passive stretch *without* altering the resistance encountered during active movement, suggesting that, in the latter case, the problem is cocontraction rather than true spasticity.[50]

Some studies failed to find positive effects on clonus[43] or deep tendon reflexes,[43,46] but these were in the minority. Most studies, however, failed to document positive drug effects on ambulation and ADL performance.[43,48] In the study by Pedersen et al.,[48] ambulation and strength deteriorated during baclofen treatment. Based on the hypothesized mechanism of action, one would predict equal clinical efficacy in complete and incomplete spinal cord lesions. This has not been extensively studied, but was confirmed in one clinical investigation.[48]

Baclofen has been studied little in spasticity of cerebral origin. No double-blind studies in this population could be identified. A review of the open trials of baclofen revealed three studies involving hemiplegic patients. Of nine patients treated with baclofen by Jones and Lance, only three showed even slight relief of spasticity.[51] Pedersen and colleagues report benefit in 6 patients with CVA, but this study involved single intravenous injections, and no raw data are available for inspection.[52] Pinto reviewed the effects of baclofen on a large sample of patients with a variety of diagnoses. CVA patients appeared to benefit less from treatment than members of other diagnostic groups, but the difference was not great. More CVA patients, however, also experienced significant side effects.[53]

Baclofen has recently been studied during intrathecal use (see Chapter 12). A baclofen solution is placed in an implanted pump, which delivers programmable quantities of the medication into the lumbar cerebrospinal fluid. Initial open trials were carried out in patients with severe spasticity who either had not benefited from oral baclofen or did not tolerate its adverse effects. A small number of patients with MS, transverse myelitis, traumatic cord injury and cerebral anoxia all showed dramatic responses.[54] Subsequent double-blind placebo controlled crossover studies with SCI and MS patients confirmed these results. Of 16 patients who received 3 days of intrathe-

cal baclofen and 3 days of intrathecal saline, all 16 showed clear reduction of spasticity on baclofen as judged by the Ashworth scale, the number of flexor spasms, and various neurophysiologic measures of resistance to stretch and evoked muscle electrical activity.[55] Functional data were not reported. Patients whose sleep was disrupted by spasms were also studied in a sleep laboratory and showed reduced night-time arousals on baclofen.

Drug side effects were few, although some patients had pump failure, catheter blockage, or surgical complications. Only one of the 16 patients required continuous increases in dosage. This patient was later switched to intrathecal morphine, and when tolerance to that also developed, was switched successfully back to intrathecal baclofen at a reduced dose. The author suggests that the greater efficacy of intrathecal baclofen is due to its tenfold higher CSF concentration as compared to oral administration, and the fact that the predominantly upward flow of CSF reduces the concentration by the time it reaches the brain to produce adverse effects.

Some questions, however, remain from this study. Patients were chosen because of their initial positive response to an intrathecal injection of baclofen. Thus, it is unclear what proportion of potential candidates were ultimately selected for pump implantation. In addition, the outcome measures primarily assessed lower extremity function. Therefore, it remains to be seen whether adequate concentrations of baclofen can be achieved in the cervical cord or the brain to affect function in quadriplegics or TBI patients, without running into the same toxicity problems seen with oral use. Indeed, in a small study of intrathecal use of baclofen, midazolam, and morphine, 2 patients who received doses of baclofen nearly 100 times larger than in the above study became unresponsive for a few hours.[56] It is possible that some of the surgical complications might be minimized by epidural rather than intrathecal administration,[57] but research comparing these two approaches is needed.

In summary, baclofen appears to be an effective drug for treatment of spasticity in patients with spinal cord injury and multiple sclerosis. It may have some advantage over diazepam in complete cord injury, although more research is needed on this question. Few data are available on the use of baclofen in cerebral spasticity, although there is some evidence that the drug is effective but may have an increased incidence of side effects. As with the other medications reviewed, its benefits in disabling positive symptoms such as spasms, clonus, and resistance to stretch are far more clear than on complex functional skills such as mobility or ADLs.

Baclofen was used in doses ranging from 30 to 100 mg/day in the literature reviewed. It is generally begun at a dose of 5 mg b.i.d. or t.i.d. and increased every 4 to 7 days by 5 mg increments until a total daily dose of 80 mg is reached. Higher doses have been used in some instances. The effect of baclofen may increase up to some critical dose and then decrease with continued dosage increments. Thus, it is important to monitor clinical symptoms between dosage increases to avoid overshooting.

Common adverse effects include drowsiness, fatigue, and muscle weakness. The latter effect may be more troublesome for the more functional patient than for the severely disabled. In one study,[48] adverse effects (primarily weakness) led to drug discontinuation in 53% of mobile patients and 25% of incapacitated patients. Other adverse effects commonly seen include nausea, dizziness, intoxication, and paresthesias. Abrupt withdrawal can lead to hallucinations, rendering this drug hazardous in patients with precarious GI function because it is not available in parenteral form.[58] Although a case report has suggested a risk of psychosis from ongoing treatment with high doses of baclofen, there were other possible explanations for the psychiatric symptoms of the reported patient.[59]

COMPARATIVE STUDIES

As is evident from the above discussion, there are three commonly used medications with some degree of efficacy across a variety of diagnoses and target symptoms. Thus it becomes particularly important to *compare* the efficacy of the various drugs in specific patient populations and clinical situations to assist the physician in rationally choosing the most appropriate medication for the individual patient. Perhaps because diazepam is the oldest medication still in clinical use, identified studies compared baclofen or dantrolene to diazepam. Unfortunately, no controlled studies comparing baclofen and dantrolene were identified.

Cartlidge et al.[60] compared diazepam in doses of 15 and 30 mg/day to baclofen in doses of 30 and 60 mg/day in 37 patients, 34 of whom had MS. Each subject was exposed to all four drug/dose conditions for two weeks. Efficacy was assessed by a clinical examination of limb spasticity and by overall patient preference. In this study, low-dose baclofen proved equivalent to low-dose diazepam in diminishing spasticity. High doses of each drug produced still greater improvements in those who tolerated the higher doses. However, 11 (baclofen) and 14 (diazepam) patients could not take the high dose because of adverse effects. Seventeen patients expressed a global preference for baclofen in comparison to 10 for diazepam. Patients with greater body weight benefited less from a given dose of baclofen, but this was not the case with diazepam, suggesting the need to adjust baclofen doses for patient size.

Two studies compared diazepam and baclofen in flexible dosage regimens. Sixteen patients with severe MS (14 nonambulatory) were treated for 4 weeks with each medication in a double-blind crossover design.[61] The first 2 weeks of each condition involved the optimization of dosage of the unknown drug with respect to clinical examination, while the subsequent 2 weeks provided the data on clinical examination of spasticity, clonus, and subjective assessments of ambulation and global drug preference. The average optimal dose of baclofen was 61.2 mg/day (range 30 to 120) and that of diazepam was 26.8 mg/day (range 10 to 40). Clinical measures of spasticity, flexor spasms, and clonus improved equally on both drugs. The only two ambulatory patients experienced deterioration of walking ability, one on each drug. No positive effects were seen from either drug on bladder function. Sedation was much more common on diazepam, whereas side effects were more varied but equal in number on baclofen. Despite the equal efficacy and number of adverse effects in this trial, patient and physician preference dramatically favored baclofen. This may reflect the different *patterns* of side effects, of which sedation is apparently the most troubling.

Another flexible dose comparison involving 13 patients with MS and SCI reported only on global preference.[62] This study showed a trend favoring diazepam in both patient and physician preference, but neither trend reached statistical significance. Sedation was more troubling with diazepam treatment.

One study compared another benzodiazepine, clonazepam (0.5 to 3 mg/day), to baclofen (30 to 90 mg/day) in a population composed mainly of MS patients.[63] Although this was an open trial, both drugs were found to be comparable in efficacy. Baclofen was more effective for patients with more severe tone in the doses used. Sedation, confusion, and fatigue were greater problems with clonazepam and more frequently resulted in drug discontinuation.

Diazepam and baclofen appear to be of comparable efficacy in patients with MS. Even this conclusion, however, is tentative because no assessments of meaningful function were included in these studies and the range of illness severity was fairly restricted. Comparative data on traumatic spinal cord injury are virtually completely lacking and would be of particular interest with respect to neurologically complete injury. Brain injury has not been assessed comparatively. It appears that baclofen may offer some advantages over diazepam in patients prone to sedation or drug abuse.

Dantrolene* and diazepam have also been compared in the MS population.[64] In a double-blind crossover design, 42 MS patients (mostly ambulatory) were treated with diazepam in doses of 12 and 20 mg/day and with dantrolene in doses of 200 and 300 mg/day. Improvement in clinically assessed spasticity was equal between the low doses of each drug. Increasing the medication dose increased the control of spasticity for dantrolene but not for diazepam. Reflexes were more effectively suppressed by dantrolene at both doses, but this is of uncertain clinical relevance. Patients experienced more weakness at both doses of

dantrolene, but more deterioration in hand coordination at both doses of diazepam. More disabled patients did better on the low dose of dantrolene, but severity of disability did not affect dose response for diazepam. Drowsiness and ataxia were more severe on diazepam. At the end of the trial, 22 patients chose to continue dantrolene treatment at a still lower dose (mean of 118 mg/day), 13 chose diazepam (10 mg/day) and 7 chose to discontinue drug treatment. After 6 months, however, the number of patients being treated with each drug had equalized.

Nogen[65] compared these two drugs in children with cerebral palsy. Unfortunately, although a variety of parameters of spasticity and ADL function were assessed in this study, only global preference for one drug over the other is reported. Thus it is impossible to draw any conclusions about the particular symptoms or functional areas in which each drug may be superior. In this study, nine children experienced greater benefit from dantrolene and seven from diazepam; four experienced equal benefit, and two showed no benefit. In a subsequent phase, eight children showed greater benefit from a combination of the two drugs. Drowsiness, a common problem, was reported to decrease over time.

A final comparison of diazepam and dantrolene was performed in a mixed population including CVA, SCI, MS, and CP patients.[66] Unfortunately, only 11 patients completed the trial, which seriously limited conclusions. In this study, global clinical assessment was best for combined treatment with both drugs, followed by either drug used alone (improvement was equivalent with the two drugs) followed by placebo. No statistical analysis was done, and the relationship between electrophysiologic and clinical parameters of spasticity was poor.

In MS, the comparison of dantrolene and diazepam suggests that both drugs may be useful,[64] in contrast to the research on dantrolene alone, which questions its role in the management of MS.[24,25] It seems safe to conclude that dantrolene must be used cautiously in this population, probably at low doses, and most successfully in patients with extreme strength or weakness. It may be the better drug, however, for MS patients with coordination problems or marginal cognitive status. In contrast, patients

---

*Manufacturer's recommended dosage not to exceed 400 mg/day.

with moderate strength may benefit more from diazepam, although even in this instance potential loss of function must be kept in mind.

More comparative research is needed on treatment of CP. There is some support for combined treatment with dantrolene and diazepam, but no cognitive or learning assessments have been conducted to determine the possible consequences of combined use of these drugs on a pediatric population. Furthermore, since the single relevant study was global in nature, it is difficult to rule out the possibility that some of diazepam's apparent efficacy was caused by its behavioral effects.

Clearly, much more research is needed in comparing the three major medications in sizeable samples of homogeneous diagnostic groups. Such research should assess response in terms of multiple indicators of spasticity and relevant functional activities as well as global preference. In this way, profiles of the types of patients most likely to benefit from each drug can be drawn. In particular, comparative research on dantrolene and baclofen is needed.

MISCELLANEOUS MEDICATIONS

A large number of medications have been tested for their effects on spasticity over the last two decades. Most of these drugs have proven relatively ineffective, have had disabling side effects, or have had no significant advantages over standard drugs to make their licensing worth pursuing. Some of these drugs are reviewed below. In most cases, the quantity of relevant research is too limited to arrive at definitive conclusions. Nevertheless, some of these drugs may have limited potential in certain patient populations, or deserve further research for specific indications. This is not a comprehensive list of drugs studied for treatment of spasticity.

ADRENERGIC BLOCKING AGENTS

Descending α-adrenergic fibers are believed to play a role in the regulation of fusimotor drive.[67] Thus, some interest has been generated in the role of α-adrenergic blocking drugs as antispasticity medica-

tions. Thymoxamine has been studied both intravenously and orally. Intravenous administration resulted in a reduction of stretch-elicited EMG activity comparable to diazepam, except in one patient with a complete spinal cord injury.[68] A sample of patients, most of whom had MS, showed reductions in ankle jerk amplitude that were greater than the reduction in H-reflex amplitude following intravenous injection.[67] Reductions in resistance to passive movement, clonus, and deep tendon reflexes were also noted. All these make sense in light of the proposed descending inhibition of spindle activity, which would be bypassed by the H-reflex or abolished in complete spinal cord injury. In a study of oral thymoxamine, no effect on spasticity was seen, although this was an open trial.[69] Thus, it may be that mode of medication delivery is critical. Of particular interest is the observation of *increased* sensitivity to flexor spasms with thymoxamine in these studies.

Beta-adrenergic blocking agents are also observed to have some influence on the upper motor neuron syndrome.[67] Propranolol, when given intravenously, did appear to induce reductions in clonus in 13 of 16 patients studied, but a postulated mechanism is speculative at best. Other signs of the UMN syndrome did not seem to be affected consistently by propranolol.

ANESTHETICS

Topical anesthesia has been studied for its potential to decrease cutaneous inputs to the spastic reflex arc. In a study of 20% topical benzocaine applied to the leg of CVA patients, H-reflex amplitude increased while ankle tendon reflex was unaffected (suggesting reciprocal changes in the activity of alpha and gamma motor neuron pools), and gait, assessed in a gait lab, was improved.[70] This study was unblinded, however. An attempt to replicate the efficacy of benzocaine in a double-blind study involving head-injured adults failed to show any effect of topical anesthesia on spasticity as measured by an increased ratio of active to passive range of motion in the spastic limb.[71] Thus, the efficacy of topical anesthesia remains unclear. Further double-blind research should be conducted particularly in populations where cutaneous stimulation is believed to play a prominent role in spasticity.

CLONIDINE

Clonidine appears to act at multiple levels of the CNS, including an α-2 agonist action in the brain and brainstem and in the substantia gelatinosa of the dorsal horns. It ultimately decreases sympathetic outflow from the brain.[72] It may inhibit afferent inputs into the spastic reflex arc. Open-trial case reports found this drug effective in reducing spasms and resistance to stretch in four patients with spinal cord pathology, when given in doses of 0.2 mg/day.[72] Postural hypotension and depressed mood, however, were prominent adverse effects, leading to drug discontinuation in two of the four patients. In a more recent open study of 55 patients with SCI, 31 were judged to have responded in the collective subjective opinions of the patient, physician, and therapist, to the addition of clonidine to their existing baclofen regimen.[73] Most of the nonresponders withdrew before reaching the maximal study dose of 0.4 mg/day because of adverse effects or disappointment in the lack of dramatic benefit. The nature of the responses was not reported. Somewhat surprisingly, quadriplegics responded more favorably than paraplegics, despite their greater risk of hypotension. Although baclofen doses were reduced in many responders, no patient was able to substitute clonidine for baclofen.

CYCLOBENZAPRINE

Cyclobenzaprine (Flexeril) is used in general practice for "muscle spasm." One study assessed its efficacy in true spasticity related to the UMN syndrome.[74] Fifteen patients with mixed diagnosis of spinal or cerebral spasticity were studied in a double-blind crossover design using 60 mg/day of the medication. Drug effects were measured in terms of EMG response elicited by muscle stretch, physical examination of reflexes and spasticity, and subjective benefit. No difference was noted in any of these parameters between drug and placebo. One

SCI patient was treated with increasing doses to 150 mg/day. A dose-response relationship was noted with increasing doses. The magnitude of the clinical effect was still small, however, suggesting that this would not be a clinically useful medication.

GLYCINE

One series of seven case reports of patients treated with oral glycine was identified.[75] The patients suffered from CP, CVA, or spinal infarction and received 3 to 4 g/day of glycine and 1 to 2 g/day of sodium bicarbonate. Subjective improvement was noted in "spasticity, tonus, and paresis" in six of the patients. No later controlled studies of glycine were identified, suggesting that its initial promise may not have been well founded.

MORPHINE SULFATE

Morphine sulfate has been studied by intrathecal administration, using an approach similar to the baclofen pump described above.[76] Four spinal cord-injured patients were treated with 1 to 1.5 mg intrathecal morphine. This resulted in dramatic reduction of spasticity. Pump implantation followed, with an ultimate daily morphine dose of 2 to 4 mg daily. One patient had increasing morphine demands, but this was mainly to control a primary pain problem; the patients with spasticity alone did not develop tolerance. No bladder atony was produced. It is not clear what, if any, advantages intrathecal morphine would have over intrathecal baclofen.

PHENOTHIAZINES

Chlorpromazine reduces decerebrate rigidity in the cat, probably by means of α-adrenergic blockade (see previous text). In a controlled study of patients with a variety of diagnoses, chlorpromazine was effective in reducing resistance to passive stretch by 18 to 83%.[77] Sedation from doses of 150 mg/day was, however, a significant problem. This study also examined the efficacy of phenytoin, which has direct spindle inhibitory activity. Six of ten patients had tone reduction from phenytoin at serum levels greater than 7 g/mL, but the magnitude was less than that induced by chlorpromazine. Of most interest was the fact that the combination of phenytoin and chlorpromazine allowed equivalent tone reduction at lower doses of chlorpromazine with fewer adverse effects.

A phenothiazine derivative, dimethothiazine, has also been evaluated in spasticity. It was hoped that this drug would produce benefits at least equivalent to those of chlorpromazine but with less sedation. An assessment of intravenous administration of 25 to 100 mg revealed a dramatic reduction in limb spasticity. Voluntary power, however, was reduced on administration of optimal doses for spasticity reduction.[78] Oral administration (in doses as high as 900 mg/day) resulted in detectable benefits, which were dramatic in 15 of 42 patients with a variety of diagnoses studied in this open trial. Another open trial found that 61% of patients reported subjective benefits in doses up to 300 mg/day.[79] In both trials, sedation was significant. In addition, patients whose extensor rigidity was abolished sometimes showed release of flexor spasms. This unmasking of flexor spasms appears to be a general effect of α-adrenergic blocking drugs; it was seen with thymoxamine as well (see previous text).

One double-blind placebo-controlled study investigated a later and more potent derivative of dimethothiazine.[80] Nine patients with mixed diagnoses were studied. Measurable reductions in spasticity were noted, but their magnitude was of little clinical significance. Although it is clear that phenothiazine drugs can influence spasticity, they tend to have significant short- and long-term adverse effects. Thus, it is unclear whether there is a patient population that benefits more from these drugs than from other agents with less serious long-term adverse effects.

PIRACETAM

Piracetam is chemically related to GABA and baclofen and effectively crosses the blood-brain barrier. A double-blind crossover study investigated its effects in 16 children with spasticity due to CP.[81] Dependent measures included resistance to passive motion, assessment of hand function, ambulation ability, and filmed behavior for standardized assessment. Improvement was statistically greater in the piracetam phase of the trial, in which 8/16 improved versus 0/16 in the placebo phase. Nevertheless, the improvements were generally mild to moderate and not of great clinical significance. Side effects were minimal.

PROGABIDE

Another drug that appears to function as a GABA agonist was studied in 14 patients with MS and 2 with hereditary spastic paraparesis in a double-blind placebo crossover design.[82,83] Given in doses up to 1800 mg/day, progabide reduced deep tendon reflexes significantly and showed a trend toward reduction of flexor spasms, clonus, and resistance to passive motion. No change in voluntary power was noted and no side effects were seen. Global improvement was categorized as important in 2, moderate in 5, and slight in 6 patients.

Another study used progabide in 30 patients with MS in a double-blind, placebo-controlled crossover design. Increasing doses to 45 mg/kg/day were given over 4 weeks, with a 2-week washout period between treatment phases.[84] No significant effects were observed in functional measures of ambulation or fine motor function, in spasm count, or in strength. Significant reduction in spasticity scores was seen, however. Subjective preferences of both clinicians and patients favored progabide and 10 of the 25 patients who completed the trial chose to continue treatment. Treatment was limited by frequent adverse effects, most commonly elevation of liver function tests, which required discontinuation of progabide in 9 of the 30 patients. Progabide appears unlikely to play a major role in the treatment of MS, given the relatively modest therapeutic benefits and the presence of adverse effects in nearly one third of patients.

TETRAHYDROCANNABINOL (THC)

Spastic patients who use marijuana recreationally often report positive effects, but it is unclear whether this is caused by general relaxation or a specific spasmolytic effect, which may be mediated by THC's inhibition of spinal polysynaptic pathways. Nine patients with MS and extensor spasticity or chronic flexor posturing were entered into a double-blind trial of oral THC in doses of 5 and 10 mg compared to placebo. EMG response to stretch was measured along with subjective gradings of several aspects of spasticity. The 10 mg dose proved superior to the 5 mg dose and both were superior to placebo.[85] The number of patients who reported feeling "high" was equivalent on THC and placebo, suggesting that alteration of consciousness and nonspecific effects are not likely explanations for the effect. Functional effects were not assessed.

THREONINE

Threonine, a precursor of glycine (see previous text), was studied in an open trial using 6 patients with genetic spasticity syndromes.[86] Decreased spasticity was noted over a 12-month trial of 500 mg/day and was greater in the lower than in the upper extremities. There was some regression 4 months after cessation of treatment. More controlled studies of amino acid supplementation are needed. In particular, it is important to study patients with static or traumatic etiologies because treatment may have an effect on the underlying genetic degenerative disease rather than on the spasticity itself.

TIZANIDINE

Tizanidine has a chemical structure unlike that of other antispasticity drugs. It is believed to inhibit spinal polysynaptic pathways, possibly presynaptically.[87] When compared to placebo in patients with MS, tizanidine was found to be significantly better in reducing resistance to passive stretch and clonus in the lower extremities, but no definite neurophysiologic, functional, or strength changes were seen.[88] Although dry mouth and sedation were more common in the treatment condition, the investigators' global preference was for tizanidine.

Several clinical trials have examined tizanidine in comparison to baclofen for treatment of spasticity in patients with MS or forms of spinal cord pathology.[87,89–96] Of the controlled studies using both clinical and functional measures, tizanidine in doses of 6 to 36 mg/day was found to be comparable or slightly superior to baclofen in doses of 15 to 90 mg/day.[90,92,94–96] One study failed to find benefits of either drug, but this investigation had only 10 patients and used very gross measures of improvement.[89] Another[93] found baclofen somewhat superior based on subjective preferences of both patients and clinicians, and isolated reduction of spasticity at the ankle and clonus at the knee, with no differences in functional measures. Tizanidine produced greater sedation than baclofen but produced less weakness. In general, both drugs were well tolerated. From this group of studies, it appears that tizanidine may be a useful drug, at least for those with MS and spinal pathology, in whom sedation is less of a concern than weakness.

Tizanidine has also been compared to diazepam, in controlled trials in patients with spastic hemiplegia caused by stroke and head trauma.[97] Tizanidine was found significantly better in terms of walking distance on flat ground and, overall, was preferred by the investigators. The two drugs were comparable in other functional and clinical measures. Tizanidine was better tolerated than diazepam, although sedation was a prominent side effect of both groups. Thus, tizanidine emerges as a potentially useful option in spasticity of cerebral origin if a close watch is kept for its sedating side effects.

SUMMARY OF MEDICATIONS

A large number of medications have been reviewed. Three drugs, diazepam, baclofen, and dantrolene, are in common use and have a large amount of research supporting their efficacy, at least in some situations. Even with these well-studied drugs, however, it is difficult to assess precisely what target symptoms are best relieved by each drug, what patient populations are best suited for each drug, and what functional benefits, if any, can reasonably be expected from each drug.

As is evident from the above discussion, many additional drugs have been tested for their spasmolytic effects. Some have been ineffective (e.g., cyclobenzaprine), whereas others have had measurable effects that were, however, clinically small and offered no obvious advantages over existing drugs (e.g., piracetam). In general, these drugs have been tested against too few patients to allow recommendations regarding particular areas in which they may offer advantages. It appears that α-adrenergic blocking drugs offer some promise, particularly if chemical modifications allow the development of nonphenothiazine forms, which produce less orthostatic hypotension. In some patients, extensor spasticity and co-existing psychiatric disturbances might argue for the selection of a neuroleptic with α-blocking properties, such as chlorpromazine. Tizanidine also appears to hold promise, although it is not dramatically superior to baclofen. Nevertheless, it provides one more effective drug when faced with adverse effects from previous medications. THC, in particular THC derivatives with fewer psychotropic properties, may also prove beneficial in the future.

CLINICAL DECISION MAKING

Pharmacologic treatment can be a useful adjunct to an integrated treatment program, but should not be viewed as the primary treatment modality. In general, patients with the UMN syndrome are disabled by a complex combination of positive and negative symptoms. One of the challenges in designing a comprehensive treatment program for such patients is the unique symptom pattern presented by each patient. For some patients, although medications may measurably improve some manifestations of spasticity, these manifestations may not be of much concern, and those that are may go untreated.

Before contemplating drug treatment of spasticity, it is wise to engage the patient and the rehabilitation team in a discussion of the problems faced by the patient and the goals of treatment. (Table 10–4) Some patients may be primarily concerned with painful spasms or sudden involuntary movements and others with improving their fine or gross motor abilities. Some goals of treatment may be unrealistic with

TABLE 10–4. CLINICAL DECISION MAKING

1. Establish the individual pattern of the UMN syndrome and how the symptoms interfere with function in each patient
2. Establish realistic goals in terms of suppression of positive target symptoms and anticipated gains in associated target functions
3. Decide on the most systematic and relevant measures with which to follow patient response to treatment: neurophysiologic, clinical, functional, global measures (some or all of these)
4. Consider the total repertoire of treatment modalities and ask if drug treatment can be useful
5. Decide which particular drug would be useful given the diagnosis, clinical presentation, and anticipated side effects
6. Perform serial drug trials with repeated assessments using the measures previously selected

currently available treatments (e.g., restoration of strength in a patient with complete spinal cord injury). Other goals of treatment should be agreed on between the patient and the treatment team. Examples of such goals are:

1. Reducing painful nighttime spasms
2. Decreasing adductor spasticity to facilitate nursing hygiene
3. Eliminating clonus to allow safe independent transfers
4. Improving speed and smoothness of gait
5. Decreasing arm spasticity to facilitate independent dressing
6. Decreasing arm spasticity to restore movement to a paralyzed arm

Goals 1 and 2 relate only to positive symptoms. Thus it is almost certain that a drug that is effective to any significant degree in reducing those symptoms will be valuable to the patient. Goal 3 is also related to a positive symptom. Here, however, unless the drug can virtually eliminate the symptom, there may not be a functional benefit. Goals 4 and 5 involve a hypothetic relationship between the positive symptoms of spasticity and performance of a functional task. That is, it is assumed that part of the basis for a slow, unsteady gait or difficulty with dressing *are* the positive symptoms of spasticity. Thus, for a drug to be of benefit here, two things must be true: the drug must successfully decrease the positive symptom *and* the positive symptom must be partly responsible for the functional deficit. Goal 6 suggests that a negative symptom (paralysis) is caused by a positive symptom (spasticity), which is unlikely to be true.

Framing the goals of treatment in this way helps the team and the patient know in advance how realistic their expectations of treatment are. In some cases, it suggests that treatment of the spasticity itself is not of great relevance and that more effort should be directed toward strengthening, coordination training, or learning of compensatory strategies. When such a formulation suggests that the goals of treatment are primarily reduction of positive symptoms, treatment outcome can be assessed in terms of those symptoms. When functional benefit is also desired, then measurement of spasticity should still be undertaken to verify that the drug is effective at that level, but the effects on function should be measured concurrently. If a drug fails to improve the positive symptoms of interest, another drug can be tried. If a drug, however, succeeds in improving the positive symptoms, but fails to provide the desired functional benefits, it is unlikely that another drug will do so.

Selection of medication treatment is influenced by a variety of factors beyond likely drug efficacy for the symptoms in question. Patients with marginal cognitive capacities, such as the severely brain-injured, may not tolerate any spasmolytic drug well, and clinicians will be directed toward physical modalities and/or multiple nerve blocks. In patients with a history of drug abuse, drugs other than benzodiazepines may be more appropriate. Patients with focal problems may want to avoid systemic medication administration, even if it would be effective, in favor of more local treatments such as phenol blocks. Furthermore, in our experience, patients with spasticity of overwhelming proportions (i.e., those whose therapists are barely strong enough to adequately perform ROM exercises) rarely have a clinically significant improvement from any medication.

Whenever a patient suffers from a sudden increase in spasticity, other reasons should be sought before simply intensifying the treatment program and raising medication doses. Acute infections, bladder or bowel distension, anxiety, skin breakdown or a new neurologic event may all exacerbate existing problems with spasticity and should be treated primarily.

When medication treatment of spasticity is indicated, selecting the best drug for an individual patient remains a challenge. This is particularly so in dealing with patients with traumatic brain injury (TBI). No pure series of 10 or more TBI patients has been studied in response to *any* antispasticity drug, although as many as 11 TBI patients are included in a variety of mixed studies. Because TBI involves brainstem as well as cerebral pathology, it is not at all clear whether extrapolations from research on CVA patients, SCI patients, or neither, are applicable.

The following is an attempt to make some generalizations regarding useful agents in various patient populations. Some recommendations come directly from research, whereas others involve attempts to apply research findings to situations that have not been directly studied (Table 10–5).

TABLE 10–5. MEDICATION SELECTION FOR SPECIFIC PATIENT POPULATIONS

	MS	SCI*/#	CVA	TBI	CP
Dantrolene	−	+/−	+	(+)	+
Diazepam	+	−/+	−	−	+
Baclofen	++	++/++	−	?	?
Alpha blockers/Phenothiazines	+	−	?	(−)	?
Investigational drugs					
Piracetam	?	?	?	?	+
Progabide	+	?	?	?	?
THC	+	?/+	(−)	(−)	(−)
Tizanidine	++	?/++	+	+	?

*/# = complete SCI/incomplete SCI
( ) = rating based on extrapolation rather than direct study

MULTIPLE SCLEROSIS

MS is among the best-studied diagnoses in terms of pharmacologic treatment of spasticity. Almost all the medications reviewed in this chapter have demonstrable efficacy in MS-related spasticity. Thus, selection of a drug is guided by various other considerations. In general, baclofen is considered the drug of choice in MS, although tizanidine shows promise of providing comparable or superior results. However, both these drugs can produce sedation and other troublesome side effects. For patients with cerebral involvement and impaired cognition, cautious use of dantrolene could be attempted, particularly if the patient's spasticity is coupled with good residual strength, or on the other hand, if weakness is already so profound that functional losses are unlikely. Diazepam is another alternative, but should probably be avoided in the face of impaired coordination, ataxia, or cognitive deficits. In the uncommon situation when a neuroleptic is indicated for psychiatric reasons, selection of one with alpha-adrenergic blocking capabilities may benefit spasticity. Patients with flexor spasms, however, may suffer exacerbations. Finally, nonjudgmental questioning regarding marijuana use may reveal that the patient is self-medicating. This may be beneficial in some situations (e.g., flexor spasms disrupting sleep), but patients using marijuana at work or school for spasticity control may benefit from substitution of a drug with fewer psychotropic actions.

SPINAL CORD INJURY

Patients with complete SCI can benefit significantly from baclofen or dantrolene. Whether they benefit equally from diazepam remains controversial. In general, it is wise to start with baclofen because it has fewer serious adverse effects than dantrolene and causes less sedation and drug dependency than diazepam. Patients who cannot tolerate baclofen may, however, benefit form dantrolene or diazepam. Patients with incomplete injury show similar response patterns to those with MS; that is, diazepam and baclofen are both effective. Dantrolene may be relatively contraindicated in those who have useful but marginal strength. Alpha-adrenergic blocking drugs, although theoretically effective, are likely to cause excessive hypotension, especially in quadriplegics, and may exacerbate flexor spasms or cause new ones.

CEREBROVASCULAR ACCIDENT

Dantrolene is generally the drug recommended for spasticity in CVA patients. It is by no means ideal, however. Weakness can be a significant problem, and the risk of adverse effects is higher in older patients, particularly women. A small amount of literature supports the use of diazepam, baclofen, and tizanidine in CVA, although it is generally acknowledged that adverse effects such as sedation are more common in this population. Thus, it probably makes sense to initiate treatment with dantrolene, but if adverse effects occur, or treatment is ineffective, the other drugs may be worth assessing, especially in alert patients. No data on the investigational drugs, with the exception of tizanidine, are available for CVA patients.

TRAUMATIC BRAIN INJURY

Clinical decisions about drug treatment in this population must rely on parallels from other patient populations and common sense until further research is available. Because dantrolene is the least sedating drug and works independently of mechanisms of spasticity, it is generally the first choice of the authors for this population. We have, however, seen individual cases in which even dantrolene proved significantly sedating in those with marginal cognitive status. Baclofen has sometimes been of benefit in those in whom liver pathology developed on dantrolene. Diazepam is generally profoundly sedating, although it may be of benefit in persistently vegetative patients beyond the point where cognitive improvements can be expected. In such patients, the drug should be tapered periodically in the remote possibility that the patient has made some cognitive recovery. Because TBI patients are among the most severely spastic patients, and yet among the most sensitive to adverse cognitive effects, further trials of intrathecal baclofen will be of interest in this population.

CEREBRAL PALSY

Treatment of spasticity in CP has been inadequately studied. The drug that has been most convincingly shown to be effective is dantrolene, although the same concern about its use in patients with significant weakness (but with residual functional strength) applies. Diazepam has been reported to be of benefit, particularly in combination with dantrolene, but the relevant research used global measures of response and seemed to attribute some of diazepam's benefits to behavioral changes. In particular, more research is needed in balancing actual effects on spasticity against cognitive effects and potential changes in school performance in the pediatric population. Piracetam shows some promise in CP, but its benefits in one small study were relatively modest. Although there are no studies of baclofen in children with CP, physicians who work with this population have found it helpful to some patients.

SUMMARY

Medications can play a useful role in the treatment of patients with disabling spasticity. Practical issues regarding dosage schedules and adverse effects are summarized in Table 10–6. The astute clinician must keep in mind that many of the disabilities of the patient with the UMN syndrome are not primarily caused by spasticity. Thus one should avoid sequential trials of multiple toxic medications in the unrealistic pursuit of a "cure" for the UMN syndrome. Clinical assessment should first address the degree to which spasticity itself contributes to the discomfort and disability experienced by the patient. Next, those problems directly attributable to spasticity should be assessed in terms of which of the many treatment modalities (relaxation, physical modalities, medications, nerve blocks, surgery, etc.) are likely to be most effective. Finally, the medication(s) most likely to be effective should be selected as soon as pharmacologic treatment seems indicated.

Even this methodical process does not eliminate the need for trial and error assessment of individual drugs. Research on comparative drug selection is lacking at present. Even if more research were available, it is unlikely that it would allow accurate preselection in all cases; each patient is unique in terms of relevant pathophysiology, degree of disability, and functional goals. In cases in which adjustment of dose is problematic, or there is disagreement among the team and patient about the degree of benefit and adverse effects from a drug, a single-case placebo-controlled trial

TABLE 10–6. ANTI-SPASTICITY MEDICATIONS: PRACTICAL INFORMATION

	Dantrolene Sodium	Benzodiazepines	Baclofen
Usual dosage schedule	Baseline LFTs Begin with 25 mg b.i.d. Increase by 25–50 mg every 5–7 days Maximal dose 200–400 mg/day	Begin with 2 mg b.i.d. Increase by 2 mg every 5–7 days Maximal dose 40–60 mg/day	Begin with 5 mg b.i.d. Increase by 5 mg every 5–7 days Maximal dose 80 mg/day
Common	Weakness (especially with marginal strength) Sedation Dizziness Paresthesias Nausea Diarrhea Hepatitis	Sedation Weakness Depression Ataxia Memory loss Drug dependence	Sedation Fatigue Weakness Nausea Dizziness Paresthesias Decreased seizure threshold Hallucinations if discontinued abruptly

for clinical purposes, with blinded ratings by the patient and team, may lead to more objective decision making.[98]

It is hoped that research in the future will include more of the following essential features:

- Homogeneous patient groups with adequate sample sizes and estimates of statistical power
- Double-blind crossover trials with adjustable dosage ranges
- Comparison of two or more drugs in a given patient population
- Concurrent measurement of physical and functional indicators
- Assessment of criterion measures of drug response
- Follow-up on long-term use of medications

As more data on currently available and newly developed drugs that satisfy these conditions become available, the task of identifying patients who will benefit from drug treatment and selecting the most appropriate drug will become more rational.

REFERENCES

1. Antel, J.P., and Arnason, B.G.W.: Multiple sclerosis and other demyelinating diseases. *In* Petersdorf, R.G., et al., eds. Harrison's Principles of Internal Medicine (10th Ed.). New York, McGraw-Hill, 1983.
2. Miller, J.D.: Early evaluation and management. *In* Rosenthal, M., Griffith, E.R., Bond, M.R., et al., eds. Rehabilitation of the Head Injured Adult, Philadelphia, F.A. Davis, 1983.
3. Young, R.R., and Delwaide, P.J.: Spasticity. N. Engl. J. Med. *304*:28–33, 96–99, 1981.
4. Whyte, J.: Outcome evaluation in the remediation of attention and memory deficits. J. Head Trauma Rehabil. *1(3)*:64–71, 1986.
5. Burke, D.: An approach to the treatment of spasticity. Drugs *10*:112–120, 1975.
6. Davidoff, R.A.: Pharmacology of spasticity. Neurology *28*:46–51, 1978.
7. Davidoff, R.A.: Drug treatment of spasticity. The Lancet *ii(683)*:1131, November 28, 1970.
8. Pedersen, E.: Clinical assessment and pharmacologic therapy of spasticity. Arch. Phys. Med. Rehabil. *55*:344–354, 1974.
9. Verrier, M., Ashby, P., and Macleod, S.: Diazepam effect on reflex activity in patients with complete spinal lesions and in those with other causes of spasticity. Arch. Phys. Med. Rehabil. *58*:148–153, 1977.
10. Cook, J.B., and Nathan, P.W.: On the site of action of diazepam in spasticity in man. J. Neurol. Sci. *5*:33–37, 1967.
11. Martenson, A.: Antispastic medication. Scand. J. Rehab. Med. *13*:143–147, 1981.
12. Ellis, K.O., and Carpenter, J.F.: Mechanism of control of skeletal-muscle contraction by dantrolene sodium. Arch. Phys. Med. Rehabil. *55*:362–369, 1974.
13. Pinder, R.M., Brogden, R.N., Speight, T.M., et al.: Dantrolene sodium: A review of its pharmacological properties and therapeutic efficacy in spasticity. Drugs *13*:3–23, 1977.
14. Monster, A.W., Herman, R., Meeks, S., et al.: Cooperative study for assessing the effects of a pharmacological agent on spasticity. Am. J. Phys. Med. *52*:163–188, 1973.
15. Mai, J., and Pedersen, E.: Mode of action of dantrolene sodium in spasticity. Acta Neurol. Scand. *59*:309–316, 1979.
16. Monster, A.W., Tamai, Y., and McHenry, J.: Dantrolene sodium: Its effect on extrafusal muscle fibers. Arch. Phys. Med. Rehabil. *55*:355–362, 1974.
17. Luisto, M., Moller, K., Nuutila, A., et al.: Dantrolene sodium in chronic spasticity of varying etiology. Acta Neurol. Scand. *65*:355–362, 1982.
18. Monster, A.W.: Spasticity and the effect of dantrolene sodium. Arch. Phys. Med. Rehabil. *55*:373–383, 1974.
19. Weiser, R., Terenty, T., Hudgson, P., et al.: Dantrolene sodium in the treatment of spasticity in chronic spinal cord disease. Practitioner *221*:123–127, 1978.
20. Basmajian, J.V., and Super, G.A.: Dantrolene sodium in the treatment of spasticity. Arch. Phys. Med. Rehabil. *54*:60–64, 1973.
21. Chyatte, S.B., Birdsong, J.H., and Bergman, B.A.: The effects of dantrolene sodium on spasticity and motor performance in hemiplegia. South. Med. J. *64(2)*:180–185, 1971.
22. Ketel, W.B., and Kolb, M.E.: Long term treatment with dantrolene sodium of stroke patients with spasticity limiting the return of function. Curr. Med. Res. Opin. *9*:161–169, 1984.
23. Haslam, R.H.A., Walcher, J.R., Lietman, P.S., et al.: Dantrolene sodium in children with spasticity. Arch. Phys. Med. Rehabil. *55*:384–388, 1974.
24. Gelenberg, A.J., and Poskanzer, D.C.: The effect of dantrolene sodium of spasticity in multiple sclerosis. Neurology *23*:1313–1315, 1973.
25. Tolosa, E.S., Soll, R.W., and Loewenson, R.B.: Treatment of spasticity in multiple sclerosis with dantrolene. JAMA *233(10)*: 1046, 1975.

26. Utili, R., Boitnott, J.K. and Zimmerman, H.J.: Dantrolene-associated hepatic injury: Incidence and character. Gastroenterology 72:610, 1977.

27. Tseng, T., and Wang, S.: Locus of action of centrally acting muscle relaxants diazepam and tybamate. J. Pharmcol. Exp. Ther. 178:350–360, 1971.

28. Davidoff, R.A.: Antispasticity drugs: Mechanisms of action. Ann. Neurol. 17:107–116, 1985.

29. Corbett, M., Frankel, H.L., and Michaelis, L.: A double blind cross-over trial of valium in the treatment of spasticity. Paraplegia 10:19–22, 1972.

30. Wilson, L.A., and McKechnie, A.A.: Oral diazepam in the treatment of spasticity in paraplegia: A double blind trial and subsequent impressions. Scott. Med. J. 11:46–51, 1966.

31. Kendall, H.P.: The use of diazepam in hemiplegia. Ann. Phys. Med. 7(6):225–228, 1964.

32. Cocchiarella, A., Downey, J.A., and Darling, R.C.: Evaluation of the effect of diazepam on spasticity. Arch. Phys. Med. Rehabil. 49:393–396, 1967.

33. Engle, H.A.: The effect of diazepam (Valium) in children with cerebral palsy: A double-blind study. Dev. Med. Child Neurol. 8:661–667, 1966.

34. Marsh, H.O.: Diazepam in incapacitated cerebral-palsied children. JAMA 191(10):797–800, 1965.

35. Lossius, R., Dietrichson, P., and Lunde, P.K.M.: Effect of clorazepate in spasticity and rigidity: a quantitative study of reflexes and plasma concentrations. Acta Neurol. Scand. 71:190–194, 1985.

36. Scharf, M.B., Hirschowitz, J., Woods, M., et al.: Lack of amnestic effects of clorazepate on geriatric recall. Clin. Psychiatr. 46(12):518–520, 1985.

37. Romney, D.M., and Angus, W.R.: A brief review of the effects of diazepam on memory. Psychopharm. Bull. 20(2):313–316, 1984.

38. Basmajian, J.V., Shankardass, K., Russell, D., et al.: Ketazolam treatment for spasticity: double-blind study of a new drug. Arch. Phys. Med. Rehabil. 65:698–701, 1984.

39. Basmajian, J.V., Shankardass, K., and Russell, D.: Ketazolam once daily for spasticity: double-blind cross-over study. Arch. Phys. Med. Rehabil. 67:556–557, 1986.

40. Ashby, P., and White, D.G.: "Presynaptic" inhibition in spasticity and the effect of B(4-chlorophenyl) GABA. J. Neurol. Sci. 20:329–338, 1973.

41. Basmajian, J.V.: Lioresal (baclofen) treatment of spasticity in multiple sclerosis. Am. J. Phys. Med. 54(4):175–177, 1975.

42. Basmajian, J.V., and Yucel, V.: Effects of a GABA-derivative (BA-34647) on spasticity. Am. J. Phys. Med. 53(5):223–228, 1974.

43. Duncan, G.W., Shahani, B.T., and Young, R.R.: An evaluation of baclofen treatment for certain symptoms in patients with spinal cord lesions. Neurology 26:441–446, 1976.

44. Feldman, R.G., Kelly-Hayes, M., Conomy, J.P., et al.: Baclofen for spasticity in multiple sclerosis. Neurology 28:1094–1098, 1978.

45. Hudgson, P., and Weightman, D.: Baclofen in the treatment of spasticity. Brit. Med. J. 4:15–17, 1971.

46. Jones, R.F., Burke, D., Marosszeky, J.E., et al: A new agent for the control of spasticity. J. Neurol. Neurosurg. Psychiatry 33:464–468, 1970.

47. Levine, I.M., Jossmann, P.B., and DeAngelis, V.: Lioresal, a new muscle relaxant in the treatment of spasticity—a double-blind quantitative evaluation. Dis. Nerv. Sys. 38:1011–1015, 1977.

48. Pedersen, E., Arlien-Soborg, P., Grynderup, V., et al.: GABA derivative in spasticity. Acta Neurol. Scand. 46:257–266, 1970.

49. Sawa, G.M., and Paty, D.W.: The use of baclofen in treatment of spasticity in multiple sclerosis. Can. J. Neurol. Sci. 6(3):351–354, 1979.

50. McLellan, D.L.: Co-contraction and stretch reflexes in spasticity during treatment with baclofen. J. Neurol. Neurosurg. Psychiatry. 40:30–38, 1977.

51. Jones, R.F., and Lance, J.W.: Baclofen (Lioresal) in the long term management of spasticity. Med. J. Aust. 1:654–657, 1976.

52. Pedersen, E., Arlien-Soborg, P., and Mai, J.: The mode of action of the GABA derivative baclofen in human spasticity. Acta. Neurol. Scand. 50:665–680, 1974.

53. Pinto, O.D., Polker, M., and Debono, G.: Results of international clinical trials with Lioresal. Postgrad. Med. J. 48(Suppl 5):18–23, 1972.

54. Dralle, D., Muller, H., Zierski, J., et al.: Intrathecal baclofen for spasticity. Lancet ii:1003, 1985.

55. Penn, R.D.: Intrathecal baclofen for severe spasticity. Ann. N.Y. Acad. Sci. 531:157–166, 1988.

56. Siegfried, J., Rea, G.L.: Intrathecal application of drugs for muscle hypertonia. Scand. J. Rehab. Med. Suppl. 17:145–148, 1988.

57. Jones, R.F., Anthony, M., Torda, T.A., et al.: Epidural baclofen for intractable spasticity. Lancet i(8584):527, 1988.

58. Reisman Mann, N., and Gans, B.M.: Hallucinations associated with acute baclofen withdrawal: Report of two pediatric cases. Poster presented at the 47th Annual Assembly of the American Academy of Physical

Medicine and Rehabilitation, Kansas City, MO, October 2, 1985.

59. Roy, C.W., and Wakefield, I.R.: Baclofen psychosis: Case report. Paraplegia 24:318–321, 1986.

60. Cartlidge, N.E.F., Hudgson, P., and Weightman, D.: A comparison of baclofen and diazepam in the treatment of spasticity. J. Neurol. Sci. 23:17–24, 1974.

61. From, A., and Heltberg, A.: A double-blind trial with baclofen and diazepam in spasticity due to multiple sclerosis. Acta Neurol. Scand. 51:158–166, 1975.

62. Roussan, M., Terrence C., and Fromm, G.: Baclofen versus diazepam for the treatment of spasticity and long-term follow-up of baclofen therapy. Pharmatherapeutica 4(5):278–284, 1987.

63. Cendrowski, W., and Sobczyk, W.: Clonazepam, baclofen, and placebo in the treatment of spasticity. Eur. Neurol. 16:257–262, 1977.

64. Schmidt, R.T., Lee, R.H., and Spehlman, R.: Comparison of dantrolene sodium and diazepam in the treatment of spasticity. J. Neurol. Neurosurg. Psychiatry 39:350–356, 1976.

65. Nogen, A.G.: Medical treatment for spasticity in children with cerebral palsy. Child's Brain 2:304–308, 1976.

66. Glass, A., and Hannah, A.: A comparison of dantrolene sodium and diazepam in the treatment of spasticity. Paraplegia 12:170–174, 1974.

67. Mai, J.: Depression of spasticity by alpha-adrenergic blockade. Acta Neurol. Scand. 57:65–76, 1978.

68. White, C. de B., and Richens, A.: Thymoxamine and spasticity. Lancet i(859):686–687, April 13, 1974.

69. Yuill, G.M., and Neary, D.: Thymoxamine ineffective against spasticity. Lancet ii:1504, Dec. 29, 1973.

70. Sabbahi, M.A., and Powers, W.R.: Topical anesthesia: A possible treatment method for spasticity. Arch. Phys. Med. Rehabil. 62:310–314, 1981.

71. Giebler, K., Inacio, C., Whyte, J., et al.: Topical anesthesia to decrease spasticity. Poster presented at Braintree Hospital's Sixth Annual Traumatic Head Injury Conference, November 24, 1985.

72. Nance, P.W., Shears, A.H., and Nance, D.M.: Clonidine in spinal cord injury. Can. Med. Assoc. J. 133:41–42, 1985.

73. Donovan, W.H., Carter, R.E., Rossi, C.D., et al.: Clonidine effect on spasticity: A clinical trial. Arch. Phys. Med. Rehabil. 69:193–194, 1988.

74. Ashby, P, Burke, D., Rao, S., et al.: Assessment of cyclobenzaprine in the treatment of

spasticity. J. Neurol. Neurosurg. Psychiatry 35:599–605, 1972.

75. Stern, P., and Bokonjic, R.: Glycine therapy in 7 cases of spasticity. Pharmacology 12:117–119, 1974.

76. Erickson, D.L., Blacklock, J.B., Michaelson, M., et al.: Control of spasticity by implantable continuous flow morphine pump. Neurosurgery 16(2):215–217, 1985.

77. Cohan, S.L. Raines, A., Panagakos, J., et al.: Phenytoin and chlorpromazine in the treatment of spasticity. Arch. Neurol. 37:360–364, 1980.

78. Matthews, W.B., Rushworth, G., and Wakefield, G.S.: Dimethothiazine in spasticity. Acta Neurol. Scand. 48:635–644, 1972.

79. Addis-Jones, C.D., Addlestone, G., Allebone, P., et al.: A phenothiazine in spasticity. Practitioner 210:429–431, 1973.

80. Burke, D., Hammond, C., Skuse, N., et al.: A phenothiazine derivative in the treatment of spasticity. J. Neurol. Neurosurg. Psychiatry 38:469–474, 1975.

81. Maritz, N.G., Muller, F.O., and Pompe van Meerdervoort, H.F.: Piracetam in the management of spasticity in cerebral palsy. S. Afr. Med. J. 53:889–891, 1978.

82. Mondrup, K., and Pedersen, E.: The effect of the GABA-agonist, progabide, on stretch and flexor reflexes and on voluntary power in spastic patients. Acta. Neurol. Scand. 69:191–199, 1984.

83. Mondrup, K., and Pedersen, E.: The clinical effect of the GABA-agonist, progabide, on spasticity. Acta Neurol. Scand. 69:200–206, 1984.

84. Rudick, R.A., Breton, D., and Krall, R.L.: The GABA-agonist progabide for spasticity in multiple sclerosis. Arch. Neurol. 44:1033–1036, 1987.

85. Petro, D.J., and Ellenberger, C.: Treatment of human spasticity with delta-9-tetrahydrocannabinol. J. Clin. Pharmacol. 21:413S–416S, 1981.

86. Barbeau, A., Roy, M., and Chouza, C.: Pilot study of threonine supplementation in human spasticity. Can. J. Neurol. Sci. 9(2):141–145, 1982.

87. Newman, P.M., Nogues, M., Newman, P.K., et al.: Tizanidine in the treatment of spasticity. Eur. J. Clin. Pharmacol. 23:31–35, 1982.

88. Lapierre, Y., Bouchard, S., Tansey, C., et al.: Treatment of spasticity with tizanidine in multiple sclerosis. Can. J. Neurol. Sci. 14:513–517, 1987.

89. Corston, R.N., Johnson, F., and Godwin-Austen, R.B.: The assessment of drug treatment of spastic gait. J. Neurol. Neurosurg. Psychiatry 44:1035–1039, 1981.

90. Hassan, N., and McLellan, D.L.: Double-blind comparison of single doses of DS103-

282, baclofen, and placebo for suppression of spasticity. J. Neurol. Neurosurg. Psychiatry 43:1132–1136, 1980.

91. Heazlewood, V., Symoniw, P., Maruff, P., et al.: Tizanidine-initial pharmacokinetic studies in patients with spasticity. Eur. J. Clin. Pharmacol. 25:65–67, 1983.

92. Smolenski, C., Muff, S., Smolenski-Kautz, S.: A double-blind comparative trial of a new muscle-relaxant, tizanidine (DS102-282), and baclofen in the treatment of chronic spasticity in multiple sclerosis. Curr. Med. Res. Opin. 7(6):374–383, 1981.

93. Bass, B., Weinshenker, B., Rice, G.P.A., et al: Tizanidine versus baclofen in the treatment of spasticity in patients with multiple sclerosis. Can. J. Neurol. Sci. 15(1):15–19, 1988.

94. Hoogstraten, M.C., van der Ploeg, R.J.O., Van der Burg, W., et al.: Tizanidine versus baclofen in the treatment of multiple sclerosis patients. Acta Neurol. Scand. 77:224–230, 1988.

95. Stein, R., Nordal, H.J., Oftedal, S.I., et al.: The treatment of spasticity in multiple sclerosis: A double-blind clinical trial of a new anti-spastic drug tizanidine compared with baclofen. Acta Neurol. Scand. 75:190–194, 1987.

96. Eysette, M., Rohmer, F., Serratrice, G., et al.: Multi-centre, double-blind trial of a novel antispastic agent, tizanidine, in spasticity associated with multiple sclerosis. Curr. Med. Res. Opin. 10(10):699–708, 1988.

97. Bes, A., Eysette, M., Pierrot-Deseilligny, E., et al.: A multi-centre, double-blind trial of tizanidine, a new antispastic agent, in spasticity associated with hemiplegia. Curr. Med. Res. Opin. 10(10):709–718, 1988.

98. Whyte, J.: Clinical drug evaluation. J. Head Trauma Rehabil. 3(4):95–99, 1988.

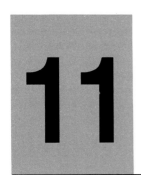

11

NERVE BLOCKS

MEL B. GLENN

If we were to try to conceive of an ideal treatment for spasticity, one of its properties would be reduction of the reflexive contractions of muscle without affecting voluntary strength. At first glance, the peripheral nervous system does not appear to be a likely site for such an intervention because, up to its most distal aspects, nerves that are involved largely with the stretch reflex run together with nerves that affect voluntary strength, and, in fact, these two neurophysiologic systems are not entirely separable. In 1957, however, Matthews and Rushworth,[1] extending a line of investigation pursued by Liljestrand and Magnus[2] in 1919, demonstrated that the injection of dilute procaine onto peripheral nerves of decerebrate cats could indeed have a selective effect on the hyperactive stretch reflex. They presented evidence to support the notion that this effect was caused by a greater sensitivity of small-diameter nerves, such as the gamma motor neurons, to procaine.[3] This information, however, did not have any practical application because of the short duration of effect of local anesthetic agents. Meanwhile, chemical neurolysis with phenol and alcohol was being used for the treatment of pain and vascular disease.[4] It was not until 1959, however, that Kelley and Gauthier-Smith[5] and Nathan[6] reported on the use of intrathecal phenol to treat spasticity. Encouraged by the speculation (later shown to be unwarranted) that they had found a sub-stance that would preferentially affect small diameter fibers over long periods of time, numerous reports emerged in the 1960s documenting the successful treatment of spasticity by nerve block with phenol[7-15] and alcohol.[16-18] Since that time chemical neurolysis has been widely, though sporadically, used to treat spasticity.

Nerve block refers to the application of chemical agents to a nerve to impair, either temporarily or permanently, the conduction along that nerve. The agents most frequently used are phenol, alcohol, and local anesthetics. Chemical neurolysis is a nerve block that impairs conduction by means of destruction of a portion of the nerve. When these agents are applied to the treatment of spasticity, the intent is to interrupt the stretch reflex arc. Although this can be achieved by means of intrathecal injection to affect the lumbar and sacral nerve roots at the level of the cauda equina, the peripheral nervous system can be approached more selectively distal to the cauda. Intrathecal neurolysis is rarely used today, and is discussed in chapter 12.

Chemical neurolysis has been performed at every level of the peripheral nervous system from the root to the motor end plate. The therapeutic result achieved and the potential side effects and complications depend to some extent on the anatomic site at which the nerve is injected. The discussion of neurolytic procedure in this chapter will, therefore, emphasize not only the chemical agent injected but the location of the injection as well.

Chemical neurolysis can be an extremely effective intervention for reducing spasticity. Although the effects have not usually been documented in controlled trials, the results are immediate and the clinical descriptions of relief of spasticity have frequently been dramatic and explicit. Many authors have described the sustained elimination of clonus beginning immediately after nerve blocks with phenol.[7,8,10,11,19−27] Others have described increases in strength or speed of active voluntary movement in antagonists of muscles blocked, and occasionally in the blocked muscle itself.[9−11,13,19,21,23,24,28] Nerve blocks have also diminished spasticity in opposite extremities, or in synergists not innervated by the nerve that was blocked.[11] Passive range of motion has often been improved when spasticity was contributing to contracture formation,[8,11,23,26,28,29] and a reduced need for passive stretching has been seen.[9] In young, preambulatory children, relief of adductor spasticity by chemical neurolysis has facilitated crawling, sitting and standing,[13,22] and nerve blocks with phenol to the gluteus maximus have improved sitting or allowed the sitting position for the first time.[17] Improvements in gait have been seen due to a reduction of hip adductor tone, with a resultant decrease in scissoring.[17,18,22,23] Halpern and Meelhuysen reported three cases of children aged 2, 3, and 6 years with spastic diplegia who ambulated for the first time a few days after chemical neurolysis, or after several weeks of ambulation training following nerve blocks.[13] Nerve blocks targeted at spastic ankle plantarflexors have contributed to improved dorsiflexion during gait, and at times allowed the use of orthotics that could not be previously applied.[9,10,17,18,21,22,25−27] Others have found that nerve blocks have facilitated proper fitting of an orthotic device.[7,8] Painful clawing of the toes has been relieved by tibial nerve blocks.[23,26] Painful spasms have been relieved,[18,26] and spasms have been reduced in patients with spinal cord injury.[7] Reduction in hip flexor spasticity by means of chemical neurolysis has been reported to reduce the compensatory lumbar lordosis.[17] Some authors have reported improvements

in activities of daily living (ADLs) following chemical neurolysis.[9−11,18,19,23−27] Chemical neurolysis has facilitated nursing care, hygiene, positioning, and prevention of decubitus ulcers.[13,22,23] Perineal nerve block with phenol resulted in a significant reduction of postvoid residual urine volumes in a man with a spastic external urethral sphincter following spinal cord injury.[11] Several authors have performed selective sacral rhizotomies with phenol or alcohol to reduce detrusor hyperreflexia or external urethral sphincter spasticity.[30−32]

Helweg-Larsen and Jacobsen[7] found that in children with cerebral palsy, 97 of 150 peripheral nerve blocks with 3% phenol reduced spasticity. Although improvements in gait were common following lower-extremity procedures, upper-extremity blocks did not usually result in functional gains.

Khalili et al.[9] rated the degree of spasticity before nerve blocks with 2 or 3% phenol on a scale of 1+ (slight) to 4+ (severe), and after blocks added flaccid and normal to the scale. Spasticity was rated 4+ in all instances before 39 nerve blocks. After blocks, spasticity was rated as normal in 19 cases, 1+ in 15, 2+ in 5, and 3+ in 1. The medial and lateral hamstrings were rated separately after one sciatic nerve block, resulting in 40 post-block ratings. After follow-up intervals varying from 6 to 233 days, 17 of 19 ratings of normal remained at normal or 1+, and 34 of 40 ratings had increased by one or less.

Meelhuysen et al.[15] reported that of 31 paravertebral nerve blocks with 3 to 5% phenol, 20 completely eliminated hip flexor spasticity, and 7 others reduced spasticity. Halpern and Meelhuysen[14] found that of 394 muscles treated with intramuscular neurolysis with 5% phenol in 95 patients, decreased spasticity resulted in functional gains or improved posture in 374. Katz et al.,[8] using 3% phenol, obtained "50% or more" relief of spasticity after 31 of 56 peripheral nerve injections.

Tardieu et al.[16,17] published the only controlled study of chemical neurolysis reported in the literature. They applied 35% alcohol to the right posterior tibial nerve of cats, and rendered them decerebrate with a midcollicular section several weeks later.

They then plotted length-tension curves for stretch of both soleus muscles. The tension elicited by passive stretch was significantly lower on the right side than on the left. No such difference was found in a group of control animals.

Although nerve blocks can, in some instances, completely eliminate hypertonicity, they can also be titrated to a certain extent by adjusting the concentration and quantity of the neurolytic agent injected, by choosing the site along the nerve tree to be injected (and thus the size of the motor branch), and by choosing the number of branches to be injected. This impression must be tempered by the poor correlation in the literature between concentration and quantity of phenol and apparent effectiveness, and the lack of controlled data in this area. The effectiveness of a neurolytic procedure is related to many variables, not the least of which are the choice of patient and the goals of the treatment.

The effect on spasticity can be localized to the specific muscle or group of muscles that are causing a problem. On the other hand, because the result is not generalized, many blocks may have to be performed to affect a widespread problem with spasticity, and some muscles may be inaccessible or difficult to block.

The duration of the effect is extremely variable. Although the effect of most neurolytic procedures lasts from several months to a few years, it is usually not permanent. This is in some ways an advantage, because the patient and family, as well as the physician performing the block and the treating team, can be reassured to some degree that if adverse effects result from the block, they are not likely to be permanent. The need to repeat nerve blocks multiple times in some individuals can, however, be a disadvantage of the procedure, although this is certainly not always necessary. The duration of effect of neurolytic procedures will be discussed in greater detail later in this chapter (see "Duration of Effect" below).

Nerve blocks can be performed at bedside, or in a clinic or office, and general anesthesia is rarely required. Morbidity is not excessive. (see "Side Effects and Complications" below)

TECHNIQUE

Nerve blocks are usually performed using a 22-gauge sterile needle that is Teflon®-coated except at the bevel, so that a pulsed electrical stimulus will be transmitted to the nerve only when it is in the proximity of the bevel itself. The hub of the needle is connected to a stimulator that delivers a square wave pulse of 0.1 msec duration once or twice per second, and which contains a rheostat to regulate the current, and, ideally, an ammeter as well. A reference electrode is attached to the surface of the skin (Fig. 11–1). An assistant is often necessary to aid in positioning the patient. The needle is inserted in the vicinity of the nerve to be injected, and pulsed stimulation delivered at a current of 5 to 10 milliamperes (mA). When a rhythmic response is observed, the physician checks to be sure that the appropriate muscle or group of muscles is contracting. Some practitioners use electromyographic recording equipment to assist in determining that only the target muscle is contracting. The amperage is then reduced, and with the muscle still contracting, but less vigorously so, a search is made by moving the needle in minute increments, in three dimensions if necessary, until a strong contraction is again observed, indicating that the bevel is now closer to the nerve. This process is continued until one mA or less is needed to produce a contraction, at which point the bevel is close enough to the nerve to inject.[7,9–15,19,20,22,23,25–28,33] If the injection is successful, the contraction will disappear almost immediately or diminish gradually within 1 or 2 minutes. At times this response is preceded by an initial increase in the force of contraction as the solution makes contact with the nerve. The use of flexible extension tubing to connect the syringe to the needle helps prevent unwanted movement during injection.

The patient can be expected to feel some discomfort during the search; individual tolerance varies greatly. The patient usually feels a burning sensation when phenol or alcohol is injected.

Peripheral nerves, their large motor branches, or electrosensitive areas of muscle where small motor branches are enter-

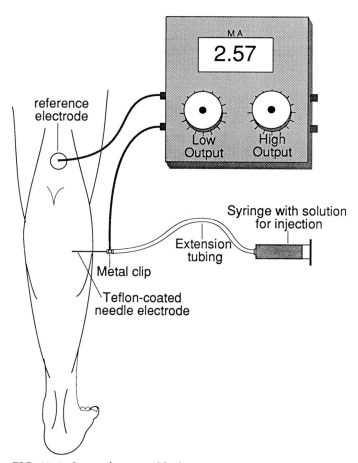

FIG. 11–1. Set-up for nerve block.

ing the muscle can all be located by surface stimulation before needle stimulation. It is useful to have a stimulator capable of delivering the current necessary for surface stimulation, generally 5–10 mA or greater.

Details of the technique specific to each type of nerve block will be discussed in the following sections.

NERVE BLOCKS WITH PHENOL

QUALITIES OF PHENOL

Phenol (carbolic acid) is a derivative of benzene with one hydroxyl group (Fig. 11–2). It is a colorless crystal that is soluble in water at room temperature at concentrations below 6.7%. At higher concentrations, it must be warmed to remain soluble.

It is also soluble in glycerine and in a number of oils. When exposed to air, it oxidizes to form compounds that lend it a reddish hue.[4]

In concentrations of 5% or more in water, phenol denatures protein, causing tissue necrosis, and it is this property that makes it valuable as a neurolytic agent. Phenol also has local anesthetic properties, even at concentrations of 1 to 2%, and has been used as a topical local anesthetic agent.[4] The local anesthetic effect is probably responsible for the transient anesthesia and weakness that are commonly seen after nerve blocks.

Phenol is rapidly absorbed through the skin, and in systemic doses of 8.5 g or more, which might occur in industrial accidents, it causes convulsions, central nervous system depression, and cardiovascular collapse.

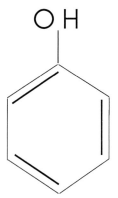

FIG. 11-2. Chemical structure of phenol.

Chronic exposure to phenol causes rash, gastrointestinal symptoms, and renal toxicity with smoky urine.[4]

Phenol is conjugated largely by the liver to form phenyl compounds. It is also oxidized to quinols or to carbon dioxide and water. The conjugated derivatives are excreted by the kidney.[4]

EFFECT OF PHENOL ON NERVES

Reports that phenol was capable of diminishing spasticity and chronic pain without impairing cutaneous or proprioceptive sensibility or strength generated considerable interest in the differential effect of phenol on nerves of varying fiber size.[5,6,34,35] Investigators hypothesized that phenol might selectively affect small gamma motor neurons, leaving alpha motor neurons intact. The sparing of sensibility to pain provoked by cutaneous stimulation was, however, difficult to explain by this theory.

Iggo and Walsh[36] studied compound action potentials in spinal rootlets of cats before, and then within minutes after, phenol was applied to the rootlets. They found that the motor α wave was the most resistant to the phenol and that the smaller, slower C fibers were more susceptible. Using natural stimuli, they found that cutaneous afferents were more susceptible to phenol than were proprioceptive afferents. They reported that 0.5% phenol dissolved in Ringer's solution was equivalent to 5% phenol in iodophenylundecylylate (Myodil). They did not,

however, look at the late effects of phenol on conduction, and therefore this study can be said to be consistent with a local anesthetic effect. Indeed, small fibers are more susceptible to the effects of local anesthetic agents.

In a 1960 report, Nathan and Sears,[37] having noted a temporary effect of phenol on sensation and strength and a lasting effect only on the chronic pain caused by malignant lesions, studied the effect of phenol in Myodil and aqueous solutions on conduction in the spinal roots of cats. They too reported the slow-conducting small fibers to be more susceptible. They noted, however, that the effect of 7.5% phenol in Myodil on the largest fibers was still partially reversible more than three hours after application, but that no recovery occurred in the small C fibers by that time. When 5% phenol in Myodil was applied for up to 50 minutes, some of the gamma fibers always recovered. They concluded that phenol has both a local anesthetic action and an irreversible effect on nerves that vary to some degree depending on the concentration of phenol, the length of time it is applied, and the solvent in which it is dissolved. They did not observe beyond 3 hours for a reversible effect, and did not study reversibility as extensively with aqueous solutions, which are considerably more effective. A 5% solution of phenol in Myodil was found to be approximately equivalent to 0.1% aqueous solution. When 0.5% aqueous solution was applied, blocking of the C fibers was complete, although not necessarily irreversibly so, in 10 seconds.

Schaumburg et al.[38] saw complete disappearance of evoked potentials in peripheral nerves of cats within two minutes of the application of 1% aqueous phenol, with partial recovery after washing with saline. However, they observed only a slightly quicker decline in the potentials from the delta and C fibers when compared to the larger, more rapidly conducting A-fibers, and felt that this did not represent a significant differential block. Fischer et al.[39] injected 3 to 6% aqueous phenol under the epineurium of rabbit sciatic nerves, and found that, within one minute, evoked potentials of both large and small diameter fibers were affected equally, with the effect still present 40 minutes after the injection. Similar results were obtained with an external application of phenol.

Histologic and electrophysiologic observations over longer periods have been helpful in clarifying the chronic effects of phenol on nerve. Nathan et al.,[40] again using Myodil in varying concentrations on spinal roots of cats, report nonselective destruction of nerve fibers of all sizes. The total number of nerves affected was correlated with the concentration of phenol applied. They observed a marked inflammatory reaction surrounding the rootlets at 6 days and complete destruction of all fibers in some parts of the root, with complete sparing in others. This localizing effect could be related to qualities of the solvent rather than the phenol itself. Fischer et al.,[41] however, found that when sciatic nerves of rabbits were injected with aqueous phenol, the effect on the evoked responses recorded in the dorsal versus the ventral roots varied

randomly, suggesting that aqueous phenol also exerts a patchy effect on nerve.

Burkel and McPhee[42] studied the effects of 5% phenol in saline on peripheral nerves of rats at multiple points in time, up to 14 weeks after the application. Again, destruction of fibers of all sizes was seen, although large axons degenerated more slowly. Coagulation of nerves at the site of injection was seen 1 hour following injection. They observed Wallerian degeneration with eventual regrowth of most axons. When phenol was dripped onto the nerve, axons in the center of the nerve were not affected. Figure 11–3 is a simulation of the possible distribution of axonal destruction when phenol is dripped onto a peripheral nerve. When Burkel and McPhee injected phenol into the nerve, all fibers were destroyed. At 14 weeks, regenerated nerves looked almost completely normal, although they noted an increase in collagen and fibroblasts in the endoneurium. They speculate

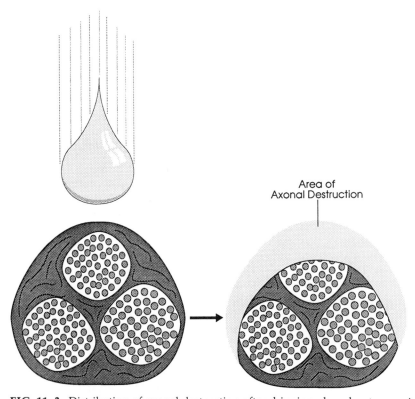

Area of
Axonal Destruction

FIG. 11–3. Distribution of axonal destruction after dripping phenol onto a peripheral nerve.

that this might make the nerve more resistant to subsequent injection. They also found occlusion of many small blood vessels, and speculate that this might account for the diminution in spasticity lasting for several years after nerve block that is seen in some cases.

Mooney et al.[43] examined rabbit peripheral nerves at various intervals following injection (into the nerve sheath) of 1 or 6% phenol or sterile water. They found the greatest amount of destruction 2 weeks after injection, but still a large amount at 8 weeks. Fibrosis in and surrounding the nerve, however, increased with time. The degree of both nerve damage and fibrosis appeared to be greater with 6% phenol. Nerves of all diameters were equally affected, as were axons and myelin. They also re-explored and sampled motor nerves from 4 patients who had had a recurrence of spasticity from 8 to 24 months following open nerve blocks with intraneural injection of phenol. Histologic examination revealed that there was still extensive destruction of nerve fibers, with equal numbers of thickly and thinly myelinated fibers among those remaining. Their impression after studying both human and animal samples was that "major amounts of reinnervation seem to be impossible, considering the degree of tissue destruction," and that reinnervation did not account for the recurrence of spasticity in their patients.

Schaumburg et al.[38] found that when 0.5% aqueous phenol was applied to peripheral nerves of cats, there was no histologic change after 30 days, although there had been an acute but reversible (after washing) disappearance of the evoked action potential. With 0.75 and 1% solutions, the predominant findings were segmental demyelination and remyelination, which were apparent by 2 or 3 weeks. By 2 months after application, shortened, remyelinated internodes were found. As the concentration of phenol and the duration of application before washing were increased, axonal destruction and Wallerian degeneration increased accordingly. They reported a relative sparing of unmyelinated and small myelinated fibers in comparison with large myelinated fibers. Electrophysiologic

studies done one month after the application of 1 or 2.5% phenol showed either complete absence of the α peak or loss of some of its components, with relative sparing of the Δ wave. When the nerve had been treated with 3 or 5% phenol for periods of 10 minutes or longer, the action potential could not be evoked one month later.

Halpern[44] studied 144 tissue samples from rats and dogs from 1 day to 10 months after intramuscular neurolysis was performed with 1 to 7% aqueous phenol. Axons of all sizes were destroyed regardless of the concentration of phenol used. In some areas, motor end-plates were partially resorbed. Neurogenic atrophy of the muscles and simultaneous evidence of collateral reinnervation and regeneration of muscle fibers were seen by 2 months, and by the third month, muscles were almost normal in specimens in which 1 to 3% phenol was used. Evidence of denervation, however, persisted at three months in specimens injected with 5 or 7% solutions.

Although these reports are not completely consistent, it is clear that phenol, when applied in solutions of sufficient strength, destroys axons of all sizes. Confirmation of its ability to cause axonal degeneration of α motor neurons has been obtained through electromyographic (EMG) examination of human subjects. Fusfeld[45] found positive sharp waves and fibrillation potentials in five of seven patients 1 month following peripheral nerve or motor point block with 3% aqueous phenol. High-amplitude polyphasic motor units were seen in a sixth subject, who had no reduction in spasticity after the blocks. The patient with normal EMG findings had an estimated reduction in spasticity of 25%. Glass et al.[46] did EMG examinations on 20 patients before and 2 weeks to 1½ years after peripheral nerve or motor point block with either 3 or 6% aqueous phenol. The 6% solution resulted in evidence of denervation in all subjects who had received peripheral nerve blocks, but in only one of those who had had motor point blocks. Five ml, the largest quantity of phenol used for motor point blocks in this study, had been applied in this instance. Neither peripheral nerve nor motor point blocks using 3% phenol resulted in EMG evidence of denervation. Clinical results were also poor with this group, and frequent repetition of blocks was necessary. The authors speculate that appropriate sampling might be more difficult when EMG is performed after motor point block because of the more localized areas affected. They did not report how EMG findings correlated with time since injection, except in one instance, in which serial studies over one and one-half years showed decreasing numbers of fibrillations and positive sharp waves despite persistent reduction in resistance to passive stretch of muscle and absence of clonus. Short duration of clinical effect and lack of evidence of denervation with 3% solution is consistent with the predominance of segmental demyelination over axonal degeneration found by Schaumberg et al.[38] with lower concentrations of phenol.

In summary, the weight of the histologic and electrophysiologic evidence is consistent with the following conclusions:

1. Phenol has a reversible local anesthetic effect on nerves, as well as the ability to destroy myelin and axons.
2. Phenol destroys axons of all sizes, probably in a patchy distribution, and more so on the outer aspect of the nerve bundle when phenol is dripped onto a peripheral nerve.
3. Axons destroyed by phenol regenerate, with some increase in fibrous tissue at the site of injection.
4. Lower concentrations of phenol may cause demyelination without axonal destruction.

SITE OF INJECTION

Mixed Sensorimotor Peripheral Nerve Blocks. The technique for performing mixed sensorimotor nerve blocks is described above (see "Technique"). Surface stimulation can be used before needle stimulation, if desired, to facilitate localization of the nerve. Fascicles containing fibers innervating specific muscles can often be differentially stimulated with the needle electrode and phenol can be injected in the proximity of the particular fascicles so targeted. Some physicians use EMG recording electrodes to ensure precise differential localization, although this can usually be adequately assessed by visual inspection of the contracting limb. Most practitioners have used aqueous phenol in concentrations ranging from 2 to 7%, although some authors have found 3% aqueous phenol to be relatively ineffective or to give results of relatively short duration.[46] The quantity injected should depend upon the concentration of the solution, the relative size of the nerve, whether the entire nerve or particular fascicles are targeted, and upon the thoroughness of block desired. Quantities of 5% aqueous phenol, for example, injected onto peripheral nerves, usually vary from one to 10 ml.[27] The effect of the block can be titrated either within a session or over multiple sessions by injecting smaller quantities, assessing the effectiveness, and reinjecting if necessary. If done within a short period of time, the possible confounding effect of the local anesthetic action of phenol upon assessment should be considered.

Mixed sensorimotor peripheral nerve blocks offer some potential advantages over motor nerve blocks. Although the issue has never been systematically studied, they can probably provide a more complete block because of the additional blocking of the cutaneous sensory fibers, which do have an excitatory influence on alpha motor neurons and therefore on muscle tone. In addition, all motor fibers are available to be blocked in one location, although it is unlikely that this could be accomplished with the quantities of phenol commonly used for neurolysis. One could, in fact, argue that, in practice, fewer fibers are actually available because the more peripheral fascicles may provide some protection for the centrally located fibers, as noted by Burkel and McPhee.[42] It is certainly true, however, that peripheral nerve blocks are generally quicker and easier procedures than blocks of the more distal branches of the motor nerve tree, and this can at times translate into a more thorough block. Although the literature does not necessarily support this assertion, some practitioners feel that peripheral neurolysis lasts longer than motor branch blocks. If axonal regeneration is the major factor in recurrence of spasticity after neurolysis, then this should indeed be the case. This subject is addressed in more detail in a later section of this chapter, Duration of Effect.

The major disadvantage of mixed sensorimotor nerve blocks with phenol is the potential for the development of pain in the distribution of the sensory component of the nerve. Complications of mixed sensorimotor neurolysis are described below in the section entitled Side Effects and Complications.

Motor Nerve Blocks. Largely motor nerves can be blocked at many levels of the peripheral nervous system, and such blocks have been given a variety of names (intramuscular neurolysis, motor point blocks, motor end-plate blocks), depending in part on the anatomic site at which the block takes place. Most frequently, motor nerves are approached within the particular muscle that is targeted. Electrosensitive sites (motor points) can be located by surface stimulation before a needle is inserted. Walthard and Tchicaloff[47] have published charts of the locations of motor points within the various muscles. Motor points are usually thought to correspond to the site at which the nerve enters the muscle or to an area where motor endplates cluster,[47] but can also represent a more proximal motor nerve as it approaches the surface of the muscle. The phenol can be injected at any of these areas, even at the motor endplate, which can be definitively identified by the characteristic pattern of EMG activity seen with an EMG needle recording electrode.[24] Motor endplates cluster at characteristic areas within each muscle ("innervation band"), as the endplate lies in the midpoint of any given muscle fiber.[48]

The more peripheral in the nervous system one goes, the smaller the branches, and therefore the more sites that need to be injected for an effective block. The patient then has to suffer more needle sticks and searches, and the physician performing the block becomes more fatigued during a longer, more tedious procedure. The more proximally one moves along the nerve tree, the easier and more effective the procedure becomes. If the practitioner knows the anatomy of the innervation of a particular muscle, he or she can locate large motor branches at the most proximal site after leaving the mixed sensorimotor nerve that is practical. Some surgeons do open nerve blocks to ensure that they are indeed injecting onto the motor branches and not onto the mixed nerve.[28,29,49-51] Some nerves, such as the obturator nerve, that are usually considered "peripheral nerves," have only a small cutaneous sensory component, and sensory complications from blocking the obturator nerve, for instance, are rare. Even at the root and plexus level, one can identify motor nerves to such muscles as the iliopsoas, quadratus lumborum, and paraspinal muscles.

The important distinction, then, is not the location of the nerve within the peripheral nervous system, but rather whether or not the nerve contains cutaneous afferent fibers. If it does not, then the risk of dysesthesias following the procedure is eliminated, and the chance of significant complications of the procedure becomes minimal in most anatomic sites commonly injected (see section entitled Side Effects and Complications, later in this chapter). "Motor nerves" do, of course, contain noncutaneous afferent fibers.

At times, the physician performing the block may choose to lyse multiple small motor branches rather than large ones so that the effect can be finely titrated. This may be a consideration when spasticity or primitive motor behaviors provide some useful function in addition to being problematic. In general, ease of titration is an advantage of motor nerve blocks over mixed sensorimotor nerve blocks. In addition, specific blocking of a single target muscle can be ensured.

Practitioners have used concentrations of aqueous phenol ranging from 2 to 7%. The quantity injected can range from 0.1 to several ml, depending on the size of the motor branch, which is best judged by the strength of contraction observed in the muscle when stimulated by the needle electrode.

Lumbosacral Paravertebral Nerve Block. Lumbar or sacral roots or elements of the lumbosacral plexus can be blocked in the paravertebral area.[15,20] Either mixed sensorimotor or motor nerves can be isolated in this area. Paravertebral blocks are discussed separately here because of the special risks and benefits associated with them. Anatomic localization is discussed in a later section of this chapter entitled Anatomic Considerations.

The technique is similar to that used for other nerve blocks with phenol, with the addition of precautions related to the risk of accidental intrathecal injection by way of the root sleeves, which are an extension of the subarachnoid space.[52] The patient should be placed in the lateral recumbent position with the trunk laterally flexed at an angle of at least 30 degrees, and should not be fully reclined until at least 15 minutes after the procedure has been completed. Alternatively, the patient can be sitting upright if this is feasible. Thus, if phenol were to be injected into the subarachnoid space, only the cauda equina would be affected. If clear fluid is aspirated, the needle should be withdrawn without injecting. As an added precaution, aspiration can be repeated after the injection of a small amount of phenol, in case a small piece of tissue lodged in the lumen of the needle had obstructed the initial aspiration, only to be dislodged by the force of the injection.

The major advantage of lumbosacral paravertebral blocks is that only in this location is there adequate access to the innervation of the iliopsoas muscles. Branches from the lumbar roots to the quadratus lumborum and to the lumbar and sacral paraspinal muscles can also be located in this area. One can also, of course, locate elements of the roots or plexus innervating most of the lower extremity musculature in this area, although this is not usually necessary because they can be blocked more distally without the additional risk of bowel, bladder, and sexual dysfunction that could ensue from accidental intrathecal injection. In addition, anatomic specificity is not always completely possible as one moves more proximally in the peripheral nervous system, although frequently one can satisfactorily isolate fascicles even at this level.

Neuropathic pain is, of course, a possibility when mixed sensorimotor nerves are blocked at the paravertebral level as well.

SIDE EFFECTS AND COMPLICATIONS

Despite extensive literature documenting nerve block effectiveness, many physicians remain reluctant to perform neurolytic procedures or to refer their patients to other physicians for nerve blocks for the treatment of spasticity. As would be expected, this is largely because of the fear of side effects or complications. Serious adverse effects are not common when nerve blocks are performed by physicians who are familiar with potential side effects and complications and know how to minimize the likelihood of their occurrence.

Motor and Mixed Sensorimotor Nerve Blocks. Other than dysesthesias, which occur only when mixed nerves are injected for the treatment of spasticity (see Mixed Sensorimotor Nerve Blocks, later in this chapter), the most common serious side effect of chemical neurolysis is the loss of useful motor function that was based on spasticity or primitive motor behaviors. While spasticity and associated motor behaviors may impair a patient's function to a degree that warrants intervention with nerve blocks, at the same time the patient may be using the increased muscle tone, abnormal posturing, or reflexive behaviors to his or her benefit in some respects. Lysing the nerves that supply the affected muscles, then, may result not only in the benefits that accrue from reducing spasticity, but also in functional losses. Instability of the hip and knee during ambulation has been reported following obturator and tibial nerve block, respectively.[26] Loss of "push-off" during ambulation has occurred following tibial nerve block in children with cerebral palsy.[22] Loss of the ability to grasp objects with spastic finger flexors can result from median nerve blocks.[26] Significant weakness developed following four of 150 peripheral nerve blocks performed in one series.[7] The muscle groups involved included the triceps surae, the quadriceps femoris, and the finger flexors. The authors, however, did not specify whether or not the involved muscle groups had been operating as part of a primitive motor pattern in these children with cerebral palsy. Nerve blocks can affect other aspects of the upper motor neuron syndrome whether spasticity is present or not.

Any reflex can be affected if either the afferent or efferent components are interrupted. A burn has been reported as a consequence of loss of a withdrawal reflex following multiple upper extremity blocks.[11] Temporary loss of reflex erection has been reported in patients with spinal cord injury after obturator nerve block with phenol.[11]

In addition to its direct effect on the muscles that are denervated, a nerve block may have kinesiologic consequences that are not obvious at first glance. For instance, blocking spastic ankle plantarflexors may cause instability at the knee if the extension moment created by the plantarflexion was being used to compensate for weak quadriceps muscles during ambulation (Fig. 11–4). Difficulty in ambulating for several days after tibial nerve blocks with phenol is relatively common.[11,22] This may be secondary to the need to adapt to a new kinesiologic dynamic or to a transient weakness that is occasionally seen.[7]

The occurrence of such motor complications is not surprising, given that motor and sometimes sensory nerves are interrupted. Most such effects can be avoided by a careful motor and functional evaluation before the block, or by the use of diagnostic blocks with local anesthetic agents or alcohol wash to evaluate the functional consequences of a more permanent procedure. Such diagnostic blocks, however, may not be totally equivalent to a nerve block with phenol, and therefore there is a degree of uncertainty involved in any neurolytic procedure in an area in which spasticity and primitive motor behaviors are providing some functional benefits. If the benefits are likely to outweigh the risk involved, the physician might recommend the procedure, but must explain the risks to the patient or guardian before obtaining consent.

Perhaps more surprising is the fact that strong, isolated, voluntary contraction of muscle is not significantly weakened by chemical neurolysis, except in the first hours or days after a nerve block, when weakness is not uncommon. The preservation of strength has been documented by

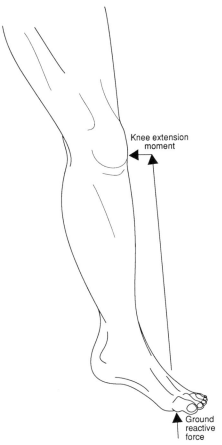

FIG. 11–4. Plantarflexion spasticity creates an extensor moment at the knee.

numerous clinical observations,[8,9,15,17,21,23,27] as well as in an animal study by Tardieu et al.[17] As described previously, these authors applied 35% alcohol to the right posterior tibial nerves of cats. They then observed that for several weeks before a midcollicular section, the cats walked, ran, and jumped normally, despite the fact that the nerve block resulted in a diminution of spasticity after decerebration. Furthermore, an electrical stimulus applied to the nerve evoked a contraction in the soleus that produced tension equal to that of the unblocked side. It should be noted, however, that their histologic and chemical studies were at variance with most studies done with phenol in that they were consistent with γ motor neuron involvement without substantial α blocking.

The relative preservation of voluntary, isolated strength in the face of dramatic reductions in spasticity is not the result of a relative immunity of α motor neurons to neurolytic agents, for, as noted previously in the section entitled Effect of Phenol on Nerves, numerous histologic and electrophysiologic studies have demonstrated that neurons of all sizes are affected when phenol is applied to nerves. Interrupting both efferents (α and γ motor neurons) and afferents (from the muscle spindle), however, may have a synergistic effect upon reflex contractions in comparison to nonreflexive contractions. The nervous system can compensate for loss of motor neurons by recruiting larger motor units when increased effort is needed. The loss of motor units may therefore be significant only when the muscle is placed under maximal stress, and even then, other muscles can help to compensate. When cutaneous afferents are also blocked in a mixed nerve, an additional excitatory influence is diminished, perhaps further enhancing the effect, and in particular affecting nociceptive reflexes such as the withdrawal reflex. Although primitive motor behaviors such as the synergistic movement patterns seen after cerebral cortical insults seem, for the most part, centrally mediated, they too receive a contribution from the muscle spindle afferents, which send facilitory fibers to muscles involved in synergistic movements.[10] In addition, they are often weaker than isolated voluntary contractions, and are probably more susceptible on this account as well. The strength of the contraction available in a given situation before a nerve block may be as important a consideration in determining whether or not it will be preserved as is the extent to which it is free from reflexive or primitive influences.

Indeed, Fischer et al.[39,41] speculate that phenol may have a greater effect on spasticity largely on the basis of its effect on efferents. They point out that partial curarization, which affects only the neuromuscular junction and not the afferents from the muscle spindle, has also been shown to reduce spasticity to a much greater degree than voluntary strength.[53] The differential effect would therefore depend largely on the numbers of motor neurons that are lysed, spasticity being affected by a relatively small reduction in motor neurons and voluntary strength being affected only when a relatively large number of fibers are destroyed. Arguing against the destruction of efferents as the predominant factor is the observation of dramatic reductions in spasticity after posterior rhizotomy (Chapter 12).

Presumably, a slight weakening, even of strong, isolated contractions after nerve blocks, is not great enough to have a functional effect under most circumstances, and this should be kept in mind. If unusual demands were made on a muscle after a nerve block, a mild weakening could be significant. A weak muscle is certainly more susceptible to further weakening by a nerve block.[10]

Another potential complication of chemical neurolysis is an unfavorable reversal of the balance of muscle groups about a joint. This is most likely to occur in the context of severe spasticity that is causing or threatening contracture. The nerve(s) supplying the responsible muscle or group of muscles is/are blocked, but if the antagonists to those muscles are also severely spastic, a contracture may begin to develop in the opposite direction. Another manifestation of this complication might be apparent weakness in the muscle or an increase in spasticity in the antagonist caused by loss of reciprocal inhibition. In either case, the situation can be remedied by blocking the nerves supplying the antagonist muscle(s). This complication can usually be anticipated during the evaluation preceding the neurolytic procedure, and plans can be made for either careful titration of the effect of the block (over more than one session if necessary) or for blocking the antagonist(s) shortly after the first procedure.

Muscle or ligament sprains can occur after nerve blocks caused by loss of reflexive protection against overstretching the muscle in which spasticity has been relieved, changes in the dynamics of ambulation, or loss of reflexive support for other soft tissues.[11] Therapists should anticipate possible difficulties in ambulation, and should be careful not to overstretch in the first days and weeks following nerve block.

Peripheral edema is not uncommon after

chemical neurolysis, particularly in the lower extremity. It can be treated with elevation of the extremity and compressive garments or elastic wrapping, and usually resolves within a week or two.

Local infection at the site of injection is, of course, always a possibility. Both alcohol and phenol, however, are bacteriocidal at the concentrations used for neurolysis,[54] so this is a rare occurrence.

There has been one report of severe, lancinating pain in the forearm following median nerve block with phenol at the level of the elbow.[7]

Overdosage with phenol causes convulsions, central nervous system depression, and cardiovascular collapse. The amount of phenol routinely used for nerve blocks, however, is well below the lethal range (8.5 grams or more).[4] For instance, 10 ml of 5% phenol contains 0.5 grams of phenol. To remain well within safe limits, no more than one gram should generally be injected on any given day (20 ml of 5% phenol).

Routine precautions, such as aspiration before injection, make intravascular injection unlikely. Neither overdosage nor accidental intravascular injection has been reported in association with phenol neurolysis. At the time when others were beginning to report on the use of phenol for direct chemical neurolysis, Cooper et al.[55] described the reduction of spasticity by perfusion of an isolated limb with 0.36% aqueous phenol for 10 to 30 minutes. Studies of animals before treatment of humans with spasticity had demonstrated that such concentrations could be perfused without damage to large or small vessel walls. Higher concentrations, however, caused necrosis of the intima of arteries and veins and thrombotic occlusion of small vessels.

Deep venous thrombosis has rarely been reported.[56] It is unclear whether this complication results from the direct effect of phenol on the vein, trauma to the vein, or the loss of muscle pumping action leaving the extremity more susceptible to thrombosis.

Complications related to arterial occlusion have never been reported with nerve blocks for the treatment of spasticity. Arterial occlusion, however, resulted in cervical spinal cord infarction in a woman who underwent stellate ganglion block with phenol in glycerine for intractable pain,[57] and a small cerebellar infarct was found at autopsy in a woman with intractable pain related to a Pancoast tumor who was treated with cervical subarachnoid injection of phenol in glycerine.[57,58] Although the media and elastica of many small arteries on the surface of the spinal cord were affected, and some thrombosed, no spinal cord infarcts were found. Demyelination and Wallerian degeneration, however, were found in the cervical spinal cord. The patient died of complications related to respiratory failure. Nerve blocks with phenol in the vicinity of the cervical spinal cord carry too great a risk to warrant their use in the treatment of spasticity.

Mixed Sensorimotor Nerve Blocks. Mixed nerve blocks with phenol carry many of the same risk factors as the other chemical neurolytic procedures described above. The major drawback to sensorimotor nerve blocks, compared with motor nerve blocks, is the additional risk of neuropathic pain, that is, dysesthesias in the sensory distribution of the nerve. The pain usually has its onset from a few days to about 2 weeks after the procedure. It is generally experienced as a continuous burning paresthesia exacerbated by light tactile stimulation, so that even a draft or a sheet moving across the affected area can be uncomfortable or even intolerable. The pain is generally experienced in only a small portion of the sensory distribution of the nerve that was blocked.[11,22,27]

The incidence of dysesthesias reported after peripheral nerve blocks with phenol has varied from 2 to 32% (Table 11–1).[7,8,19,20,22,27] This wide variation may reflect to some degree the experience and technique of the individual physician performing the procedure, but is probably partly due to variation in the method of followup, the frequency with which obturator nerve blocks were included, and the patient population. Dysesthesias following obturator nerve blocks have not been reported, and patients with complete sensory loss do not suffer from this complication.

The majority of patients with neuropathic pain following chemical neurolysis experience a mild to moderate burning sen-

TABLE 11–1. INCIDENCE OF DYSESTHESIAS AFTER
PERIPHERAL NERVE BLOCKS

Author	D/N (%)	N(Obt)	%/ml Phenol
Brattstrom	8/25(32%)	0	2%/1.5–6 ml
Helweg-Larsen*	4/150(3%)	58	3%/0.5–2 ml
Khalili	?/267(13%)	?	2–3%/0.5–5 ml
Moritz	?/90(<10%)	11	2–3%/0.5–6 ml
Petrillo	8/33(24%)	0	5%/2–10 ml
Spira*	7/136(5%)	40	5%/2–5 ml

D/N = Number of blocks resulting in dysesthesias/total number
N(Obt) = Number of obturator nerve blocks
*Nerve blocks performed on children

sation that lasts from several days to more than 3 months, though several weeks is most typical.[7,11,19,22,23,27] Helweg-Larsen and Jacobsen[7] reported 12 months of pain and tenderness on the sole of the foot following tibial nerve block with phenol in a child with cerebral palsy. The etiology of neuropathic pain following chemical neurolysis is unknown, although some physicians feel that it is related to the effects of mechanical trauma to the nerve caused by the needle.[11,20] The lack of such complications from local anesthetic blocks argues against this conclusion. This phenomenon may be similar to that experienced by patients with incomplete sensory neuropathies of other etiologies or regrowth of sensory axons following traumatic lesions. Local inflammation may play a role. Some physicians feel that the incidence of pain has diminished as they have become more experienced with chemical neurolysis.[26] Although never studied in a controlled manner, a survey of the literature does not reveal a relationship between the concentration or quantity of phenol used and the incidence of dysesthesias. The two studies including only children had an incidence of dysesthesia of 5% or less (Table 11–1).

Because this complication is usually temporary, treatment is generally aimed at managing the pain until it disappears of its own accord. Reassurance that the pain is likely to resolve within a few weeks will reduce the intensity of concern on the part of the patient. A uniformly applied compressive garment such as a sock, glove, or elastic wrap minimizes cutaneous stimulation and decreases edema if present. Transcutaneous electrical nerve stimulation (TENS) can be very effective for reducing dysesthesias in some patients. Acetaminophen or nonsteroidal anti-inflammatory drugs sometimes provide some temporary relief, although it is not usually dramatic. Low-dose amitriptyline can be helpful in more severe cases. When the pain is severe and unremitting, a short course of steroids may aid in its resolution. If all else fails and the patient is finding the pain intolerable, reblocking the nerve with phenol usually brings relief.[27] However, both patient and physician are likely to experience some trepidation about employing as treatment that which caused the problem to begin with. Braun et al.[29] employed surgical neurolysis to resolve persistent dysesthesias caused by median nerve blocks in two patients.

As with complications related to loss of voluntary, isolated strength, the physician who performs nerve blocks is likely to be surprised to find that functional loss of sensation is an unusual occurrence following mixed sensorimotor nerve block with phenol. Presumably, the number of sensory axons affected by chemical neurolysis as it is commonly performed is not great enough to have a significant effect. In the first hours or days following the procedure, sensory loss is common,[27] presumably because of the local anesthetic action of phenol or the early inflammatory reaction that occurs. This almost invariably resolves, however. Katz et al.[8] reported that, in 56 peripheral nerve blocks performed using 3% phenol, there was one instance of hypesthesia lasting for two months following ulnar nerve block, and persisting at the time of their writing. Most authors have found no loss of sensation.[9,19,21,23,45] One would, however, have to presume that minor, perhaps subclinical, sensory loss can occur, but that it is of little significance to most patients. Further studies are needed in this area.

Motor Nerve Blocks. The only additional side effect involved with the blocking of motor nerves with phenol is that, if the block is performed at multiple sites within the muscle itself, local pain, swelling, and induration may be present for a few days or occasionally longer.[13,28] Tender nodules may appear in the muscle one to three weeks after the injection.[33] Halpern[44] found local necrosis of muscle and an associated inflammatory reaction of the fascia and subfascial tissue in specimens taken from dogs and rats that had undergone intramuscular neurolysis with aqueous phenol. This reaction began within days of the procedure and intensified by the end of 2 weeks, when it began to resolve.

The application of ice, acutely, and later heat, elevation of the extremity, and administration of analgesic medications can be helpful in instances in which pain, swelling, or nodule formation is prominent. These measures can be applied prophylactically if desired. The administration of analgesics is warranted as a prophylactic measure in the patient who, for physical or cognitive reasons, has difficulty communicating his or her needs.

Intramuscular neurolysis with phenol performed within the calf muscles occasionally causes a local reaction that can mimic deep venous thrombosis. Calf pain and swelling, and sometimes peripheral edema, may be present, and impedance plethysmography may be consistent with deep vein thrombosis. The venogram, however, is negative in these cases.

Lumbosacral Paravertebral Nerve Blocks. As noted previously in the section entitled Technique, lumbosacral paravertebral nerve blocks with phenol carry the additional risk of accidental intrathecal injection, which could cause cauda equina or even spinal cord injury. The special precautions described previously are necessary when injecting in this area. Lumbosacral paravertebral blocks should be reserved for treating spasticity in muscle groups that are otherwise inaccessible, such as the iliopsoas, quadratus lumborum, and paraspinal muscles, or when more peripheral approaches have been unsuccessful.

DURATION OF EFFECT

The issue of duration of effect of nerve blocks with phenol remains an unresolved enigma. Although one might imagine that the distance that the axon must regrow before reinnervating the muscle or the time it takes for collateral sprouting to take place would be the most important factors in the duration of effect of neurolysis with phenol, the literature does not necessarily support this contention (Table 11–2).

Khalili[20] completed follow-up in a series of 94 *peripheral* nerve blocks using 2 to 3% phenol and reported that they lasted anywhere from 10 to 850 days, with an average of 317 days. Petrillo[27] found that tibial nerve blocks with 5% phenol were still effective at a follow-up of 9 to 22 months, with an average follow-up time of 12.9 months after the procedure. Spira[22] reported that "good relief" of spasticity was still present in 31% and "some relief" in another 31% at 3 to 6 months following 136 peripheral nerve blocks with phenol in children. He found sustained relief was less likely in muscles with severe spasticity. Moritz[26] reported relief of spasticity lasting from a few days to more than 1 year, with an average duration of effect of 8 months. When spasticity reappeared, it was generally not as pronounced. Copp and Keenan[23] have observed abolition of clonus for as long as 3 years. Katz et al.,[8] however, found that of 31 effective peripheral nerve blocks (out of 56 performed using 3% phenol), only nine lasted for longer than one month. Meelhuysen et al.[15] performed paravertebral blocks with 3 to 5% phenol and reported that, whereas some lasted only 1½ months, others were still effective at follow-up 10 months after the procedure. Sixty-seven percent of the blocks lasted 4 months or more.

Easton,[33] however, reported similar vari-

TABLE 11-2. DURATION OF EFFECT OF NERVE BLOCKS

Type	Range	Average OR% >	% Phenol
Peripheral			
(Khalili, 1984)	10–850 days	317 days	2–3%
(Petrillo, 1980)	>9–22 mos.	Average >12.9 mos.	5%
(Katz, 1967)		29%>1 mo.	3%
Paravertebral			
(Meelhuysen, 1968)	1½–>10 mos.	67%>4 mos.	3–5%
Intramuscular			
(Easton, 1979)	1–36 mos.		5%
(Halpern, 1967)	1–>14 mos.	60% >6 mos.	5%
Endplate			
(Delateur, 1972)	3–6 mos.		5%
Open motor			
(Garland, 1982)		6 mos.	3%
(Braun, 1973)		23% >1 yr.	3–5%

ability in the duration of effect of *intramuscular* neurolysis with 5% phenol, with effects lasting from 1 to 36 months. In a series of 394 procedures, Halpern and Meelhuysen[14] found the range of duration before return of spasticity was 1 to at least 14 months, with some blocks still effective at the final 14-month follow-up time. Of these, 84% lasted longer than 4 months and 60% longer than 6 months. Garland et al.[49] did open motor branch blocks with 3% phenol at a site more proximal than most intramuscular procedures and reported the duration of effect to be about 6 months. Braun et al.[29] also did open intraneural motor nerve blocks in 18 adults, using 3 to 5% phenol. Of the 17 who had a good result, 6 lasted for more than 6 months, and 4 for longer than 1 year. DeLateur[24] performed motor end-plate blocks with 5% phenol and found the effect to last for 3 to 6 months.

Although at first glance these data are somewhat surprising, it is difficult to come to any conclusions about the relative duration of effect based on this literature. No controlled comparisons of the effect of the site of the block on outcome have been done, and in fact few of the studies even indicate on what basis they have judged the spasticity to have returned.

It is probable that factors other than the length of axon growth affect the duration of the block, for, as noted previously in the section entitled Effect of Phenol on Nerves, several histologic studies found regrowth of

axons or collateral reinnervation taking place within a few months. The technique of the person performing the block and the quantity and concentration of solution may influence the number of axons affected, although it is not clear that this should affect the duration as much as the effectiveness of the block unless formation of endoneural fibrous tissue or destruction of vasculature are important factors. A greater loss of axons, however, may limit the degree to which collateral sprouting can compensate. Halpern[44] did find that the histologic evidence of reinnervation was still present at 3 months in animals injected with 5 or 7% phenol, whereas reinnervation was complete at this time when intramuscular neurolysis was performed with more dilute solutions. The influence of afferent and gamma motor denervation on the muscle spindle itself is another unknown factor. The degree of spasticity and other central neurophysiologic factors may have an influence as well. A relative consistency in the quality and duration of block in different muscles in the same individual supports the possibility of individual neurophysiologic influences.[14] Neurologic recovery over time may diminish the central factors contributing to spasticity.

Although most of the histologic evidence leads one to wonder why spasticity does not return more quickly than it frequently does, Mooney et al.[43] found little evidence of regrowth of axons in four patients who had had a return of spasticity following phenol neurolysis. They proposed that the anterior horn cells not destroyed by phenol "develop an ability to operate at a new level of sensitivity."

Treatment variables may have an important influence on the duration of spasticity reduction after chemical neurolysis. If the muscle is effectively stretched after nerve block, spasticity may be further reduced, and a long-term benefit could ensue. If the antagonist to the muscle blocked is strengthened in the interim, this may have a long-lasting inhibitory effect on the agonist. Braun et al.[29] felt that the presence of selective motor control before neurolysis was associated with a longer duration of effect. Roper[50] noted that, among 46 patients treated with open intraneural injection of 3% phenol in glycerine, the 3 who had permanent resolution of spasticity all had selective motor control in the muscles supplied by the *treated* nerve prior to the block. He found a greater incidence of "long-term improvement" among those patients with selective control than those without such control.

Finally, the manner in which one evaluates the degree of spasticity influences the results of any study on this subject.

EFFECT OF REPEATED NERVE BLOCKS WITH PHENOL

Limited data are available on the effect of repeating nerve blocks with phenol after the recurrence of spasticity. Halpern and Meelhuysen[14] reported that repeating intramuscular neurolysis once in 57 muscles, and twice in 14 produced results similar to those achieved on the first occasion. Localization of motor branches by electrical stimulation was more difficult. Helweg-Larsen and Jacobsen[7] achieved similar effects and duration of effect on repeat of peripheral nerve blocks. Awad[25] found that in some patients a permanent reduction in spasticity was achieved after repeating intramuscular neurolysis with phenol three or four times. He speculates that necrosis of muscle leads to fibrosis, which protects against complete reinnervation. After several procedures, there is a cumulative effect that is clinically significant.

NERVE BLOCKS WITH ALCOHOL

QUALITIES OF ETHANOL AND EFFECT ON NERVES

Ethyl alcohol (ethanol), a potent neurolytic agent, has not been used as extensively as phenol for the treatment of spasticity. Ethanol has been used mostly for sympathectomy and for the treatment of pain. Its use in spasticity has probably been more limited because of the popularity of phenol and by early reports of a relatively high incidence of dysesthesias and hyperesthesias. It is not clear, however, whether or not the occurrence of this complication is in fact any higher than with phenol, and there are no reports on the treatment of spasticity by mixed motor and sensory nerve block with alcohol.

Animal studies of the effect of ethanol on nerves have generally shown destruction of both axons and myelin, but the extent of damage has been variable regardless of the concentration of ethanol used, with the exception of absolute alcohol, which, in a study by May,[59] always caused degeneration of neurons with extensive fibrosis and partial regeneration. With lower concentrations, however, May found axonal destruction in some cases but not others. The duration of paralysis varied considerably, but the animals always recovered. With 50% ethanol, no weakness was seen. Gordon[60] found varying degrees of neuronal degeneration and surrounding fibrosis after application of 80% alcohol. Some weakness usually occurred when motor nerves were injected, but none of the animals were completely paralyzed. Labat[61] injected alcohol into the sciatic nerve of dogs. He used 48% alcohol in some animals and 95% in others, and found a temporary paralysis with both. The duration of effect did not correlate with the concentration of solution used, and was usually less than two months. Tardieu et al.[17] found lesions of the myelin, mostly in small fibers, but no axonal damage 3 weeks after application of 35% ethanol to the posterior tibial nerve of cats. Cholinesterase activity was reduced in the endplate of the muscle spindle on the side treated with alcohol, but was normal in the spindle on the untreated side, as well as in the extrafusal muscle fibers bilaterally. The tension produced by the stretch reflex was reduced, but the tension elicited by stimulation of the tibial nerve itself was not, and voluntary movement was normal. These findings suggest a selective effect of the less concentrated solution on small-diameter gamma motor neurons.

Fischer et al.[39] found that 35 to 47% ethanol had a nonselective effect on the evoked response of fibers of various diameters in the early minutes after exposure. It is unclear whether this represents a nonselective but reversible local anesthetic effect or lasting damage to the nerve, and is therefore not necessarily at odds with the selective small fiber damage seen by Tardieu et al.[17] several weeks after the block. Alcohol can act as a local anesthetic in concentrations as low as 5 or 10% by decreasing sodium and potassium conductance.[62]

MOTOR NERVE BLOCK WITH ALCOHOL

Tardieu et al.[16,17] have injected 45% alcohol "in the neighborhood of the motor nerve endings" to treat spasticity in children. They injected 1 to 1.5 ml at each point. Spasticity was reduced in most cases, with the effect usually lasting from 6 to 12 months, although occasionally as long as 2 or 3 years. Voluntary strength was not reduced.

INTRAMUSCULAR ALCOHOL WASH

O'Hanlan et al.[18] modified the technique of Tardieu et al. Rather than specifically localizing motor nerves, they injected large quantities of 45% alcohol into multiple locations within the target muscles of patients with a variety of diagnoses resulting in spasticity. They injected about 20 to 30 ml of alcohol into three sites in the biceps brachii muscle of an adult, 30 to 40 ml into the gastrocnemius and soleus through six sites, and less into the wrist and finger flexors. In children with cerebral palsy, they injected about 10 ml of alcohol into the hip adductors on each side. They had a significant reduction of spasticity with functional gains

in the 10 cases reported. There was no loss of voluntary motor power or sensation. They did not report the duration of effect.

Carpenter and Seitz[63] and Carpenter[64] used a similar procedure and coined the term "intramuscular alcohol wash." A large muscle such as the gastrocnemius was divided into quadrants and 2 to 6 ml of 45 to 50% alcohol injected into each quadrant. In 130 children with cerebral palsy in whom alcohol was injected into the gastrocnemius-soleus muscles, all but two had a complete elimination of equinus gait for periods lasting from 7 to 20 days. In other muscles, results were not as consistently good. Overall, in 211 children, the effect lasted from 1 to 6 weeks.

If confirmed by other studies, the procedure's limited duration of effect could be useful for diagnostic purposes when a longer period of evaluation is necessary than can be provided by a local anesthetic agent, and for therapeutic purposes when longer-lasting procedures are unnecessary or undesirable. Another advantage of this procedure is that, because precise localization of nerves is not necessary, it can be performed quickly in situations where speed is a consideration, for example in agitated and combative patients and in children. Carpenter and Seitz[63] used general anesthesia nonetheless.

The limited duration of effect of this procedure may be related to the relatively low concentration of ethanol used. Although the literature is inconclusive, it may be that, as with phenol, lower concentrations result largely in demyelination as opposed to axonal destruction with Wallerian degeneration. The anatomically imprecise nature of the procedure might also play a role in the limited duration of effect. This imprecision could, theoretically, result in inconsistent strength and duration of effect.

The only complications noted have been a burning sensation in the muscle, usually lasting no more than 24 hours, and local hyperemia lasting from 24 to 36 hours. In six patients in whom muscle biopsies were performed at the time of surgery 4 to 6 weeks after the injection, only a small amount of round cell infiltrate was seen in the muscle, but no fibrosis. Dysesthesias should not be a problem with an intramuscular procedure. O'Hanlan et al.[18] reported phlebitis occurring when they used "state store" alcohol mixed with sterile water. When they began using solutions prepared by the pharmacist, this complication no longer occurred.

Inebriation could result from the injection and subsequent absorption of large amounts of alcohol. This should be considered in patients with a history of untoward reactions to alcohol and in those on sedating medications or with respiratory compromise, or shortly after a central nervous system injury. In these cases, alcohol intoxication might theoretically interfere with neurologic recovery.[65]

NERVE BLOCKS WITH LOCAL ANESTHETIC AGENTS

QUALITIES OF LOCAL ANESTHETICS AND EFFECT ON NERVES

Although phenol and alcohol have local anesthetic properties, local anesthetic agents are defined here as drugs that, when applied directly to a nerve, reversibly block conduction without causing structural damage to the nerve. They do so by acting on the membrane to decrease the transient increase in permeability to sodium ions that normally occurs when the membrane is depolarized. In general, they affect small-diameter fibers more rapidly than large, and their blocking action lasts longer on small fibers as well. This is probably because of the smaller internodal distances of small diameter fibers, which can be covered more rapidly by the diffusing local anesthetic. Once the agent has been allowed to diffuse, however, there may be no differential effect, although this point has not been en-

tirely clarified.[66] Local anesthetic agents, if absorbed systemically in high enough concentrations, can cause central nervous system stimulation, manifested by restlessness, tremor, and convulsions, followed by central nervous system depression. With some agents, such as lidocaine and procaine, sedation and unconsciousness may not be preceded by stimulation. In addition, myocardial conduction, and therefore contraction, can be depressed, usually only in concentrations that have produced central nervous system effects. Rarely, cardiovascular collapse and death have resulted from infiltration of small amounts of a local anesthetic. Hypersensitivity reactions, including fatal anaphylaxis, rarely occur, and do so more commonly with agents that have an ester link, such as procaine and tetracaine. The maximal quantities of various local anesthetic drugs without epinephrine that can be safely infiltrated in an adult are presented in Table 11–3.[66] The amount needed for a diagnostic nerve block to evaluate the effect on spasticity is usually only a few milliliters, well below this limit.

The duration of effect of local anesthetics varies considerably from agent to agent (Table 11–3).[66] Lidocaine is commonly used for a relatively short action, as is bupivacaine for a longer duration.

NERVE BLOCKS WITH LOCAL ANESTHETIC AGENTS

The technique for performing nerve blocks with local anesthetics is similar to that for performing nerve blocks with phenol. Local anesthetic agents can be injected at any level of the peripheral nervous system. Because intramuscular blocks require a longer, more painful procedure, most physicians prefer to do local anesthetic blocks

TABLE 11–3. PRACTICAL USE OF LOCAL ANESTHETIC AGENTS IN ADULTS

Agent	Maximal Amount	Duration of Action
Procaine 0.5%	1.4 ml/kg	<1 hour
Lidocaine 1%	0.45 ml/kg	1–2 hours
Bupivacaine 0.25%	1 ml/kg	7 hours

at more proximal motor branches or at mixed motor and sensory nerves. When local anesthetic agents are injected at the paravertebral level, there is a risk of diffusion into the intrathecal space by way of root sleeves, so that smaller doses can result in central nervous system side effects more than if absorbed systemically.

A new technique that would allow easy access for repeated nerve blocks is currently under investigation.[51] As it is currently used, a Silastic catheter is surgically implanted into the axillary sheath. It is connected to a subcutaneous reservoir on the lateral aspect of the arm, which is injected with a local anesthetic agent several times a week. During the time when the anesthetic is still effective, range-of-motion exercises can more easily be performed. If the patient improves to the point where he or she can be involved in active therapies, the device can be removed. Alternately, it can be left indefinitely if necessary, and family members can be taught to inject the reservoir if the patient is to be discharged to home.

Nerve blocks with local anesthetics are usually performed as diagnostic procedures. A discussion of their clinical use can be found in the following section entitled Clinical Applications.

CLINICAL APPLICATIONS

INDICATIONS FOR NERVE BLOCKS

The decision to perform a nerve block should be based on both a neuromuscular-kinesiologic evaluation and an assessment of the functional or potential functional implications of the disordered muscle tone. The possibility of functional gains resulting from chemical neurolysis must be weighed against the potential for functional losses or other complications and side effects. For purposes of evaluation, functional considerations can be classified as involving active motor control or passive positioning. Contractures can play an important role in both.

Spasticity most commonly inhibits active motor control when hyperactive stretch reflexes in antagonist muscles resist the motion of the agonists. When the agonists appear to have sufficient strength for func-

tional purposes if freed from the hyperactive antagonists, nerve blocks are often useful.

For instance, if toe drag or toe-heel gait is resulting from spasticity of the plantarflexors of the ankle in the face of the ability to actively dorsiflex the ankle, either in an isolated fashion or as part of a flexor synergy, blocking the posterior tibial nerve or its branches to the gastrocnemius and soleus can remedy the problem. The effect of the block on other joints should be considered, in particular the effect of the decreased extension moment on the stability of the knee (see Fig. 11–4). If increased inversion of the foot is also present, an attempt should be made to determine whether this is caused by increased tone in the tibialis anterior or in the tibialis posterior muscle. This can be difficult to determine by observation alone, and polyelectromyography or diagnostic nerve blocks can be helpful in this situation. Sometimes inversion during swing phase results from the inability of the tibialis anterior to "fight" spastic or contracted plantarflexors, so that all of its contractile force goes toward inversion rather than dorsiflexion. In such cases, nerve blocks affecting the plantarflexors or remediation of contractures will resolve the situation. If a spastic tibialis posterior is felt to be responsible for excessive inversion, the branch or fascicles of the posterior tibial nerve to the tibialis posterior can be blocked as well. As the tibialis posterior helps to support the arch of the foot, the possibility of pes planus resulting from such a block should be considered.

Although spasticity itself is the most likely condition to be affected by a nerve block, other motor disorders associated with the upper motor neuron syndrome, such as cocontractions and primitive motor behaviors, can adversely affect function by overpowering an agonist with or without the presence of significant spasticity. If an increase in tone is present only during active motion or is associated with position but not stretch, nerve blocks may still be helpful, although not as consistently. Mooney et al.[43] found that two of eight patients with upper extremity synergy patterns had a weakening of the pattern following phenol neurolysis of motor branches of the median nerve. Easton et al.[33] had less satisfactory results with intramuscular blocks in children with dystonic athetosis, decerebrate rigidity, and hypertonia related to disinhibited vestibular, tonic neck, or spinal reflexes than in children with pure spasticity. Khalili[20] reported on the use of phenol nerve blocks in a patient with dystonia musculorum deformans who developed superimposed spastic right hemiplegia following a neurosurgical procedure. Although a tibial nerve block relieved ankle clonus, dystonic and voluntary contraction of the plantarflexors was not affected. Halpern and Meelhuysen,[13] however, reported reduction in muscle tone in three children with tension athetosis. Rigidity is also less susceptible to the influence of neurolysis with phenol, although Halpern and Meelhuysen[13] also reduced rigidity of the sternocleidomastoids and hip adductors in two patients with Parkinson's disease, with subsequent improvements in posture and ambulation. Similarly, Kjellberg et al.[67] observed improvements in gait in about half of their patients following intrathecal injection of 5% phenol in glycerine. As noted in a previous section in this chapter entitled Side Effects and Complications, reductions in abnormal motor responses of any kind can result in functional losses when the motor response was being used for functional purposes. Therefore, the careful clinician should take an inventory of any such activities when considering a patient for nerve block so that the risks and benefits can be carefully weighed before proceeding.

Less frequently, spasticity masks the voluntary strength of the very muscle in which tone is increased. A nerve block, then, may result in increased strength in the muscle denervated. Such a result is difficult, if not impossible, to predict, except by the use of a diagnostic block with a local anesthetic agent, for instance. More often, it is the unanticipated by-product of a nerve block performed for other reasons, and can be accepted as a gift. It is a particularly pleasant surprise when the innervation of the finger flexors is being blocked to facilitate finger extension, and the strength of both improves.

Although the result of a nerve block is likely to have a greater effect on function when active control is at stake, the reduction of passive posturing because of spasticity or primitive motor behaviors can also have significant functional implications. In the case of increased plantarflexion and inversion tone described above, a good result can be obtained even in some instances where no active dorsiflexion or eversion can be seen. Similarly, if hypertonicity of the toe flexors is causing a painful grabbing during stance phase, blocking the branch of the posterior tibial nerve to the flexor digitorum muscles can be beneficial whether active toe extension is present or not. The benefit of an orthosis can be improved by a nerve block that allows it to do its job more effectively, for instance, when plantarflexion or inversion tone prevents proper fitting of an ankle-foot orthosis.

Proper passive positioning in a wheelchair, bed, or other device can result in greater patient comfort and can improve communication, alertness, respiration, upper extremity use, hygiene and skin care and otherwise facilitate function or nursing care. Thus, obturator nerve blocks that alleviate excessive hip adduction can help produce more comfortable sitting or facilitate perineal hygiene. Similarly, hygiene of the axilla, palm of the hand, or antecubital fossa can be improved by nerve blocks that relax the muscle that prevents adequate access. Powerful lower extremity extensor synergies that cause a patient to slide out of even well-constructed wheelchairs can be reduced by blocking the innervation of the primary muscles involved, usually the gluteus maximus, quadriceps femoris, and/or spinal extensors. Ankle clonus that causes positioning problems during transfer, for instance, can be eliminated with blocks of the posterior tibial nerve or its branches. Opisthotonus can be reduced by blocking the innervation of spinal extensor muscles. Hypertonicity in any accessible muscle or muscle group that results in discomfort or dysfunctional positioning can be considered for treatment with nerve blocks.

Contractures can prevent active motion or proper passive positioning, and nerve blocks can be used to prevent contractures of potential functional significance when their development is associated with spasticity. If spasticity has already caused contracture, remediation of the contracture by means of range-of-motion exercises, serial casting, or other means can be greatly facilitated by nerve blocks. Recurrence of contracture can be prevented by prophylactic nerve blocks that allow range-of-motion exercises to be performed more easily and less painfully, and that permit the proper fitting of bivalved casts or other orthoses. They can be useful for preventing the recurrence of contractures that have been surgically remedied as well.

The clinician considering chemical neurolysis as a treatment alternative must consider the time since onset of the upper motor neuron lesion and the prognosis for improvement. If a nerve block with phenol is performed prematurely, and a patient improves more dramatically than expected shortly after the block, potential function based on primitive motor behaviors may be lost, or strength of already weak muscles reduced. In addition, if the pattern of hypertonicity changes, contracture or loss of function may develop in the direction opposite that initially anticipated. On the other hand, if a nerve block is avoided because of such risks, and the anticipated contractures develop, the consequences are also likely to be significant. Clinicians should make every attempt possible to prevent contractures if there is even a small possibility of a good outcome.

Alcohol wash represents an alternative approach to nerve blocks with phenol. Although the literature is limited, it indicates that the effect is likely to last only for several weeks after which longer-lasting blocks with phenol can be reconsidered or alcohol wash repeated if necessary. Even when the physician is confident that enough time has elapsed to warrant the use of phenol, the patient or family member may be unconvinced. In such situations, they may more readily accept an alcohol wash because of the shorter duration of effect, and later, having seen the benefits, consent to a nerve block with phenol. Local anesthetic blocks can also be used to help prevent contractures early after an injury, though they may need to be repeated frequently, and this can be impractical. The benefit of a local anesthetic block can, how-

ever, be stretched by placing the extremity in a cast that inhibits the return of hypertonicity and prevents contracture formation.[51] The limb must be carefully observed because the return of forceful spasticity within the cast could cause skin breakdown.

The usual indication for local anesthetic block, however, is for diagnostic purposes. Local anesthetics can be used to help determine whether or not there is a component of spasticity at end range in the presence of severe contracture. They can be used to determine which muscle is contributing to a pathologic posturing, as in the case of inversion of the foot described previously. They are probably most useful, however, in situations where it is uncertain if a nerve block will cause more harm than good, particularly when significant function based on primitive motor behaviors or spasticity is at stake, or when blocks may affect more than one aspect of a function such as ambulation. The clinician evaluating such a situation should keep in mind, however, that the local anesthetic block, although frequently helpful, is not likely to reproduce exactly the effect of a nerve block with phenol. This is particularly true when mixed sensorimotor nerves are blocked with local anesthetics, in which case the resulting sensory loss may have significant functional consequences. Alcohol wash can also be used if several weeks may be needed to evaluate fully the potential effects of a block.

Chemical neurolysis must be considered in light of the other treatment alternatives, and when practical, more conservative approaches tried first. In some instances, spasticity is so powerful, or contracture developing so rapidly, that nerve blocks may of necessity be resorted to before other less invasive treatments are tried. The question of which of two interventions is more conservative can be a matter of subjective opinion, and judgment must be exercised. For instance, although many clinicians consider medications more conservative than chemical neurolysis, in an elderly person or a patient with brain damage secondary to trauma, cerebrovascular accident, multiple sclerosis, or other causes, medications that impair cognition can cause significant time loss from a rehabilitation program even when the problem is recognized, and if it is unrecognized, they may permanently impede recovery.

Another important consideration is the possible need to repeat nerve blocks because of the frequently limited duration of their effect. When the time comes to consider repetition, this should not be done reflexively. The possibility that other approaches that were previously unsuccessful might now prove beneficial, or that medications that might previously have been contraindicated might now be acceptable, should be considered. The lack of availability of physicians who perform nerve blocks in the area to which the patient might be discharged may make nerve blocks a poor choice for treatment if it appears that they will need to be repeated. Frequent need for repetition of blocks may also make them less acceptable. In such situations, an attempt to find an appropriate systemic pharmacologic alternative should be pursued, and potentially longer-lasting procedures such as radiofrequency rhizotomy, selective posterior rhizotomy, or musculotendinous releases with or without neurectomy may be indicated. Chemical neurolysis can be useful to facilitate the effectiveness of musculotendinous procedures performed in the presence of spasticity.

CHOICE OF SITE FOR A NERVE BLOCK

Although some physicians prefer to perform almost exclusively either motor or mixed sensorimotor nerve blocks, the physician who has the ability and willingness to perform nerve blocks at a variety of sites in the peripheral nervous system will be in a better position to meet the needs of his or her patients and their families.

The physician should consider a variety of factors when deciding upon the site at which to do a nerve block. First of all, the size and accessibility of the muscle should be considered. The psoas major muscle, for example, is so large that a long and difficult procedure would be necessary to block the many small intramuscular branches. Therefore, it is more practical to block the large muscular branches more proximally where they leave the lumbar roots. If the quadra-tus lumborum is targeted as a muscle in need of blocking, a similar site can be chosen, not because of the size of the muscle, but rather because of its proximity to the peritoneal cavity and the kidney, which could be accidently punctured during the procedure. At the paravertebral level, however, the peritoneal cavity is well protected by the combined depth of the paraspinal and psoas muscles (Fig. 11–5).

Usually the major consideration in choosing the site of a neurolytic block is whether or not it is worth taking the risk of dysesthesias following a mixed sensorimotor nerve block. All else being equal, it would clearly be better to perform motor nerve blocks and avoid the possibility of this complication. Many physicians who perform nerve blocks, however, feel that a more effective block is possible at the more proximal site, and that the duration of effect is longer as well. Therefore, if spasticity is particularly severe, or if a long duration of action is particularly important, mixed nerve blocks may be relatively more indicated. On the other hand, it is not clear to what extent these factors are influenced by the inclusion of the sensory portion of the nerve in the block. It is possible that the distance of the site from the muscle and the number of fascicles available for lysis in the more proximal mixed nerve are more important. Therefore, an alternative to a mixed neurolytic block might be to perform the procedure at the most proximal portion of the motor branch as possible. These branches can usually be located by means of surface or needle stimulation, given a familiarity with the usual anatomy of a nerve. Open nerve blocks can be performed to ensure that only motor branches are being blocked, but this involves placing the patient under anesthesia and making an incision that might temporarily restrict the use of the extremity, and is usually not necessary.

Other factors may enter into this decision. In some cases, a long duration of action may not be desired. As discussed above, relatively early after the onset of a central nervous system disorder, the prognosis may be uncertain, and a short-acting block may be desired. Alcohol wash, an intramuscular procedure, may be the best

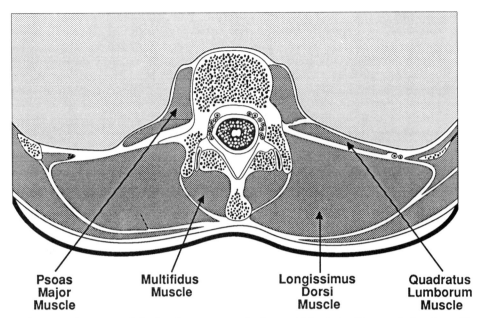

Psoas	Multifidus	Longissimus	Quadratus
Major	Muscle	Dorsi	Lumborum
Muscle		Muscle	Muscle

FIG. 11-5. Anatomy of the lumbar paravertebral area (Adapted with permission from Goodgold, J.: Anatomical Correlates of Clinical Electromyography. Baltimore, Williams and Wilkins, 1974, p. 94).

choice in this situation. Similarly, one may want to preserve some of the hypertonicity of a muscle when it serves a useful purpose. In such instances, the physician and other members of the treatment team can more easily titrate the effect of the block if distal motor branches are lysed.

If the patient is likely to have difficulty tolerating the procedure to the degree that it may be difficult or impossible to perform, sedation is often sufficient to make a long and unpleasant intramuscular procedure possible. There are occasions, however, particularly with aggressive brain-injured patients or young children, when general anesthesia is the only way to ensure completion of such a block. Some physicians have used general anesthesia for neurolysis in children.[7,22,33,68] Another alternative to consider would be a nerve block at a more proximal site, perhaps at a mixed nerve, to attain an effective reduction in spasticity with a relatively quick procedure. This should not, of course, be done routinely for the purpose of ensuring compliance, but rather should be reserved for selected situations.

The physician should also consider the patient's ability to perceive pain. If a patient

has permanently lost sensation in the distribution of a nerve under consideration for chemical neurolysis, a mixed nerve block can be performed without fear for the development of dysesthesias. If a patient is in a vegetative state, one might be tempted to assume that he or she cannot experience pain. There is, however, evidence to support the possibility that such people can experience pain,[69] although this probably cannot be known with any certainty. It is best to consider it a possibility when making decisions regarding the site of a nerve block.

Psychologic considerations are important as well. Motor nerve blocks are preferred in patients with a poor tolerance for pain. In addition, clinicians should attempt to identify in advance inidividuals for whom a mild pain problem might become the source of significant disability related to secondary gain, or the focal point for the displacement of other anxieties. Sensorimotor neuroloysis should be avoided in such cases.

There is no clear-cut protocol for deciding whether to do a mixed nerve or motor branch block. If all else is equal, however, one approach that is practical is to do motor branch blocks the first time a nerve block is performed to reduce spasticity in a given muscle or muscle group. If the block is successful and lasts for a long time, if it ever needs to be repeated, a similar block can be performed again. If the block is not as complete as was hoped, however, or if spasticity recurs in a relatively short period, a mixed sensorimotor nerve block can then be considered more strongly.

Until more data are available on the efficacy and duration of effect of chemical neurolysis, and on the etiology and treatment of dysesthesias following mixed nerve blocks, the individual physician's own experience with these factors is an important consideration in the choice of the site at which a neurolytic procedure is performed.

ANATOMIC CONSIDERATIONS

A brief description of the anatomic approach to some of the more commonly blocked peripheral nerves is presented in the following paragraphs. A complete discussion of the anatomy is beyond the scope of this chapter. The physician performing nerve blocks should be familiar with the local anatomy relevant to any nerve block he or she is performing, to avoid the puncture of major arteries or other structures, the perforation of which could cause untoward complications.

In addition to the nerves described in this section, other nerves and their branches can be approached, given a proper understanding of the anatomy. Although the emphasis is on the larger peripheral nerves, motor branches can be located within any muscle, and the larger motor branches, in particular, can be located if the anatomy of a peripheral nerve and its muscular branches is known. The identification of small motor branches can be facilitated by the use of charts that depict the usual location of motor points within a given muscle.[47]

OBTURATOR NERVE

The obturator nerve divides into anterior and posterior branches before exiting through the obturator foramen. The anterior branch lies between the adductor lon-gus and adductor brevis muscles, and usually innervates the adductor longus and brevis muscles, as well as the gracilis. The posterior branch lies between the adductor brevis and adductor magnus, and innervates the obturator externus and adductor magnus.[52,70,71] Two approaches to blocking the obturator nerve are commonly used. For both approaches, the patient lies supine, and the prominent adductor longus tendon is identified where it arises from the body of the pubis. In the medial approach, the needle is inserted one to two fingerbreadths distal to the origin of the tendon, along the posterior aspect of the muscle. To locate the anterior branch, the needle is directed laterally, parallel to the inguinal ligament, to a depth of about 2 cm. To locate the posterior branch, the needle is withdrawn and redirected laterally, but now tilted posteriorly at a 45-degree angle.[70] Felsenthal[71] suggests a slightly different approach to this branch. The needle is inserted parallel to the coronal plane, and directed cephalad at a 30-degree angle to the midsagittal plane, to a depth of about 2 cm.

In the patient with severe adductor spasticity or contracture, the obturator nerve is more easily approached anteriorly (Fig. 11–6). The femoral vessels are located to be certain they are not pierced. The needle is inserted along the lateral border of the adductor longus muscle, 1 to 2 cm distal to its origin. It is directed posteriorly, perpendicular to the coronal plane. The anterior branch can be located at a depth of about 2 cm.[71] The two branches lie in approximately the same saggital plane; if the needle is inserted another 1 or 2 cm, the posterior branch will be found. With this method, one can be more confident of avoiding the femoral vessels.

In a significant number of people, an accessory obturator nerve is also present. It gives a branch to the pectineus muscle before feeding into the anterior branch. Because it joins the anterior branch distal to the usual site at which it is blocked, the anterior branch block may be less than optimally effective if the accessory obturator nerve is present. This nerve can be located by inserting the needle into the anterior aspect of the adductor longus muscle, about two fingerbreadths distal to its origin. The

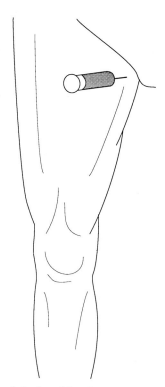

FIG. 11-6. Approach to the obturator nerve.

needle is directed cephalad toward the superior ramus of the pubis at a 30-degree angle to the midsagittal plane.[52,71]

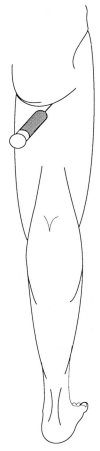

FIG. 11-7. Approach to the sciatic nerve.

SCIATIC NERVE

The sciatic nerve or its branches to the hamstring muscles can be blocked to alleviate hamstring spasticity. The sciatic nerve itself can be blocked at the point bisecting a line drawn between the ischial tuberosity and the greater trochanter (Fig. 11-7).[70] This is preferable to blocking at the level of the sciatic notch, where the fibers to the hamstrings are more widely dispersed throughout the nerve.[71] Motor branches to the hamstring muscles can usually be found at or slightly below the level of the ischial tuberosity. The sciatic nerve can be located at this level using needle stimulation, and then the needle gradually inched medially. If only the medial or lateral hamstrings continue to contract after moving 1 or 2 cm from the point of insertion, one can be rea-sonably certain to be stimulating a motor branch rather than the sciatic nerve itself. A large branch to the medial hamstrings can usually be found at this point. If a branch to the lateral hamstrings is not found at this level, sometimes it can be located by stimulation lateral to the sciatic nerve at this level, although it may be necessary to search for large intramuscular branches. These can be located using a surface stimulator before inserting the needle, if desired. Because branches to the hamstrings may exit the sciatic nerve at multiple sites along the nerve, it may be necessary to search for several intramuscular branches to both the medial and lateral hamstrings if blocking at the level of the ischial tuberosity does not produce the optimal effect. The hamstrings can also be blocked at the paravertebral level.

TIBIAL NERVE

The tibial nerve runs through the popliteal fossa, which is a diamond-shaped area bounded superiorly by the medial and lateral hamstrings, and inferiorly by the two heads of the gastrocnemius. The tibial nerve can be blocked at either the apex of the fossa between the medial and lateral hamstrings (Fig. 11–8) or at the popliteal crease, where it can be located slightly lateral to the midline. The fibers to the gastrocnemius have already exited at the level of the popliteal crease, however, and so motor branches to the gastrocnemius would also have to be located to obtain an effective block at this level.[70,71] Large motor branches can be found at this level just medial and lateral to the nerve, or within the gastrocnemius itself. Several large motor branches can usually be found two or three fingerbreadths below the popliteal crease within the belly of the medial and lateral heads. When blocking at the apex of the popliteal fossa, the practitioner should be aware of the close proximity of the common peroneal nerve to the tibial nerve and the origin of the sural nerve at this level.[52,70]

Branches of the tibial nerve to the tibialis posterior and to the flexor digitorum longus muscle can be isolated in the calf, 5 to 8 cm below the popliteal crease. To locate the branch to the tibialis posterior, the needle is inserted just lateral to the midline and directed anteriorly. The branch to the flexor digitorum muscles is approached just medial to the midline, again directing the needle anteriorly. Both the gastrocnemius and soleus muscles must be penetrated to locate these branches.[70]

FEMORAL NERVE

The femoral nerve is easily located 1 cm lateral to the femoral artery, just below the inguinal ligament.[70] The branches to the quadriceps femoris muscles arise from the posterior division of the femoral nerve, and one can sometimes isolate motor branches to the rectus femoris, and to the vastus lateralis, intermedius, and medialis respectively, by inching down carefully from this level while stimulating with the needle electrode. The sartorius is innervated by the intermediate femoral cutaneous nerve (from the anterior division), and therefore, to locate purely motor branches, one must insert the needle into the muscle itself.[52]

PARAVERTEBRAL BLOCKS

The paravertebral approach is most important for locating the nerve supply to the psoas major muscle, but the innervation of the quadratus lumborum, paraspinal muscles, hamstrings, hip adductors, and other lower extremity musculature can be blocked at this level as well. The approach described here is intended to facilitate location of elements of the lumbosacral plexus rather than the nerve roots themselves, to diminish the possibility of intrathecal injection. The great depth of combined paraspinal muscles and psoas major muscles is adequate to prevent penetration of the peritoneum (see Figure 11–5).[70]

A line drawn between the two iliac crests crosses the midline between the L4 and L5 spinous processes. The needle is inserted at the desired level, 1 to 1½ inches lateral to the midline, and advanced through the

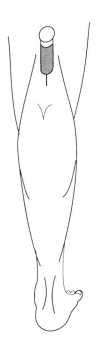

FIG. 11–8. Approach to the tibial nerve.

paraspinal muscles and into the psoas muscle, within which the plexus lies. A 75 mm needle may suffice for a relatively thin individual, but a longer needle may be necessary for others. At the L4-L5 level, contraction of the hip flexors or adductors, or knee extensors or flexors may be seen. One is likely, however, to have to tilt the needle downward past the level of the L5 spinous process or reinsert it at this level to locate the elements innervating the hamstrings. One can often locate the innervation to the hip adductors and flexors, as well as the knee extensors at the L3-L4 level, but it may be necessary to go to the L2-L3 level to adequately block the hip flexors.[15,52,70] While one is searching for a response, the needle can be safely tilted rostrally and caudally, but more than slight lateral redirection of the needle should be avoided to ensure maximal protection by the iliopsoas muscle. Innervation of the quadratus lumborum muscle can be located at L2-3 or at L1-2, and can generally be found more superficially, just deep to the paraspinal muscles.

THORACODORSAL NERVE

The thoracodorsal nerve can be located between the mid and posterior axillary lines as it descends from the posterior cord of the brachial plexus to innervate the latissimus dorsi muscle. The needle is inserted anterior to the outer border of the scapula, at the midpoint of a line connecting the inferior angle of the scapula with the apex of the axilla, or four fingerbreadths below the apex of the axilla between the mid and posterior axillary lines. It is pointed in a rostral direction, inclined at a slight angle toward the thorax, but almost parallel to the sagittal plane to avoid entering the intercostal space (Fig. 11–9).[70]

MUSCULOCUTANEOUS NERVE

There are two commonly used approaches to the musculocutaneous nerve. In the axillary approach, the patient lies supine with the shoulder held at about 90 degrees of abduction and external rotation. The axillary artery is palpated in the axilla, and the needle is inserted about 1 cm above the artery, just behind the tendon of the pectoralis major, close to its insertion to the humerus. It is advanced in the direction of the coracoid process until a contraction of the biceps is seen. The median nerve may be stimulated before the musculocutaneous nerve is located (Fig. 11–10).[70]

As an alternative, the musculocutaenous nerve can be approached at a more distal site in the upper arm. The brachial artery is palpated about two fingerbreadths distal to the insertion of the pectoralis major in the humerus. The needle is inserted anterior to the artery, perpendicular to the arm, and is advanced laterally until a contraction of the biceps muscle is seen.[70]

FIG. 11–9. Approach to the thoracodorsal nerve.

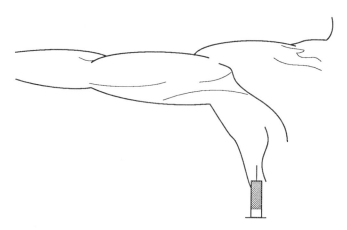

FIG. 11-10. Approach to the musculocutaneous nerve.

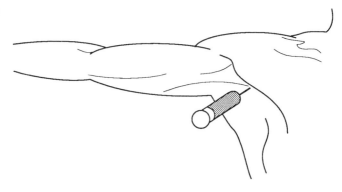

MEDIAN NERVE

The median nerve can be approached in the axilla, as noted above in the discussion of the musculocutaneous nerve, and, in fact, the two nerves may run together at this level.[52] It is, however, usually approached just distal to the antecubital fossa as it courses between the two heads of the pronator teres muscle. The needle is inserted perpendicular to the forearm, 1 inch distal to the midpoint of a line drawn between the medial epicondyle and the biceps tendon (1 inch below and 1 inch anterior to the medial epicondyle) (Fig. 11-11).[70,72]

Branches to the pronator teres leave the median nerve at the antecubital fossa. Therefore a median nerve block that is to include the fascicles to this muscle must be done at or above the antecubital fossa. It should be kept in mind that the brachial artery runs just lateral to the median nerve at both levels, but that there is a somewhat greater separation at the forearm site.[70]

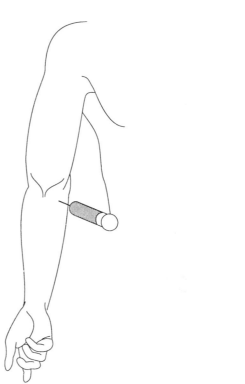

FIG. 11-11. Approach to the median nerve.

REFERENCES

1. Matthews, P.B.C., and Rushworth, G.: The selective effect of procaine on the stretch reflex and tendon jerk of soleus muscle when applied to its nerve. J. Physiol. *135*:245–262, 1957.
2. Liljestrand, G., and Magnus, R.: Uber die wirkung des novakains auf den normalen und den tetanusstarren skelettmuskel und uber die entstehung der lokalen muskelstarre beim wundstarrkrampf. Pflugers Arch. *176*:168–208, 1919.
3. Matthews, P.B.C., and Rushworth, G.: The relative sensitivity of muscle nerve fibres to procaine. J. Physiol. *135*:263–269, 1957.
4. Wood, K.E.: The use of phenol as a neurolytic agent: A review. Pain *5*:205–229, 1978.
5. Kelly, R.E., and Gauthier-Smith, P.C.: Intrathecal phenol in the treatment of reflex spasms and spasticity. Lancet *ii*:1102–1105, 1959.

6. Nathan, P.W.: Intrathecal phenol to relieve spasticity in paraplegia. Lancet *ii*:1099–1102, 1959.

7. Helweg-Larsen, J., and Jacobsen, E.: Treatment of spasticity in cerebral palsy by means of phenol nerve block of peripheral nerves. Dan. Med. Bull. *16*:20–25, 1969.

8. Katz, J., Knott, L.W., and Feldman, D.J.: Peripheral nerve injections with phenol in the management of spastic patients. Arch. Phys. Med. Rehabil. *48*:97–99, 1967.

9. Khalili, A.A., Harmel, M.H., Forster, S., and Benton, J.G.: Management of spasticity by selective peripheral nerve block with dilute phenol solutions in clinical rehabilitation. Arch. Phys. Med. Rehabil. *45*:513–519, 1964.

10. Khalili, A.A., and Benton, J.G.: A physiologic approach to the evaluation and the management of spasticity with procaine and phenol nerve block. Clin. Orthop. *47*:97–104, 1966.

11. Khalili, A.A., and Betts, H.B.: Peripheral nerve block with phenol in the management of spasticity: Indications and complications. JAMA *200*:1155–1157, 1967.

12. Khalili, A.A., and Betts, H.B.: Isolated block of musculocutaneous and perineal nerves in the management of spasticity with special reference to the use of a nerve stimulator. Anesthesiology *28*:219–222, 1967.

13. Halpern, D., and Meelhuysen, F.E.: Phenol motor point block in the management of muscular hypertonia. Arch. Phys. Med. Rehabil. *47*:659–664, 1966.

14. Halpern, D., and Meelhuysen, F.E.: Duration of relaxation after intramuscular neurolysis with phenol. JAMA *200*:1152–1154, 1967.

15. Meelhuysen, F.E., Halpern, D., and Quast, J.: Treatment of flexor spasticity of hip by paravertebral lumbar spinal nerve block. Arch. Phys. Med. Rehabil. *49*:36–41, 1968.

16. Tardieu, C., et al: Fondement experimental d'une thérapeutique des raideurs d'origine cérébrale. Arch. Fr. Pediatr. *21*:5–23, 1964.

17. Tardieu, G., Tardieu, C., Hariga, J., and Gagnard, L.: Treatment of spasticity by injection of dilute alcohol at the motor point or by epidural route. Dev. Med. Child Neurol. *10*:555–568, 1968.

18. O'Hanlan, J.T., Galford, H.R., and Bosley, J.: The use of 45% alcohol to control spasticity. Virginia Med. Monthly *96*:429–436, 1969.

19. Brattstrom, M., Mortiz, U., and Svantesson, G.: Electromyographic studies of peripheral nerve block with phenol. Scand. J. Rehabil. Med. 2:17–22, 1970.

20. Khalili, A.A.: Physiatric management of spasticity by phenol nerve and motor point block. *In* Current Therapy in Physiatry. Ed. A.P. Ruskin. Philadelphia, W.B. Saunders, 1984.

21. Copp, E.P., Harris, R., and Keenan, J.: Peripheral nerve block and motor point block with phenol in the management of spasticity. Proc. R. Soc. Med. *63*:937–938, 1970.

22. Spira, R.: Management of spasticity in cerebral palsied children by peripheral nerve block with phenol. Dev. Med. Child Neurol. *13*:164–173, 1971.

23. Copp, E.P., and Keenan, J.: Phenol nerve and motor point block in spasticity. Rheum. Phys. Med. *11*:287–292, 1972.

24. DeLateur, B.J.: A new technique of intramuscular phenol neurolysis. Arch. Phys. Med. Rehabil. *53*:179–185, 1972.

25. Awad, E.A.: Intramuscular neurolysis for stroke. Minn. Med. *8*:711–713, 1972.

26. Mortiz, U.: Phenol Block of Peripheral Nerves. Scand. J. Rehabil. Med. *5*:160–163, 1973.

27. Petrillo, C.R., Chu, D.S., and Davis, S.W.: Phenol block of the tibial nerve in the hemiplegic patient. Orthopedics *3*:871–874, 1980.

28. Garland, D.E., Lilling, M., and Keenan, M.A.: Percutaneous phenol blocks to motor points of spastic forearm muscles in head-injured adults. Arch. Phys. Med. Rehabil. *65*:243–245, 1984.

29. Braun, R.M., et al.: Phenol nerve block in the treatment of acquired spastic hemiplegia in the upper limb. J. Bone Joint Surg. *55A*:580–585, 1973.

30. Westgate, H.D.: Selective percutaneous sacral root blockade with phenol in neurovesical dysfunction. Can. Anaesth. Soc. J. *17*:456–463, 1970.

31. Susset, J.G. Zinner, N., and Archimbaud, J.P.: Differential sacral blocks and selective neurotomies in the treatment of incomplete upper motor neuron lesion. Urol. Int. *29*:236–248, 1974.

32. Simon, D.L., Carron, H., and Rowlingson, J.C.: Treatment of bladder pain with transsacral nerve block. Anesth. Analg. *61*:46–48, 1982.

33. Easton, J.K.M., Ozel, T., and Halpern, D.: Intramuscular neurolysis for spasticity in children. Arch. Phys. Med. Rehabil. *60*:155–158, 1979.

34. Maher, R.M.: Neurone selection in relief of pain: further experiences with intrathecal injections. Lancet *ii*:16–19, 1957.

35. Brown, A.S.: The treatment of intractable

pain by subarachnoid injection of carbolic acid, Lancet *ii*:975–978, 1958.

36. Iggo, A., and Walsh, E.G.: Selective block of small fibres in the spinal roots by phenol. J. Physiol. *146*:701–708, 1959.

37. Nathan, P.W., and Sears, T.A.: Effects of phenol on nervous conduction. J. Physiol. *150*:565–580, 1960.

38. Schaumburg, H.N., Byck, R., and Weller, R.O.: The effect of phenol on peripheral nerve. A histological and electrophysiological study. J. Neuropathol. Exp. Neurol. *29*:615–630, 1970.

39. Fischer, E., et al.: Evoked nerve conduction after nerve block by chemical means. Am. J. Phys. Med. *49*:333–347, 1970.

40. Nathan, P.W., Sears, T.A., and Smith, M.C.: Effects of phenol solutions on the nerve roots of the cat: An electrophysiological and histological study. J. Neurol. Sci. *2*:7–29, 1965.

41. Fischer, E., et al.: Recovery of nerve conduction after nerve block by phenol. Am. J. Phys. Med. *50*:230–234, 1971.

42. Burkel, W.E., and McPhee, M.: Effect of phenol injection into peripheral nerve of rat: Electron microscope studies. Arch. Phys. Med. Rehabil. *51*:391–397, 1970.

43. Mooney, V., Frykman, G., and McLamb, J.: Current status of intraneural phenol injections. Clin. Orthop. *63*:122–131, 1969.

44. Halpern, D.: Histologic studies in animals after intramuscular neurolysis with phenol. Arch. Phys. Med. Rehabil. *58*:438–443, 1977.

45. Fusfeld, R.D.: Electromyographic findings after phenol block. Arch. Phys. Med. Rehabil. *49*:217–220, 1968.

46. Glass, A., Cain, H.D., Liebgold, H., and Mead, S.: Electromyographic and evoked potential responses after phenol blocks of peripheral nerves. Arch. Phys. Med. Rehabil. *49*:455–459, 1968.

47. Walthard, K.M., and Tchicaloff, M.: Motor points. *In* Licht, S. (ed.): Electrodiagnosis and Electromyography, 3rd Ed. New Haven, Licht, 1971.

48. Zack, S.I.: The Motor Endplate. Philadelphia, W.B. Saunders, 1971.

49. Garland, D.E., Lucie, R.S., and Walters, R.L.: Current uses of open phenol nerve block for adult acquired spasticity. Clin. Orthop. *165*:217–222, 1982.

50. Roper, B.: Evaluation of spasticity. The Hand *7*:11–14, 1975.

51. Keenan, M.A.E.: The orthopedic management of spasticity. J. Head Trauma Rehabil. *2(2)*:62–71, 1987.

52. O'Rahilly, R.: Gardner-Gray-O'Rahilly Anatomy: A Regional Study of Human Structure. 5th Ed. Philadelphia, W.B. Saunders, 1986.

53. Burman, M.S.: Therapeutic use of curare and erythroidine hydrochloride for spastic and dystonic states. Arch. Neurol. Psychiat. *41*:307–327, 1939.

54. Felsenthal, G.: Pharmacology of phenol in peripheral nerve blocks: A review. Arch. Phys. Med. Rehabil. *55*:13–16, 1974.

55. Cooper, I.S., et al.: Specific neurotoxic perfusion: a new approach to selected cases of pain and spasticity. Neurology (Minneap.) *15*:985–993, 1965.

56. Macek, K.: Medical News: Venous thrombosis results from some phenol injections. JAMA *249*:1807, 1983.

57. Superville-Sovak, B., Rasminsky, M., and Finlayson, M.B.: Complications of phenol neurolysis. Arch. Neurol. *32*:226–228, 1975.

58. Holland, A.J.C., and Youssef, M.: A complication of subarachnoid phenol blockade. Anaesthesia *34*:260–262, 1978.

59. May, O.: The functional and histological effects of intraneural and intraganglionic injections of alcohol. Br. Med. J., Aug. 31, 1912:465–470.

60. Gordon, A.: Experimental study of intraneural injections of alcohol. J. Nerv. Ment. Dis. *41*:81–95, 1914.

61. Labat, G.: The action of alcohol on the living nerve: Experimental and clinical considerations. Anesth. Analg. (Current Researches) *12*:190–196, 1933.

62. Ritchie, J.M.: The aliphatic alcohols. *In* Goodman and Gilman's The Pharmacological Basis of Therapeutics, Seventh Edition. Ed. A.G. Gilman, L.S. Goodman, T.W. Rall, and F. Murad. New York. Macmillan, 1985.

63. Carpenter, E.B., and Seitz, D.G.: Intramuscular alcohol as an aid in the management of spastic cerebral palsy. Dev. Med. Child Neurol. *22*:497–501, 1980.

64. Carpenter, E.B.: Role of nerve blocks in the foot and ankle in cerebral palsy: therapeutic and diagnostic. Foot Ankle *4*:164–166, 1983.

65. Sparadeo, F.R., and Gill, D.: Effects of prior alcohol use on head injury recovery. J. Head Trauma Rehabil. *4(1)*:75–82, 1989.

66. Ritchie, J.M., and Greene, N.M.: Local anesthetics. *In* Goodman and Gilman's The Pharmacological Basis of Therapeutics, Seventh Edition. Ed. A.G. Gilman, L.S. Goodman, T.W. Rall, and F. Murad. New York. Macmillan, 1985.

67. Kjellberg, R.N., et al.: Gait improvement in Parkinsonian patients by gamma motor

neuron suppression. Trans. Am. Neurol. Assoc. *86*:126–130, 1961.

68. Griffith, E.R., and Melampy, C.N.: General Anesthesia Use in Phenol Intramuscular Neurolysis in Young Children with Spasticity. Arch. Phys. Med. Rehabil. *58*:154–157, 1977.

69. Doherty, D.L.: Can vegetative patients feel pain? (Abstract) Arch. Phys. Med. Rehabil. *69*:721, 1988.

70. Labib, K.B., and Gans, B.M.: Chemical neu-rolysis: technique and anatomical considerations (videotape). Boston, Dept. of Rehabilitation Medicine, New England Medical Center, 1984.

71. Felsenthal, G: Nerve blocks in the lower extremities: anatomic considerations. Arch. Phys. Med. Rehabil. *55*:504–507, 1974.

72. Delagi, E.F., and Perotto, A.: Anatomic Guide for the Electromyographer: The Limbs, 2nd Ed. Springfield, IL, Charles C Thomas, 1980, 1981.

12 NEUROSURGICAL APPROACHES

DAVID L. KASDON
JOEL N. ABRAMOVITZ

Spasticity is defined in this text as a persistent increase in the resting tone of a muscle and a velocity-sensitive increase in the resistance to passive stretch (hyperreflexia), often with clonus and mass reflex spread. The control of tone in the central nervous system is the result of a delicate balance of facilitation and inhibition modulated by input in many areas of the central nervous system. These include the pyramidal and extrapyramidal systems and the reticular activating system. Within the spinal cord, the rich synaptic input of interneurons on the anterior horn cells and gamma and alpha output to the striated muscle and spindle afferents play major roles.

The central nervous system surgical approaches to spasticity are traditionally in the domain of the neurosurgeon. Neurosurgical interventions have also been directed toward interrupting the monosynaptic stretch reflex in a variety of ways. Anterior rhizotomies provide denervation of the muscle whereas posterior rhizotomies interrupt the IA and IB afferents from the muscle spindle. In addition, interruption of the spindle afferents over many segments of the cord has been performed with the T-myelotomy approaches of Weber and Bischof. Modification of descending facilatory pathways with techniques such as spinal cord stimulation has been attempted. Cerebellar stimulation perhaps increases the activity of descending inhibitory pathways. Recently, intrathecal drug therapy has been used to manipulate spinal cord receptors with neuropeptide-like drugs, and has opened a new phase in the treatment of spasticity.

This chapter reviews the neurosurgical approaches to spasticity and discusses the advantages and disadvantages of each approach.

HISTORICAL TREATMENT OF SPASTICITY

In 1919, Liljestrand and Magnus reproted that injection of a local anesthetic (procaine) into the muscles of decerebrate cats would transiently abolish their extensor tone.[1] In 1924, Walshe injected procaine into the muscles of spastic patients and demonstrated a temporary absence of spasticity.[2] The effects of muscle injection last only as long as the local anesthetic effect is present in the muscles, and probably depends to a large extent on interrupting the afferent signal from the muscle spindle and the gamma motor neurons innervating the spindle, as local anesthetics affect small-diameter fibers more readily than large.

Peripheral nerve injections with caustic substances such as phenol and alcohol were early treatments of spasticity and are still in use. Phenol injections are described elsewhere in this text (see Chapter 11) and are

259

used extensively by physiatrists in rehabilitation settings. The technique and indications for peripheral nerve injections will not be reviewed in this chapter.

OPERATIVE ANTERIOR AND POSTERIOR RHIZOTOMY

Posterior rhizotomy was performed in patients with spasticity by Otfrid Foerster in 1913.[3] Foerster spared some roots in order to avoid total anesthesia and should be considered to have performed only partial posterior rhizotomies on this basis. His patients showed early transient improvement and then increasing tone over time. In 1948, Freeman and Heimberger studied a large series of patients with partial posterior rhizotomies and had similar poor long-term results that were very similar to Foerster's experience.[4,5]

Anterior rhizotomy for spasticity was reported by Munro in 1945 in 42 patients with severe lower extremity spasticity.[6] Munro cut all anterior roots from T11 through S1 and had excellent relief of spasticity in 39 of his 42 patients. This experience with anterior rhizotomy was confirmed by Freeman and Heinberger who noted successful improvement in the long term of all of their patients with complete anterior rhizotomy. The primary advantage of the anterior rhizotomy approach is that it is long-lasting and effective, and spares bladder function because the sacral roots are left intact. The disadvantages of the anterior rhizotomy are that it is an extensive operation requiring a multiple level laminectomy, and that the potential for improvement in voluntary motor activity is lost.

If spasticity is reduced, some patients are found to have a surprising degree of voluntary motor activity that was unrecognized because it had been impeded by their increased tone and antagonistic muscle groups. The early investigative work with spinal cord regeneration using peripheral nerve grafts and nerve growth factors in laboratory animals is an additional reason to avoid an anterior rhizotomy approach, which would preclude any future clinically useful spinal cord regeneration techniques.

The early, encouraging results of electrical stimulation to produce rudimentary walking lead to the same conclusion.

SELECTIVE POSTERIOR RHIZOTOMY

In 1982, Sindou et al. reported the results of selective posterior rhizotomy in the treatment of spastic paraplegia secondary to multiple sclerosis.[7] Sindou subsequently reported his extension of this selective posterior rhizotomy technique to the upper extremity in 16 hemiplegic patients in 1986.[8] All of this group of 16 patients had spasticity and 12 of the 16 had pain. Spasticity was relieved on a long-term basis in 15 of the 16 patients and pain relieved in 9 of the 12. This procedure consisted of cervical laminectomy with selective stimulation of posterior rootlets with the bipolar forceps and a microsurgical lesion both of the abnormal posterior rootlets and of the dorsal root entry zone.

The dorsal root entry zone is a portion of the posterior horn of the cord including the substantia gelatinosa of Rolondo which seems to have a major input on pain and spasticity. Nashold and Ostdahl reported dorsal root entry zone lesions for pain relief in 1979.[9] These were primarily used for deafferentation pain syndromes. Sindou extended the selective lesion of rootlets that led to an abnormal motor response by also making lesions of the dorsal root entry zone. This approach for the upper extremity was almost as successful as his early report of selective rhizotomy in the lower extremity, leading to a functional improvement in 93% of patients. One-half of the patients had noticeable sensory diminution by the selective posterior rhizotomy approach. Laitinen et al. reported a similar experience with selective posterior rhizotomy for the treatment of spasticity in the lower extremities.[10]

The value of selective rhizotomy has been reported by Peacock and Eastman in a large series of pediatric patients.[11] Most of these patients had cerebral palsy. This report expanded on an earlier series reported by Peacock and Eastman in 1981.[12] This approach consists of a laminectomy of the lumbar area up to the conus. With a special nerve hook electrode attached to a nerve stimulator, rootlets are stimulated selectively with electromyographic feedback from the lower extremities and sphincters. Some portions of the root lead to an abnormal motor response and are sectioned, whereas those portions of the root leading to either no motor response or a "normal motor response" are left intact. This approach has not caused significant sensory loss and has provided decrease in spasticity with improvement in voluntary motor activity and ambulation in the majority of patients with cerebral palsy. The selective rhizotomy using intraoperative stimulation is presently most useful in patients with partial motor function who are ambulatory or partially ambulatory. In the patient with a completed spinal cord injury and no distal voluntary function, a selective procedure of this nature is probably not ideal since it requires an extensive laminectomy. The patient with no voluntary function and severe spasticity may best be helped by percutaneous rhizotomy technique.

PERCUTANEOUS RADIOFREQUENCY RHIZOTOMY

In 1974, Umatsu reported a technique of percutaneous radiofrequency rhizotomy for various pain states.[13] In 1977, Kenmore reported his experience with percutaneous radiofrequency rhizotomy in the management of spasticity in patients with spinal cord and brain injuries.[14,15] This procedure is performed under general anesthesia unless patients are insensitive below the thoracic level because of a spinal cord injury.

FIG. 12-1. Guide needles positioned in lumbar foramina for percutaneous radiofrequency rhizotomy.

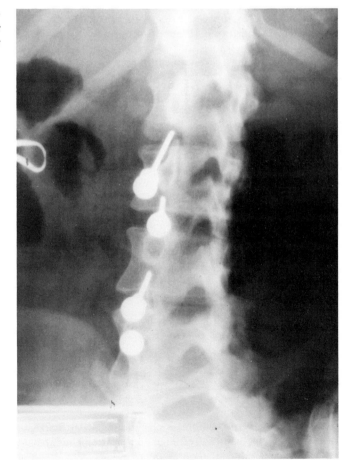

Percutaneous rhizotomy is performed in the x-ray department under fluoroscopic control or in the operating room using C-arm fluoroscopy. A thermistor electrode (Radionics Inc., Burlington, MA) is placed under fluoroscopic control through a large-bore spinal needle at multiple levels. The electrode is positioned so that it lies in the neural foramen (Fig. 12–1). Levels T12 through S1 are treated in most patients. A paraspinal approach is used from L5 through the T12 roots and an interlaminar approach is performed at S1. At each root level, the root is stimulated using the thermistor electrode in the stimulation mode. The stimulation threshold is noted and must be less than 0.5 volts if the lesion is to be effective. If the stimulation threshold is higher than 0.5 volts, the needle position must be adjusted to be closer to the root. Using the radiofrequency lesion generator and the thermistor tip, a heat lesion is made (usually for 120 seconds at 90°C) and the electrode allowed to cool to body temperature. The root is then restimulated. If the stimulation threshhold has not been increased by at least 0.2 volts, the root le-

sion is inadequate and the lesion is repeated (Fig. 12–2).

Kasdon and Lathi performed a prospective study of 25 patients with either brain or spinal cord injury and spasticity.[16,17] In this group of patients with post-traumatic spasticity, an average time of 2 years had elapsed between the patient's injury and the radiofrequency rhizotomy. Preoperative goals, as well as detailed examination and recording of muscle tone and range of motion, were reported before the performance of the radiofrequency rhizotomies. In this study, with all patients followed for more than a year postoperatively, all or most of the prospectively identified goals were accomplished in 24 of 25 patients. The recurrence rate has been approximately 10% over time following radiofrequency rhizotomy. In these cases a repeat procedure has usually been successful. Complications have been minimal with this technique, and bladder and reflex sexual functions are not threatened because the lower sacral roots are not involved. The improvement in tone was much greater than the improvement in range of motion. In a

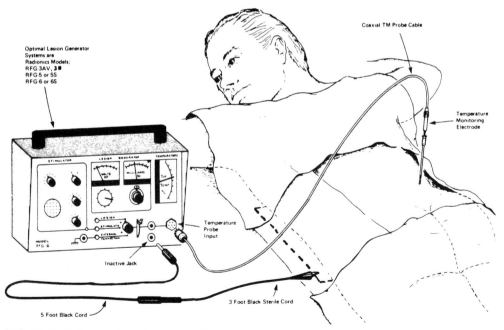

FIG. 12–2. Patient and equipment positioned for percutaneous radiofrequency rhizotomy (with permission from Shealy, C.N.: Technique for percutaneous spinal facet rhizotomy. Procedure Technique Series. Burlington, MA, Radionics, Inc.).

number of patients, orthopedic releases of contracted tendons and joints were very successful after rhizotomy had been performed.

Herz et al. reported a similar experience primarily with post-traumatic spasticity in 1983.[18] The advantages of this procedure include a high rate of efficacy, no permanent loss of voluntary function, and minimal sensory loss. The risk to sphincter and sexual function is negligible. In addition, the procedure is inexpensive, does not require an open operation, and can be performed as an outpatient surgical procedure. Decubitus ulcers do not prohibit its performance, and most patients in whom decubitus ulcers are a manifestation of the spasticity find that they heal quickly after the spasticity has been relieved. The disadvantages of the percutaneous rhizotomy technique have included a variable sensory loss and a modest rate of recurrence of spasticity.

CORDOTOMY

Cordotomy of the anterior funiculus (presumably interrupting the facilatory vestibulospinal and reticulospinal tracts) was reported by Hyndman in 1943[19] and expanded by Schurmann in 1949.[20] This technique required a laminectomy of the cervical or high thoracic area. Spasticity was usually abolished promptly by the procedure, but recurred within 2 years in almost all patients. The extensor spasm component was less likely to recur than the flexor component.

In 1951, Bischof[21] reported the value of myelotomy for the treatment of spasticity. This experience with "T-myelotomy" was expanded by Weber in 1955.[22] The "T-myelotomy" is performed through a midline incision in the posterior aspect of the spinal cord. Once the midportion of the cord is reached, the lesion is then extended toward either side at a right angle in a "T-like" fashion. This procedure interrupts the reflex arcs that connect the posterior and anterior horns of the spinal cord. This procedure was highly effective in relieving spasticity and in several patients preserved voluntary movement. Its primary disadvantage is that it is an extensive operative procedure requiring a laminectomy over multiple segments. The myelotomy was often associated with voiding difficulties and moderate sensory disturbance. Because of the extensiveness of the operative procedure and the availability of alternatives of a lesser magnitute, "T-myelotomy" for spasticity is rarely performed in the United States today.

INTRATHECAL CHEMOTHERAPY

The treatment of spasticity with intrathecal medications has undergone a renaissance because of the development of continuous flow and programmable infusion devices. Ablative chemotherapy (primarily with intrathecal phenol or alcohol) has been used for many years in the treatment of spasticity. Five percent phenol in glycerin is hyperbaric and can be manipulated within the spinal fluid by alterations in the patient's position. If phenol is to be used, the appropriate target roots are placed in a relatively dependent position with the patient on a tiltable radiologic table. Scott et al. improved the precision with which phenol could be manipulated in the spinal fluid by replacing Pantopaque with metrizamide.[23] The older technique of Pantopaque mixed with phenol and glycerin was quite useful, but was limited by the difficulty in keeping the Pantopaque droplets together and in suspension with the phenol in glycerin. By substituting a water-soluble contrast agent for Pantopaque, the phenol in glycerin can be manipulated under fluoroscopic control so that the target roots are heavily treated with limited involvement of adjacent roots. The procedure is performed without anesthesia, placing the desired target roots in the most dependent position. Progressive aliquots of approximately 0.4 ml of 5% phenol in glycerin are added until the desired decrease in tone is obtained. The procedure with alcohol is performed somewhat differently in that alcohol is hypobaric and therefore the desired target roots must be placed in the superior position. The disadvantages of intrathecal ablative chemotherapy are the difficulty of control in uncooperative patients and a higher risk of bowel and bladder dysfunction than with other procedures. There is also a moderate risk of voluntary motor weakness. On the other hand, the advantage of intrathecal chemotherapy consists of the ease and low cost with which the procedure can be performed. This procedure can usually be done on an outpatient basis. There is, unfortunately, a fairly high recurrence rate, but repeated instillations of intrathecal phenol or alcohol can be easily performed. In our experience, the procedure has been most valuable in patients with multiple sclerosis who already have indwelling bladder catheters and virtually no hope of return of voluntary function.

The development of implantable infusion devices has recently produced considerable experimental interest in the use of pharmacologic agents to manipulate spinal cord receptors and thereby decrease spasticity. The use of implantable infusion devices has already been developed for many applications including insulin administration for diabetes mellitus, intrahepatic infusions of chemotherapy for metastatic disease and intracarotid infusions for malignant gliomas, chronic heparin administration, and treatment of pain of malignant origin with intrathecal opiates. This technology depends on the types of pumps available.

TYPES OF PUMPS AVAILABLE

Rate-Constant (Infusaid Corp, Randolph, MA). (Fig. 12–3) This pump has two chambers. One is the drug chamber and is usually filled with preservative free morphine in 1 or 2 mg/cc concentrations. The pump has a 50 ml reservoir and is filled percutaneously through a silastic port. The other chamber is filled with freon gas. The two chambers are separated by a metal bellows, which is displaced as the drug chamber is filled, compressing the freon gas. The freon gas expands at a constant rate at body temperature, causing the drug chamber to empty at a constant infusion rate of approximately 2 to 3 cc/day. The pump egress tubing is connected to either an epidural or subarachnoid catheter placed by means of a Touhey needle with or without fluoros-

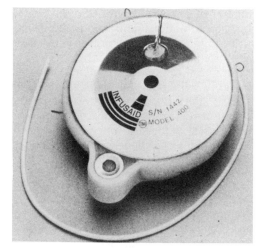

FIG. 12–3. Implantable rate-constant pump (Infusaid Corp.).

copy. The tubings are connected with a metal connector provided with the pump and the pump incision and lumbar incisions are connected subcutaneously with a tunneling instrument.

We do these operations in the lateral position under local anesthesia. The pump must be anchored to the abdominal fascia with nonabsorbable sutures to prevent it from flipping over so that its refill port remains accessible. Typically this pump is refilled every 2 to 3 weeks, depending on the flow rate for each pump. This has been a highly reliable system. Because the delivery rate is constant, drug dosage can be varied only by varying drug concentration.

Rate-Variable Pumps. Two rate-variable pumps have been developed that can be externally reprogrammed without removal.

At present, one rate-variable pump is available for clinical use. The Medtronic pump (model 8610) has a 20 ml reservoir and is percutaneously refillable. It is battery-powered and has a rotary pump that can be programmed by the physician using an external programming unit and an RF transmitter and receiver in the implanted pump. The Pimms pump is also under development in conjunction with Johns Hopkins University but is under investigational use only.

CLINICAL APPLICATIONS

At this time, two drugs have been used as intrathecal treatment for spasticity by implantable pumps.

In 1985, Erikson et al.,[24] reported serendipitous findings of improvement in spasticity by intrathecal morphine in patients with spinal cord injury and arachnoiditis in whom it was administered (1 to 2 mg doses) for the treatment of pain. Three patients subsequently had a pump placed for intrathecal delivery of morphine, with prolonged improvement in their spasticity. The site of action of morphine is thought to be the dorsal horn neurons, where it decreases multisynaptic reflexes associated with A delta and c fiber activity. Follow-up reports of four more patients with spinal cord injury treated with long-term intrathecal morphine showed no evidence of morphine tolerance, for as long as 17 months in one patient. The Tufts experience confirms this finding. The degree of flaccidity is often very remarkable.

Penn and Kroin,[25] Penn,[26,27] Parke et al.,[28] and Penn[29] reported the use of baclofen by a rate-variable (Medtronic) pump in spasticity. Doses of 12 to 749 μg/day for up to 33 months in patients with spinal cord injury or multiple sclerosis resulted in a great reduction in muscle tone to normal, and elimination of spontaneous spasms. Oral baclofen had either failed to help or produced intolerable side effects in these patients. Some need for increasing dose with time occurred.

The advantages of intrathecal pharmacologic treatment of spasticity are the lack of any ablation and the ability to titrate desired reduction in tone by manipulation of drug dosage and rate of administration. The disadvantages include the need for refilling, potential drug toxicity, and the high cost of the pump. Promising results have been obtained with intrathecal morphine and baclofen in the relief of spasticity. While at this time the FDA has not approved intrathecal use of baclofen, it is likely within the next few years. The study of other potential neurotransmitter-like drugs that may be more effective and safer has just begun.

SPINAL CORD AND CEREBELLAR STIMULATION

Spinal cord stimulation, reported by Waltz,[30] and cerebellar stimulation, reported by Waltz and Pani[31] and by Nakamura and Tsubokawa[32] have been effective in reducing spasticity in selective patients. Barolat-Romana[33] has also reported a small series of selected patients with excellent spasticity relief by spinal cord epidural stimulation. The implantation of stimulating electrodes over either the cerebellum or dorsal spinal cord presumably stimulates inhibitory pathways and inhibits facilatory pathways. Long-term follow-up studies have not been encouraging, largely because of equipment failure and electrode impairment by fibrosis. These methods do not interfere with voluntary movement and do not affect sphincter function. The disadvantages of this kind of procedure include a high long-term failure rate, requirement for either a posterior fossa exploration or cervical laminectomy, and the considerable expense of the stimulating device. Double-blind studies are impossible to perform because spinal cord or cerebellar stimulation is perceived by the patient.

Barolat-Romana et al.[33] did report electrode placement with a percutaneous approach. Stimulation trials can be performed on a temporary basis, bringing the electrode percutaneously through the skin to a temporary stimulator. The complete apparatus with implantable receiver is implanted only if the temporary trial produces the desired reduction in tone.

CONCLUSION

At the present time, no ideal surgical treatment exists for all patients with spasticity. An ideal procedure would be low in cost and extremely safe, requiring a small operation with complete relief of spasticity, yet producing total preservation of voluntary movement and normal sensation while sparing all sphincter and reflex sexual function. At present, each patient must be individually examined and the relative merits and risk of the procedures discussed in this chapter considered. With the development of selective rhizotomy techniques and of neuromodulatory transmitter-like drug delivery systems, we are moving into an exciting period in spasticity therapy that hopefully will bring us closer to the ideal treatment.

REFERENCES

1. Liljestrand, G. and Magnus, R.: Uber die wirkung des novokains auf den normalen und den tetanusstarren skelettmuskel und uber die enstehung der lokalen muskelstarre beim wunstarrkrampf. Pflugers Arch. *176*:168–208, 1919.

2. Walshe, A.E.: Observations on the nature of the muscular rigidity of paralysis agitans, and on its relationship to tremor. Brain *47*:159–177, 1924.

3. Foerster, O.: On the indications and results of the excision of posterior spinal nerve roots in men. Surg. Gynecol. Obstet. *26*:463–475, 1913.

4. Freeman, L.W. and Heimburger, R.F.: The surgical relief of spasticity in paraplegic patients I. Anterior Rhizotomy. J. Neurosurg. *5*:555–561, 1948.

5. Freeman, L.W. and Heimburger, R.F.: The surgical relief of spasticity in paraplegic patients. II. Peripheral nerve section, posterior rhizotomy and other procedures. J. Neurosurg. *4*:435–443, 1947.

6. Munro, D.: The rehabilitation of patients totally paralyzed below the waist: With special reference to making them ambulatory and capable of earning their living. I. Anterior rhizotomy for spastic paraplegia. N. Engl. J. Med. *223*:453–461, 1945.

7. Sindou, M., Millet, M.F., Mortamis, J., and Eyssette, M.: Results of selective posterior rhizotomy in the treatment of painful spastic paraplegia secondary to multiple sclerosis. Appl. Neurophysiol. *45*:335–340, 1982.

8. Sindou, M., Misfud, J.J., Boisson, D., and Goutelle, A.: Selective posterior rhizotomy in the dorsal root entry zone of hyperspasticity and pain in the hemiplegic upper limb. Neurosurgery *18*:587–595, 1986.

9. Nashold, B.S., Jr., and Ostedahl, R.H.: Dorsal root entry zone lesions for pain relief. J. Neurosurg. *51*:59–69, 1979.

10. Laitinen, L.V., Nilsson, S., and Fugl-Meyer, A.R.: Selective posterior rhizotomy for treatment of spasticity. J. Neurosurg. *58*:895–899, 1983.

11. Peacock, W.J. and Eastman, R.W.: The neurosurgical management of spasticity in cerebral palsy. S. Afr. Med. J. *62*:119–124, 1982.

12. Peacock, W.J., and Eastman, R.W.: The neurosurgical management of spasticity. S. Afr. Med. J. *60*:849–850, 1981.

13. Umatsu, S., et al.: Percutaneous radiofrequency rhizotomy. Surg. Neurol. *2*:319–324, 1974.

14. Kenmore, D.: Management of spasms and spasticity in the spinal cord and brain injured patients by percutaneous radiofrequency rhizotomy. Presented at the 45th Annual Meeting of the American Association of Neurological Surgeons, Toronto, Ontario, April 24–28, 1977.

15. Kenmore, D.: Radiofrequency neurotomy for peripheral pain and spasticity syndromes. Cont. Neurosurg. *58*:895–899, 1983.

16. Kasdon, D.L., and Lathi, E.S.: A prospective study of radiofrequency rhizotomy in the treatment of posttraumatic spasticity. Neurosurgery *15*:526–529, 1984.

17. Kasdon, D.L.: Controversies in the surgical management of spasticity. Clin. Neurosurg. *33*:523–529, 1986.

18. Herz, D.A., Parsons, K.C., and Pearl, L.: Percutaneous radiofrequency foraminal rhizotomies. Spine *8*:729–732, 1983.

19. Hyndman, O.R.: Physiology of the spinal cord. II. The influence of chordotomy on existing motor disturbances. J. Nerv. Ment. Dis. *98*:343–358, 1943.

20. Schurmann, K.: Die durchschneidung der pyramidenvordestrange und benachbarter extrapyramidaler bahen bei spastichen zustanden und unwillkurlichen bewegungsstorungen. Zentralbl. Neurchir. *9*:136–141, 1949.

21. Bischof, W.: Die longitudinal myelotomie. Zentralbl. Neurochir. *2*:79–88, 1951.

22. Weber, W.: Die behandlung der spinalen paraspastik unter besonderer berücksichtigung der longitudinalen myelotomie (Bishof) Med. Monatsschr. *9*:510–513, 1955.

23. Scott, B.A., Weinstein, Z.R.W.: The neurosurgical management of spasticity. S. Afr. Med. J. *60*:849–850, 1981.

24. Erickson, D.L., Blacklock, J.B., Michaelson, M., Spurling, K.B., and Lo, J.N.: Control of spasticity by implantable continuous flow

morphine pump. Neurosurgery *16*:215–217, 1985.

25. Penn, R.D., and Kroin, J.S.: Continuous intrathecal baclofen for severe spasticity. Lancet *ii*:125–127, 1985.
26. Penn, R.D.: Drug pumps for treatment of neurological diseases and pain. Neurol. Clin. *3(2)*:439–451, 1985.
27. Penn, R.D., and Kroin, J.S.: Intrathecal baclofen alleviates spinal cord spasticity. Lancet *i*:1078, 1984.
28. Parke, B. et al.: Functional outcome after delivery of intrathecal baclofen. Arch. Phys. Med. Rehabil. *70*:30–32, 1989.
29. Penn, R.D.: Intrathecal baclofen for severe spinal spasticity. N. Engl. J. Med. *320*:1517–1521, 1989.
30. Waltz, J.M.: Computerized percutaneous multi-level spinal cord stimulation in motor disorders. Appl. Neurophysiol. *45*:73–92, 1982.
31. Waltz, J.M., and Pani, K.C.: Spinal cord stimulations in disorders of the motor system. *In* Proceedings of the Sixth International Symposium on the External Control of Human Extremities. Belgrade, Yugoslav Committee for Electronics and Automation, 1978, pp. 545–556.
32. Nakamura, S., and Tsubokawa, T.: Evaluation of spinal cord stimulation for postapoplectic spastic hemiplegia. Neurosurgery *17*:253–259, 1985.
33. Barolat-Romana, G., Myklebust, J.B., Hemmy, D.C., et al.: Immediate effects of spinal cord stimulation in spinal spasticity. J. Neurosurg. *62*:558–562, 1985.

13

ORTHOPEDIC PROCEDURES

CLIFFORD L. CRAIG
SEYMOUR ZIMBLER

HISTORICAL PERSPECTIVE

Orthopedic surgery has played an important role in the development of the treatment of spasticity. An equinovarus foot deformity, most likely secondary to poliomyelitis, initially interested William Little of England (1810–1894) in pursuing a medical career. Ultimately he had a consultation with George Stromeyer in Germany, who had performed a subcutaneous heel cord tenotomy. Impressed by the success of his own case, Little extended this technique to other deformities produced by tendon contracture. In 1838, he established the "Orthopaedic Institution," which ultimately became the Royal National Orthopaedic Hospital. Because he saw a large number of patients with spasticity who required tenotomies, Little became interested in determining the causes of cerebral palsy (CP). This resulted in the publication of a monograph that for the first time linked prematurity, prolonged labor, and anoxia with CP.[1]

The development of aseptic technique and more reliable anesthesia allowed expansion of surgical options to more complex procedures, including neurectomies, fasciotomies, osteotomies, and arthrodeses. In 1913, Stoffel publicized and popularized the use of selective neurectomies as an alternative to tenotomy. Initially this involved geographic localization of "nerve trunks" within peripheral nerves, but was ultimately refined to division of appropriate muscular branches. The early period of expanding surgical procedures, however, was followed by reappraisal and criticism of surgery in spasticity. Understanding of the importance of preoperative assessment and postoperative care had not kept pace with technology.

Winfield Phelps, after completing his training in orthopedics, devoted his career to treating cerebral palsy. He established a clinic model at the Children's Rehabilitation Institute of Baltimore, and helped to develop similar clinics throughout the United States. The clinic concept resulted in a broader diagnostic and therapeutic approach, including neurologic assessment, physical therapy, and bracing. This culminated in the founding of the American Academy of Cerebral Palsy in 1947, with Phelps as its first president.[2] The restoration of surgery to a prominent role in the treatment of spasticity was due in large part to William T. Green of Boston. He stressed the importance of careful preoperative assessments, selection of appropriate operative procedures, and extensive and prolonged postoperative care.[3] Documentation of long-term results of patients treated following these principles helped to reverse the surgical pessimism held by many even into the 1950s.[4]

GOALS OF SURGICAL TREATMENT

The goals of orthopedic surgery in both cerebral palsy and acquired spasticity are to increase mobility, decrease the use of external aids, correct or prevent deformity, and ultimately maximize function. Chronic spasticity may lead to fixed soft tissue or bony deformities. When these do not respond to conservative measures such as manual stretch and serial casting, and are of functional significance to the patient, surgical treatment is warranted. Surgery also has a role in the treatment of spasticity in the absence of fixed deformity. A neurectomy can decrease spasticity through interruption of the reflex arc. Procedures that separate the spastic muscle from its insertion or lengthen its tendon can eliminate its action on the limb or reduce its mechanical advantage. Furthermore, such procedures may, by reducing the stretch on the muscle, decrease the spindle afferent impulses and the resulting spasticity. The specific techniques described in this chapter include tendon lengthening, tendon transfer, neurectomy, osteotomy, resection arthroplasty, and arthrodesis. Joint realignment (osteotomy) and resection or fusion (arthrodesis) are required when joint or bony deformity has developed. Tendon lengthening is used to rebalance agonist-antagonist muscle groups, or correct musculotendinous unit contractures. Tendon transfers have limited indications because of the difficulty in assessing the strength and volitional control of spastic muscles. The joint that is to be mobilized by the tendon transfer should have a full passive range of motion preoperatively to maximize the success of the procedure. Neurectomies are mostly limited to the hip (anterior obturator neurectomy) or nonfunctional limbs because an irreparable lesion is created.

SURGICAL CRITERIA

The following guidelines maximize the benefit from surgery.[5]

1. For procedures requiring active therapy postoperatively, the patient should be developmentally or cognitively at a level to allow adequate cooperation.

2. For procedures intended to improve gait, the patient should demonstrate enough trunk control to stand with minimal assistance. Deformities alone do not usually prevent walking.

3. Compliance with a preoperative program of exercises and night splinting minimizes the chance of recurrence.

4. A stable supportive home or institutional setting should be present to ensure proper postoperative care and follow-up.

PATIENT POPULATION

Although most commonly used with children with CP, the procedures discussed in this chapter can be applied to children and adults with acquired spasticity as well. The specific cause of the CNS pathology is not often directly relevant to the selection of treatment. The cause, however, may be informative about a number of issues that play a role in treatment planning:

1. Is the CNS pathology static, e.g., CP; progressive, e.g., multiple sclerosis (MS); or improving, e.g., early cerebrovascular accident (CVA) or traumatic brain injury (TBI)? The answer will clarify the functional prognosis both with and without intervention, and assist in the appropriate timing of surgery.

2. Is the patient developmentally or cognitively able to cooperate and participate in pre- and postoperative treatment regimens?

3. Are developmental changes to be expected that may influence the success and timing of surgery? (Examples are bone growth and maturation of the hip joint.)

After TBI or CVA, muscle tone peaks two to three months postinjury and usually decreases over the next year. Therefore, nonoperative techniques are used during this interval.[6] Hip flexion and adduction contractures that progress despite passive stretching and positioning, however, should be released early surgically to prevent dislocation. In children, leg lengths need to be monitored closely because a significant leg length discrepancy can develop even in an initially uninjured extremity.[6] Epiphyseal arrest can then be carried out at the appropriate age to achieve equalization.

PROCEDURES FOR THE FOOT AND ANKLE

Although the positions of the trunk, hips, knees, and feet influence each other in gait and stance, deformities at each level are more effectively reviewed separately. The most common problems at the feet and ankle are equinus, calcaneus, valgus, varus, cavus, hallux valgus, and toe deformities.

EQUINUS

Indications for surgical correction of equinus in the ambulatory patient are:

1. A fixed contracture of the heel cord that prevents passive ankle dorsiflexion to neutral, with the knee extended and the hindfoot inverted in a valgus foot, or neutral in a varus foot.
2. Persistence of toe/heel or toe/toe gait, in the absence of a fixed contracture, which interferes with balance and ambulation despite a non-operative program. Such a gait may be caused by spasticity and/or primitive motor behaviors such as a positive support response.

In nonambulatory patients, fixed equinus that interferes with comfortable foot placement in a wheelchair or prevents pivot transfers is also appropriate for surgical intervention. In patients who can actively dorsiflex the ankle to the limit of the heel cord contracture, a heel/toe gait pattern without bracing can be anticipated postoperatively. In patients with active dorsiflexion limited by plantar flexor spasticity, a Marcaine tibial nerve block can be used preoperatively to demonstrate the anticipated effect of heel cord lengthening on the gait pattern.

Many procedures are available for lengthening and reducing the stretch reflex of the gastrocnemius and soleus muscles. These include tibial neurectomy, gastrocnemius lengthening, gastrocnemius origin recession, Achilles tendon lengthening, and Achilles tendon translocation. Our preference has been for the sliding heel cord lengthening described by White[7] and popularized by Banks and Green.[8] The rotation of the two bundles of tendon fibers is identified, the anteromedial bundle is sectioned distally, and the posteromedial bundle is sectioned proximally. Passive dorsiflexion results in the sliding of the tendon fibers (Fig. 13–1). A controlled sliding lengthening can be carried out so that the ankle can be dorsiflexed 5 degrees beyond neutral with one finger. Few sutures are required for the tendon edges and minimal dissection is needed. For patients who have had previous heel cord lengthenings, the Vulpius technique of aponeurotic lengthening at the musculotendinous junction is used.[9]

Preoperative assessment and establishment of compliance with a nonoperative program are essential. The presence of hip and knee flexion contractures should be determined preoperatively by the Thomas test and by evaluating passive knee extension. Failure to correct such fixed contractures

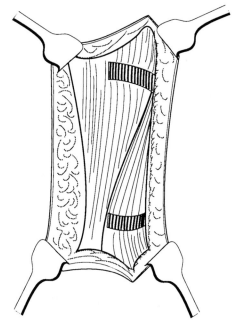

FIG. 13–1. Sliding heel cord lengthening (adapted with permission from Tachdjian, M.O.: Pediatric Orthopedics, W.B. Saunders Co., Philadelphia, 1972, p. 797). See text.

before heel cord lengthening frequently results in recurrent equinus. In patients with growth remaining, a preoperative physical therapy program of strengthening exercises for the gluteus medius, quadriceps, and ankle dorsiflexors, as well as heel cord stretching, should be done daily to establish patient compliance. Night splinting with a fiberglass long-leg bivalved cast, with the ankle at neutral when possible and the knee extended as tolerated, should be routine. Unless there is a significant fixed heel cord contracture, an ankle-foot orthosis (AFO) should be worn. Failure to require such a routine preoperatively, with the understanding that it will be needed postoperatively, significantly increases risk of recurrent deformity.[10]

Postoperatively, a long leg cast is used with the knee in full extension and the ankle at neutral. The cast is bivalved and made removable to initiate active ankle motion as soon as the patient is comfortable, usually within three days, although longer periods of solid casting may be necessary when compliance is in question. If the patient was ambulatory preoperatively, ambulation can be resumed within a week in the cast. The bivalved long-leg cast is worn full time for 6 weeks, then used at night for the remainder of growth or for at least 6 months. The use of an AFO is initiated during the day 6 weeks postoperatively, and maintained for at least 6 months. If cerebral control of ankle dorsiflexion is obtained, bracing can be discontinued or used only intermittently. The exercise program established preoperatively is continued indefinitely. Follow-up care should be continued for at least 2 years or until growth is completed.

CALCANEUS

Calcaneus deformity of the foot and ankle is most commonly caused by overlengthening of the heel cord. It results in a spectrum of gait abnormalities from poor push-off to a heel-heel gait. Functionally, it is even more disabling than equinus, and it is not easily braced or surgically corrected. It can be prevented by appropriately correcting hip and knee flexion contractures

before Achilles tendon lengthening, and by meticulously following intra- and postoperative technique. Initial treatment should focus on exercises, splinting, and bracing to improve ankle plantarflexion and limit dorsiflexion. Hip flexors, hamstrings, and ankle dorsiflexors should be passively stretched; hip extensors, quadriceps, and ankle plantarflexors should be strengthened. An AFO with a solid anterior calf band, and the ankle fixed in 3 to 5 degrees of equinus (floor reaction orthosis) should be worn during the day. At night the ankle should be splinted in plantarflexion, the knee in extension, with prone positioning. Tenodesis of the heel cord has been described, but significant numbers with long-term follow-up are not available. Lack of treatment in the growing child causes a valgus deformity at the ankle, further complicating an already difficult problem.[5,10]

VALGUS

Peroneal spasticity and the lateral insertion of the Achilles tendon combine to produce the spastic flatfoot. Both the midfoot and forefoot are pulled into abduction with consequent loss of support for the talus. This results in a plantarflexed talus, which frequently becomes painful or causes shoe fitting problems. Plantarflexion of the calcaneus, secondary to heel cord spasticity or contracture, may be a contributing factor. Persistence of medial deviation of the talar neck has also been implicated.[11] Figure 13–2, A and B, illustrates a progressive valgus foot deformity in a child with hemiplegia. Six years after a subtalar arthrodesis, the deformity remains corrected, as shown in Figure 13–2C.

Indications for surgery include progressive valgus deformity despite bracing and physical therapy, skin irritation or pain because of a prominent talus, and difficulty with shoe fitting. Ideally, correction should be done before development of secondary deformity such as hallux valgus and fixed forefoot abduction. Before surgery, accurate x-ray evaluation should be obtained, including weight-bearing anteroposterior and lateral views of the feet and ankles. If a subtalar arthrodesis is contemplated, a lateral

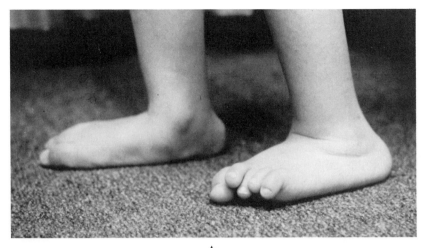

A

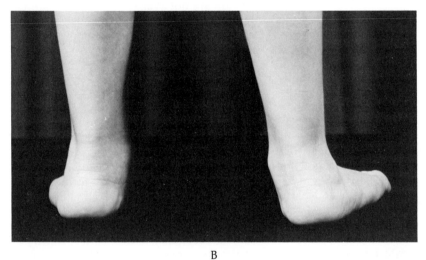

B

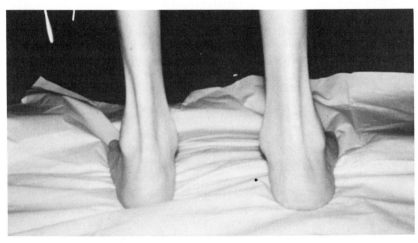

C

FIG. 13–2. Pes valgus. A and B, before and C, after subtalar arthrodesis. See text.

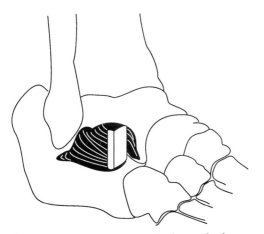

FIG. 13–3. Grice extra-articular subtalar arthrodesis (adapted with permission from Tachdjian, M.O.: Pediatric Orthopedics, W.B. Saunders Co., Philadelphia, 1972, p. 807).

4. Using a proximal tibial graft and positioning its longitudinal axis parallel to the tibia.
5. Following a postoperative regimen of nonweight bearing in a long-leg cast for 8 weeks, weight bearing in a short-leg cast for up to 4 weeks, and AFO bracing for 6 months.
6. If a valgus deformity of more than 10 degrees is present at the ankle, correcting it with a distal tibial osteotomy. If a subtalar arthrodesis alone is performed, the ankle valgus will progress.

Valgus deformity in the skeletally mature spastic foot usually has little flexibility and has secondary forefoot abduction with hallux valgus. Surgical intervention at this point is best achieved by triple arthrodesis—fusion of the calcaneocuboid, talocalcaneal, and talonavicular joints. Figure 13–4, A and B, demonstrates the forefoot and hindfoot deformities before and after removal of the bone wedges. In Figure 13–4C, the lines of the arthrodesis in final position are shown. The results of triple arthrodesis are not as satisfactory as in the younger age group because of the increased deformity.[11,13,14] Removal of bone from the subtalar joint decreases foot height which may result in impingement of the malleoli on the shoes. Inflexibility of the foot frequently makes correction of the plantarflexed and prominent talus difficult. A medial incision has been routinely used by the authors, not only to ensure adequate decortication of the talonavicular joint, but also to reduce the medial prominence of the talus. Iliac graft is also used routinely to ensure more rapid and certain arthrodesis. The use of a strut graft in the sinus tarsi to dorsiflex and support the talus has been described, and may be helpful.[11]

"corrected view" should be taken with the foot plantarflexed, inverted, then dorsiflexed. This will document whether or not plantarflexion of the talus can be corrected.

Several procedures have been reported for correction of spastic pes valgus. These include peroneal tendon lengthenings, calcaneal osteotomy, subtalar arthrodesis for the skeletally immature foot, and triple arthrodesis for the adult foot. A recent long-term follow-up study confirmed our preference for the Grice extra-articular subtalar arthrodesis, in which a tibial bone graft is used to elevate and fix the talus, as shown in Figure 13–3.[12] Twenty-one feet in 11 patients were reviewed, and only one foot had less than a good result. Bracing was eliminated in eight patients. No significant degenerative changes were seen at the ankle or midfoot. Several critical factors in achieving a successful result were identified:

1. Lengthening the heel cord if the ankle cannot be dorsiflexed to neutral in inversion.
2. Avoiding overcorrection by taking an intraoperative anteroposterior x-ray of the foot and decreasing the graft height if the talocalcaneal angle is less than 20 degrees.
3. Stabilizing the talocalcaneal joint with threaded wire fixation for 8 weeks.

VARUS

Varus deformity is significantly less common than valgus in children with CP. It is usually seen in patients with hemiplegia or after traumatic brain injury and is frequently associated with equinus. Treatment approaches depend on whether there is midfoot adduction or hindfoot varus, and

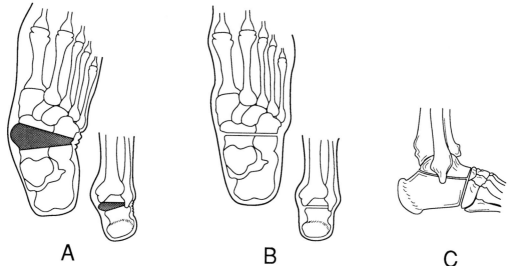

FIG. 13–4. A through C. Triple arthrodesis (adapted with permission from Tachdjian, M.O.: Pediatric Orthopedics, W.B. Saunders Co., Philadelphia, 1972, p. 1001; and Drennan, J.C.: Neuromuscular disorders. *In* Lovell, W.W., and Winter, R.B. (Eds.) Pediatric Orthopedics, Philadelphia, J.B. Lippincott, p. 283). See text.

whether passive correction is possible. Hindfoot varus is created primarily by spasticity of the posterior tibialis. Midfoot adduction occurs primarily because of peroneal weakness. Spasticity may also be present in the anterior tibialis. To avoid structural changes, surgery should be considered in children over 4 years old with varus in either the swing or stance phase of gait. Before surgery there should be an adequate trial of physical therapy, day bracing, and night splinting. Nerve blocks can also be helpful. Posterior tibialis lengthening is the easiest and most reliable technique available to correct flexible hindfoot varus.[11,14,15] This is a "Z" lengthening (Fig. 13–5) carried out proximal to the medial malleolus, with the tendon reapproximated while the foot is held in neutral. Heel cord lengthening should be done if equinus is also present. A short-leg walking cast is used for 6 weeks if only the posterior tibialis is lengthened. This is combined with an "overcylinder" bivalved cast at night for patients who have had a previous heel cord lengthening. Subsequently, night splinting until completion of growth or for at least 6 months is combined with the use of an AFO for at least 6 months. Posterior tibialis

transfer is not as predictable as lengthening and may result in overcorrection into valgus.[16–18]

Gait polyelectromyography is useful in treatment of flexible or fixed midfoot adduction, to determine the activity of the posterior tibialis during the gait cycle. Split anterior tibialis transfer (SPLATT), moving the lateral half of the anterior tibialis tendon to the cuboid, works well when the anterior tibialis is firing during the swing phase of the gait cycle. If the deformity is fixed and the posterior tibialis is also firing during the entire cycle, it should be fractionally lengthened (dividing the tendon fibers only, just proximal to the musculotendinous junction), or "Z" lengthened. The heel cord is lengthened if equinus is present.[19] Postoperative care is similar to posterior tibialis lengthening.

Fixed hindfoot varus as defined by a talocalcaneal angle of less than 15 degrees on a standing AP x-ray of the foot can be corrected by a closing lateral wedge calcaneal osteotomy as shown in Figure 13–6A (before) and 13–6B (after). This is combined with posterior tibialis lengthening and if equinus is present, with heel cord lengthening. Triple arthrodesis is indicated in pa-

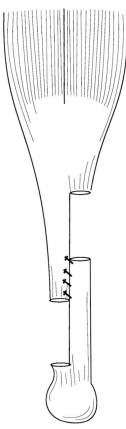

FIG. 13–5. Z-lengthening of a tendon (adapted with permission from Tachdjian, M.O.: Pediatric Orthopedics, W.B. Saunders Co., Philadelphia, 1972, p. 1303).

tients over 12 with fixed hindfoot varus. Posterior tibialis lengthening and, if indicated, heel cord lengthening are done simultaneously. An iliac bone graft is used to accelerate arthrodesis. A long-leg cast is used for 8 weeks nonweight bearing. This is followed by a weight-bearing short-leg cast and overcylinder night splint for 4 weeks. Subsequently, day bracing is used for 6 months, or indefinitely if there is inadequate ankle dorsiflexion in gait.

CAVUS

Pes cavus can be defined clinically as forefoot equinus exceeding the usual range of plantarflexion of the metatarsals. Radiographically, on a lateral weight-bearing view, the axis of the first metatarsal should normally make an angle of 140 to 160 degrees, with the horizontal axis of the calcaneus.[20] Cavus can then be defined as a decrease in this angle below 140 degrees. The cause of pes cavus is not completely resolved but relates, at least in part, to spasticity of the intrinsic muscles of the foot. If detected before skeletal adaptation has developed, plantar fasciotomy and release of short toe flexors is indicated. Postoperative AFO support with metatarsal pad and night splinting should be used to avoid recur-

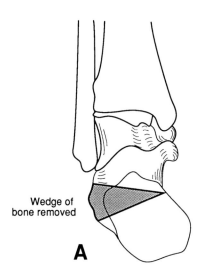

Wedge of bone removed

A

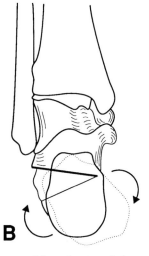

B

FIG. 13–6. A and B, Closing lateral wedge osteotomy of the calcaneus (adapted with permission from Tachdjian, M.O.: Pediatric Orthopedics, W.B. Saunders Co., Philadelphia, 1972, p. 1395). See text.

rence during the growth period. Significant fixed deformity usually causes forefoot pain in the metatarsal heads. Closed dorsal wedge osteotomy through the cuneiforms, although shortening the foot, gives a good functional and cosmetic correction.[11]

HALLUX VALGUS AND TOE DEFORMITIES

Hallux valgus (lateral deviation of the great toe at the metatarsophalangeal joint) is usually produced by spasticity of the adductor hallucis combined with a valgus force on the great toe secondary to the forefoot abduction of the valgus foot. This deformity is illustrated in Figure 13–7A. Hallux valgus is a preventable deformity if hindfoot valgus is controlled early by subtalar arthrodesis.[12] A flexible deformity can be corrected by adductor hallucis tenotomy. More fixed deformity may require lateral capsular release at the metatarsal phalangeal joint, reattachment of the adductor to the first metatarsal neck, and medial capsular plication, as shown in Figure 13–7B.[21] If the first metatarsal is adducted or deviated medially, a dorsal dome (curvilinear) or medial opening wedge osteotomy may

be required. Hammer-toe deformities can often be treated with extra-depth shoes and metatarsal pads. Surgical correction can be obtained by extensor tendon transfers to the metatarsal necks and interphalangeal arthrodeses. Flexor tendon lengthening can also be added.[22]

PROCEDURES FOR THE KNEE

Flexion is the most common deformity seen in the spastic knee, although hyperextension, patella alta, and chondromalacia can also occur.

FLEXION

Knee flexion may be caused by hamstring spasticity or secondary to hip flexion and/or equinus deformities. Contractures at the hip and ankle should be corrected before or simultaneously with correction of knee flexion deformity. Frequently, the joint primarily responsible for the crouch gait may be difficult to discern clinically. A cylinder cast can be applied to evaluate the effect of knee extension, and if the patient can stand

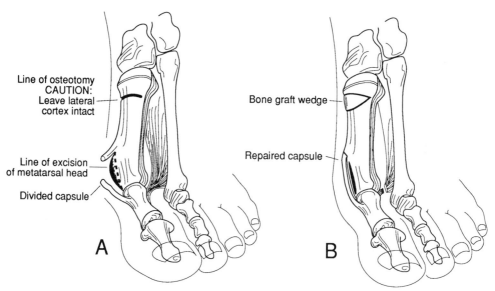

Line of osteotomy
CAUTION:
Leave lateral
cortex intact

Line of excision
of metatarsal head

Divided capsule

Bone graft wedge

Repaired capsule

A

B

FIG. 13–7. Hallux valgus. A, Before and B, after treatment (adapted with permission from Tachdjian, M.O.: Pediatric Orthopedics, W.B. Saunders Co., Philadelphia, 1972, p. 1345). See text.

erect, it suggests that the hamstrings should be lengthened. Similarly, if short leg casts allow erect stance, ankle equinus should be corrected.[11] Frequently, however, the patient is unable to stand with either cast because of multilevel deformities. In younger patients with hamstring spasticity in the absence of knee flexion contractures, we have preferred to correct hip flexion/adduction and equinus deformities before lengthening the hamstrings. A significant number of patients subsequently develop enough quadriceps strength that rebalancing hamstring spasticity is not required.

Preoperatively, quadriceps strength and spasticity should be assessed. If the knee can be actively extended against gravity through a range similar to its passive motion, sufficient quadriceps strength is present to maintain knee extension in stance and gait. The presence of quadriceps spasticity is useful, in that it will help maintain the postoperative correction. It can be grossly quantitated by measuring the angle of flexion where the quadriceps stretch reflex occurs with rapid knee flexion with the patient prone and hip extended.

If knee flexion is greater than 15 degrees in the stance phase of gait, in the absence of hip or ankle deformity, hamstring lengthening should be considered if more conservative measures have failed. This is based on studies indicating that at 15 degrees of flexion, 75% of the load across the hip joint is taken up at the knee. This figure triples at 30 degrees of knee flexion.[23] Quadriceps force is also significantly increased with increasing knee flexion. All of these factors combine to produce a significant incidence of premature degenerative arthritis of the patellofemoral joint. In patients without active lower extremity function, knee flexion contractures should be corrected if they interfere with transfers or comfortable positioning.

The hamstrings can be lengthened proximally or distally, tenotomized, or transplanted anteriorly. Our preference has been to "Z"-lengthen the semitendinosus, and fractionally lengthen the tendinous fibers of the semimembranosus and biceps femoris distally, in patients with hamstring contractures and/or spasticity.[24] Straight leg raising to 70 degrees should be obtainable under anesthesia after lengthening, at least in the ambulatory patient. In children without fixed contracture, usually only the medial hamstrings need to be lengthened. Differential medial and lateral hamstring tone can be determined by palpation preoperatively during straight leg raising. If the knee cannot be fully extended in the supine position preoperatively, the need for posterior capsulotomy should be anticipated. Long-standing contractures, especially in quadriplegic patients, may involve contracture of the neurovascular bundle. Forceful knee extension under anesthesia should be avoided in this setting, and the need for a dorsal closing wedge osteotomy of the distal femur anticipated. Knee flexion will be lost with this procedure in direct proportion to the amount of flexion contracture corrected, as illustrated in Figure 13–8A (preoperative) and 13–8B (postoperative).[11]

Despite recent enthusiasm for proximal hamstring lengthening,[25] concerns about overcorrection (recurvatum) and development of lumbar lordosis, combined with the relative ease, control, and good results with distal fractional lengthening, have prevented us from adopting this technique.[24] Postoperatively solid cylinder casts are used for 3 weeks in patients with isolated hamstring lengthening. Ambulation can begin as soon as comfort and leg control allow. Casts are bivalved and motion

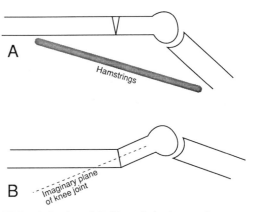

FIG. 13–8. A and B, Dorsal closing wedge osteotomy of the femur. See text.

started at 3 weeks. Until sufficient quadriceps strength is restored, cylinder casts may be needed for ambulation. Night splinting should be used until completion of growth or for a minimum of 6 months to avoid recurrence.

HYPEREXTENSION

Recurvatum at the knee in gait can be caused by unbalanced quadriceps spasticity, or plantar flexor contracture or spasticity. In all cases studied by Simon, recurvatum resulted from forward motion of the femur over a tibia held stationary by excessive plantar flexor spasticity or maximal ankle dorsiflexion.[12] Accurate patient assessment is essential to proper treatment because the approach varies with the cause. Plantar flexor spasticity can be treated by the program described earlier. A rigid plastic AFO with the ankle fixed in slight dorsiflexion helps to decrease the extensor moment at the knee. Patients with a spastic quadriceps or a gait EMG that demonstrates not only hyperextension of the knee in stance, but also decreased knee flexion in the swing phase, may benefit from a proximal rectus femoris release. Before surgery, an attempt should be made to stretch the quadriceps and develop reciprocal hip and knee flexion in gait. We prefer to reserve this procedure for patients with at least 20-degree hip flexion contractures to avoid excessively weakening hip flexion. Only the direct (straight) head of the rectus is released. Postoperatively, the patient may be treated in a spica cast with hips extended and knees slightly flexed. Another alternative is long leg casts and traction. In this instance, the patient is alternately positioned prone and supine with the legs suspended off the end of the bed in traction. This allows maximization of hip flexion and extension during the postoperative phase, but requires greater patient cooperation. Motion is initiated at 10 to 14 days and weight bearing at 2 to 3 weeks. Night splinting in the prone position is maintained indefinitely with long-leg bivalve casts and a bar to maintain hip extension, control recurvatum, and prevent recurrence of deformity.

PATELLA ALTA AND CHONDROMALACIA

Rectus femoris contracture commonly produces a proximally positioned patella. As patients are followed into adulthood, the problem of chondromalacia secondary to incongruity of the patellofemoral joint is seen more frequently. With early recognition, before x-ray changes such as fragmentation of the inferior pole of the patella, this problem can be treated by release of the direct head of the rectus femoris. Patellofemoral mechanics can be assessed arthroscopically during the same anesthesia, before and following rectus release, to evaluate patellar tracking and debride the patellar surface as needed. Untreated, severe patellofemoral arthritis can develop, necessitating patellectomy with potentially significant compromise in lower extremity function.

PROCEDURES FOR THE HIP

Problems relating to spasticity of muscles acting on the hip joint have been the subject of many studies in the last decade. The distribution and severity of the spasticity determine the deformity. In cerebral palsy, hemiplegic patients infrequently have hip deformity except for increased femoral anteversion. Flexion, adduction, and internal rotation abnormalities are frequently seen in spastic diplegia and may interfere with gait efficiency and progress to subluxation or, rarely, dislocation. Soft tissue contractures of the hip adductors and flexors are frequent in patients with quadriplegia, and commonly produce hip dislocation, affecting sitting balance.[26]

ADDUCTION

The function of the hip adductors has been the subject of much discussion. Gait electromyograms in normal patients show that the adductors fire at the end of stance phase.[27] This suggests that they act to keep the femur slightly adducted to allow maximal function of the hip abductors.[11] The adductors are probably only weak internal rotators. Adductor spasticity is manifested by a narrow base of support and short stride or, if more severe, by actual scissoring. In nonambulatory patients, the legs may actually rest in a scissored position. Both the amount of passive hip abduction and the point where the hip adductors "catch" with rapid abduction should be noted. The degree of abduction where the stretch reflex is triggered demonstrates the amount of abduction which will be seen in gait. Hip flexion contractures can be demonstrated by stabilizing the pelvis, fully flexing the contralateral hip onto the abdomen, and measuring the angle formed by the table top and the maximally extended thigh (Thomas test). Spasticity or contracture of the iliopsoas and/or rectus femoris are the most frequent causes of hip flexion contractures. If the degree of hip flexion contracture produced by the Thomas test is unchanged by flexing the knee, the iliopsoas is usually the cause of the deformity.[11]

Surgery is indicated for ambulatory patients when abduction of each hip is limited to 30 degrees or scissoring occurs during gait. If doubt exists about the effect of adductor surgery, the anterior division of the obturator nerve can be blocked with Marcaine (unless a contracture is the limiting factor). This allows not only a clinical assessment with adductor tone decreased, but also a gait evaluation by the physician and family. The number of adductors to release, and whether to section the anterior division of the obturator nerve, are at present debatable issues. This is primarily because of concern about overcorrection or a hyperabducted gait. In ambulatory patients with increased adductor tone, without significant contracture, release of the adductor longus and gracilis or transfer of the origin of the adductor longus, brevis, and gracilis to the ischium is sufficient. In our experience, if there is a fixed adduction contracture that allows only 30 degrees of abduction or less pre-operatively, myotomies of the longus, brevis, and gracilis, with neurectomy of the anterior division of the obturator nerve should be done to obtain adequate correction. Combined abduction and flexion of the hips to 120 degrees should be obtained under anesthesia following the myotomies. Postoperative care may be as important

in preventing recurrent adduction, or hyperabduction, as which muscles or nerves are sectioned. Our approach includes a bilateral long-leg spica cast, with the hips abducted combined 90 degrees, and in neutral rotation, the knees extended, and ankles at neutral. The cast is bivalved and lined for motion and strengthening exercises at 3 to 5 days. Limited sitting and time out of the spica are allowed at 4 weeks, and ambulation is resumed at 6 weeks. Night splinting, usually with long-leg casts and a bar to maintain 90 degrees' combined abduction, is used until growth is completed or for 6 months.[5] Close monitoring and adjustment of the exercise program are carried out indefinitely.

FLEXION

The iliopsoas is the primary flexor of the hip. The adductors are only weak flexors, as is the rectus femoris, which is more effective with simultaneous knee flexion. Compensation for hip flexion contracture varies depending on whether the hamstrings or quadriceps have the predominant tone. If hamstring spasticity is predominant, the pelvis inclines posteriorly, the lumbar spine is flattened, and the hips and knees are flexed. If quadriceps spasticity is dominant, the hips are flexed, the knees remain extended and a lumbar lordosis develops. This can be documented by a standing lateral radiograph that includes the lumbar spine and hips. A sacral femoral angle, less than 50 degrees indicates overactivity or contracture of the hip flexors in stance.[26,28]

Surgical correction of a hip flexion contracture is indicated if it exceeds 20 degrees in the ambulatory patient. Iliopsoas recession to the anterior hip capsule is the procedure of choice. This is best done through a separate anterior iliofemoral approach. Weakness of hip flexion may result from tenotomy if the distal margin of the iliopsoas retracts into the pelvis. This has the potential of causing difficulty with activities such as stair climbing.[11] Postoperative care of iliopsoas tenotomy or recession is usually the same as for adductor myotomy since they are frequently done together.

INTERNAL ROTATION

The anterior portion of the gluteus medius has been established as the main internal rotator of the hip by both anatomic and clinical studies.[27,29] Gait electromyograms have failed to demonstrate any difference in phasic activity of the gluteus medius in a normal child compared to a child with spasticity.[30] Similarly, electromyograms have failed to conclusively determine a major role for the semitendinosus, adductors, tensor fasciae latae, or iliopsoas.[11]

Excessive femoral anteversion appears to be the one consistent deformity associated with internal rotation gait in spasticity. In children with CP or early-onset acquired spasticity, this appears to represent lack of remodeling of newborn femoral anteversion, secondary to persisting hip flexion contracture.[11] In the past, femoral anteversion was measured by indirect radiographic techniques.[31,32] The development of CT and MRI scans, however, allows direct calculation, with cuts taken through the femoral neck and femoral condyles.

Adductor myotomies or transfers may correct internal rotation, but results are unpredictable. Gluteus medius and minimus transfer was successful in 80% of patients in one series, but the other 20% developed a more severe Trendelenberg gait.[29] Iliopsoas recession done before age 7 years improved internal rotation gait in one series, but this was in a small number of patients.[28] For patients over 8 years with persistent intoed gait and passive internal rotation of the hip to 80 degrees, with external rotation limited to 30 degrees in extension, a derotational femoral osteotomy should be done. This involves cutting the femur transversely and rotating the distal segment on the proximal one to achieve distal realignment. The osteotomy is usually done at the level of the lesser trochanter and combined with an iliopsoas recession to preserve hip flexor strength. We have used a two-piece screw and plate fixation (Coventry) with a spica cast for smaller patients, a compression screw for larger patients, with a spica cast if cooperation is a problem. Care should be taken to preserve 30 degrees of internal rotation. In older patients, compensatory external tibial torsion may be present, and may require corrective tibial osteotomy if greater than 35 degrees.

EXTENSION

Significant extensor spasticity of the hip is rare in cerebral palsy, and is seen only in quadriplegics following hip flexor and adduction releases, or in patients with rigidity or athetosis. It is more common in patients with brain injuries who develop extensor posturing. If mild, it can be controlled by passive stretching and contoured seating that keeps the hips flexed. If severe, it prevents sitting and may progress to anterior dislocation of the femoral head. Success has been reported in one series by proximal hamstring release, release of the gluteus maximus insertion and, if needed, release of the external rotators. Muscle releases were carried out until 90 degrees of hip flexion could be achieved. If the sciatic nerve was tight, femoral shortening was done. Posterior capsular release should be done cautiously, because it can result in posterior hip dislocation. Postoperatively, patients are managed in a spica cast with the hips and knees flexed from 4 to 6 weeks.[33]

TREATMENT OF HIP SUBLUXATION AND DISLOCATION

The incidence of hip dislocation in patients with spasticity varies from 2.6% to 28%, depending on the degree of spasticity.[34] Nonambulatory quadriplegic patients are more at risk for this problem. In a study of 284 patients with CP and hip dislocation, 90% had quadriplegia.[30] Sixty percent of patients classified as "dependent sitters" had subluxed or dislocated hips.[35] Statistics for subluxation are less well documented, but equally significant.[36]

ANATOMY

Hip dislocation in cerebral palsy is an acquired lesion, progressing from a normal hip configuration to lateral subluxation to complete dislocation. Unlike congenital hip dislocation, acetabular dysplasia does not occur primarily, but only after loss of contact with the femoral head. This process is similar in cases of acquired spasticity that occur in early childhood, before maturation of the hip joint. Spasticity of the iliopsoas and adductors is felt to initiate this process.[11] Increased tone in the iliopsoas causes persistence of fetal hip flexion contracture and femoral anteversion. In addition, it compresses the medial capsule, pushing the femoral head laterally. Lack of or delayed ambulation decreases the development of adequate "balancing" abductor strength. This allows overpull of the adductors to contribute further to lateral subluxation. The axis of hip rotation gradually shifts from the center of the femoral head to the lesser trochanter (iliopsoas insertion).[37,38] Flexion, lateral displacement, and anteversion cause the femoral head to push anteriorly and laterally on the joint capsule producing subluxation. If subluxation progresses to complete lateral dislocation, further flexion results in the femoral head being positioned against the superior and lateral portion of the ilium.[11] As Bleck has outlined, the ambulatory status of the patient appears to influence the degree to which this scenario develops. Dislocation is the usual result in nonambulatory patients, subluxation in those who are crutch-dependent, and internal rotation gait in independent ambulators.[11]

In early-onset acquired spasticity, a similar sequence of events may occur. If spasticity occurs after full maturation of the acetabulum and femoral neck-shaft angle, however, subluxation, if it occurs, is not associated with bony deformity. This has implications for the type of surgical treatment that may be required.

NATURAL HISTORY

Untreated hip subluxation ultimately progresses to premature degenerative arthritis, as in patients with hip dysplasia from causes other than spasticity. Hip dislocation not only can affect ambulatory status adversely, but can have negative effects on nonambulators as well. Pain, difficult positioning, poor perineal hygiene, loss of sitting endurance, and skin breakdown have been reported in most of these patients.[39,40] Pain alone has been documented in from ⅓ to ½ of non-ambulators with complete hip dislocation.[39,41–43] This pain is felt to be on the basis of unremitting muscle spasticity and/or secondary degenerative changes in the joint. In one series, all patients with pain had femoral head defects, consisting of superior or lateral flattening. The flattening appeared from the first to the third decade, and was felt to be the result of spasticity compressing the femoral head against the capsule, or ligamentum teres.[43]

The relationship between hip subluxation or dislocation, pelvic obliquity, and scoliosis remains to be clarified. Letts et al. have postulated a temporal sequence of hip dislocation, pelvic obliquity, and scoliosis. This progression is illustrated in Figure 13–9. Figure 13–9 is a radiograph of a quadriplegic patient with progressive hip subluxation. In Figure 13–9B, progression to complete dislocation, pelvic obliquity, and scoliosis is evident. Letts et al. documented the incidence of "windblown hip syndrome" (hip adduction contracture with contralateral hip abduction contracture) to be 13% in an institutionalized teen-age population.[39] An inciting role was proposed for the iliopsoas, based on its origin in the thoracolumbar spine producing ipsilateral hip dislocation and pelvic obliquity and a contralateral convex scoliosis. A review of a similar patient population by Lonstein and Beck, however, failed to substantiate this interrelationship. They found no correlation between hip dislocation and the high side or amount of pelvic obliquity.[35]

RADIOGRAPHIC CRITERIA

Because the structural changes of spastic hip dislocation do not parallel those of congenital hip dislocation, a new definition of subluxation and dislocation had to be developed. Hip subluxation can be reproducibly defined as greater than 33% femoral head migration, lateral to Perkin's line, on an anteroposterior pelvis x ray; dislocation

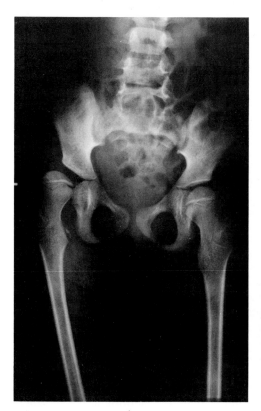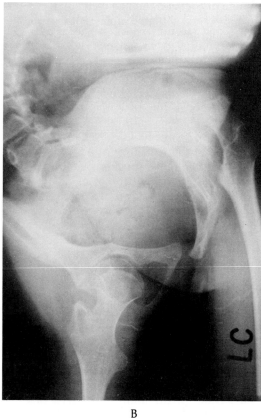

A   B

FIG. 13-9. Progression of untreated hip subluxation. See text.

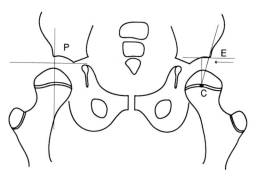

FIG. 13-10. Radiographic criteria for hip subluxation and dislocation.

extremity positioning.[45] The center of rotation of the hip is defined as the center of the cartilaginous femoral head ("C" in the right side of Figure 13-10), and is at a point along the physis equidistant from the superior and inferior borders of the femoral neck.[46] The angle between the edge of the acetabulum ("E") and a vertical line drawn through "C" is the CE angle. An angle from 0-10° can be defined as subluxed, less than 0° as severely subluxed or dislocated.[45]

SOFT TISSUE PROCEDURES

The success of adductor myotomies, iliopsoas release or recession, and anterior branch obturator neurectomy in reduction of hip subluxation and prevention of dislocation have been documented by many authors.[11,46-49] A discussion persists as to

as greater than 80% migration.[44] This is shown on the left side of Figure 13-10. The vertical line marked "P" is Perkin's line. The center edge (CE) angle of Wiberg, as modified by Massie and Howorth, can also be reliably used and isn't affected by lower whether and when to do iliopsoas release or recession, at what age soft tissue procedures alone are sufficient, whether postoperative splinting is important and for what duration, and if there is a role for adductor transfers. There is increasing support for adding iliopsoas recession in ambulatory patients and tenotomy in nonambulators. The role proposed for this muscle in the mechanism of subluxation and dislocation would seem to make this essential, although studies exist that document reversal of subluxation with adductor releases and obturator neurectomy alone.[46,48] In children with CP or early onset of acquired spasticity, the upper age limit for successful use of soft tissue procedures alone has been variously reported as from 5 to 8 years.[11,50] After this age, a bony procedure is likely to be required. However, in later onset cases of spasticity, soft tissue procedures may suffice regardless of age. The duration of postoperative splinting reported has ranged from 3 weeks to "long term."[45,49] Two recent reviews of adductor transfers showed no advantage over myotomies.[47,48] A persisting problem that makes evaluation and comparison of various studies difficult is that patients are categorized according to peripheral manifestations of their heterogeneous diagnoses. Definitions such as diplegia and quadriplegia are more qualitative than quantitative, often lacking reproducibility within the same medical center.

A recent review of our long-term results has indicated the importance of age, pelvic obliquity, and the degree of subluxation. Hip subluxation was reduced in a high percentage of patients below age 5 unless greater than 50% subluxation and greater than 10% pelvic obliquity were present.[50]

Our approach is to perform adductor myotomies and anterior branch obturator neurectomies on hips subluxed greater than 33%, sectioning the adductor longus, brevis, and gracilis. Iliopsoas tenotomy is added in patients with greater than 20 degrees of hip flexion contractures who are nonambulatory; recession or transfer to the anterior capsule is added for ambulatory patients. A solid spica cast in 90-degree combined abduction and usually full extension is maintained for 3 to 6 weeks, depending on hip stability. Abduction splinting with a pelvic band to prevent obliquity is used through the growth period. In hypotonic patients with minimal adductor tone, iliopsoas release alone is performed. In patients with "the windswept syndrome" and unilateral subluxation, care must be taken not to "over-release" the abducted or contralateral hip, or to neglect it. Depending on the degree of hip flexor and adductor tone and the age of the patient, we have done adductor longus tenotomy and partial anterior branch obturator neurectomy, with iliopsoas tenotomy if the hip flexion contracture is greater than 20 degrees. Close follow-up with consistent splinting is important to avoid hyperabduction[51] or progressive dislocation[52] of the "covered hip." If there is greater than 50% subluxation and greater than 10 degrees of pelvic obliquity, a supplemental bony procedure is usually done.

FEMORAL OSTEOTOMY

Indications and techniques for proximal femoral varus derotational osteotomy (reduction of femoral neck-shaft angle and anteversion) are varied. In general, it is advised for hip subluxation greater than 33%, persisting or progressing after soft tissue releases, which is felt to be due primarily to femoral anteversion and/or coxa valga.[11,34] It has also been reported to be appropriate for subluxation caused by coxa valga and femoral anteversion in patients over 3 years of age.[34] Femoral anteversion can be calculated radiographically by several techniques,[11] and by CT or MRI scan. Pins in plaster, compression screws, and compression nail plate have been used for fixation.[11,34]

Our indications for femoral osteotomy include those previously mentioned, as well as patients over 5 years of age with greater than 40% subluxation and for whom femoral head coverage can be obtained with a neck-shaft angle of 125 degrees. A tracing of the proximal femur can be made from an anteroposterior x ray of the internally rotated hip, using transparent plastic. The amount of coverage achievable and the size wedge needed to obtain a given neck-shaft angle can then be estimated. If the neck-shaft angle must be reduced to less than 125 degrees, a pelvic or combined pelvic/femoral osteotomy is indicated. Reducing the neck-shaft angle below 125 degrees can cause abductor insufficiency and excessive shortening in ambulatory patients, as well as limited abduction in nonambulators. Screw plate fixation is used in smaller patients, compression screw plate in heavier patients. A closing wedge based medially is made at the level of the lesser trochanter, with the distal cut perpendicular to the femoral shaft. The wedge size is determined from a preoperative cut-out as described above. The distal fragment is externally rotated to correct anteversion, leaving at least 30 degrees of internal rotation. Adductor myotomies are done if there is less than 30 degrees of abduction preoperatively, and iliopsoas recession or tenotomy is also performed when the osteotomy is cut. Spica cast immobilization is routine for 6 weeks. The cast is then bivalved and therapy initiated to restore strength and motion. Weight bearing is resumed only when leg control and upper extremity strength have been regained.

FEMORAL AND PELVIC OSTEOTOMY

Treatment of a completely dislocated, proximally migrated femoral head, requires a combined pelvic osteotomy and femoral varus, derotational, and shortening osteotomy. Associated pelvic obliquity and structural scoliosis are frequently present. Spinal deformity should usually be corrected before hip surgery. This reduces the pelvic obliquity, making acetabular reconstruction less formidable. The results of the combined pelvic and femoral osteotomy are illustrated in Figure 13–11. Figure 13–11A is a radiograph of a quadriplegic patient with bilateral progressive hip subluxation. In Figure 13–11B, the same patient is seen 2 years after bilateral pelvic and femoral osteotomies. Because of the amount of acetabular coverage which can be gained, especially posteriorly, we have preferred the Chiari osteotomy,[53] although equally good results have been described with the slotted acetabular augmentation.[54] In the Chiari, an osteotomy is made just above the capsule into the sciatic notch, and the capsule and distal fragment are pushed medially. A roof is produced for the head underneath the lateral (superior) fragment with the capsule interposed. A capsular arthroplasty is produced. Up to 70% of the width of the pelvis can be displaced if a supplemental graft is used. Preoperative assessment of the acetabular configuration and femoral head cartilage is necessary, and both can be obtained with an MRI scan. Degeneration of the femoral head cartilage is an absolute contraindication to relocation. If there is less than 30 degrees abduction preoperatively, adductor releases should also be done. Important technical details in performing the Chiari osteotomy include:

1. Doing a capsulotomy before stripping the ilium, so that if cartilage degeneration is seen on the femoral head, a muscle pedicle graft can be used for hip fusion if desired.
2. Making the osteotomy cut just superior to the lip of the true acetabulum. This frequently requires peeling redundant capsule off the lateral ilium down to the labrum.
3. Making the posterior portion of the cut with a curved osteotome to follow the contour of the posterior acetabulum and ensure posterior coverage.
4. Sliding a curvilinear cortical cancellous graft between the superior pelvic fragment and the capsule. A graft of this shape is easily obtained from the ilium and fills in the small gap which is always present.
5. Placing a bone graft medially to promote union and laterally to provide extra shelf coverage.

Important technical points of the femoral osteotomy include:

1. Obtaining a neck-shaft angle close to 125 degrees.
2. Adequately shortening the femur to decompress the joint and decrease the risk of avascular necrosis.
3. Correcting femoral anteversion but retaining 30 degrees of internal rotation.

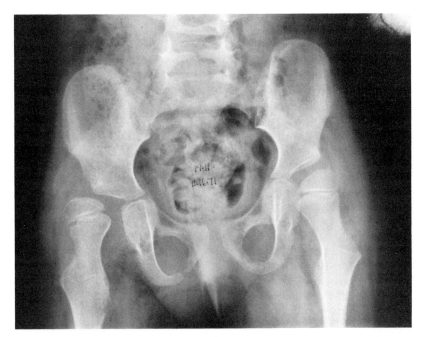

A

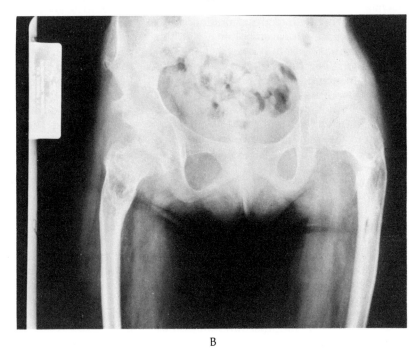

B

FIG. 13–11. A and B, Combined pelvic and femoral osteotomy. See text.

Postoperatively, a hip spica cast, bivalved and lined, is used to initiate motion at 3 weeks. As satisfactory healing progresses and motion improves, sitting is allowed in a chair with a reclining back. Abduction splinting is maintained for a minimum of 6 months, or until growth is completed. Ambulation is allowed, if appropriate, once leg control is regained.

A slotted acetabular augmentation is a modified "shelf" procedure described by Staheli.[55] It is designed to create a congruous extension of the acetabulum and appears to be a potential alternative to the Chiari.[54] A 1-cm-deep slot is placed at the lateral acetabular margin. Strips of corticocancellous bone are placed into the slot and extend laterally for the distance needed to create a center edge angle of 35 degrees (determined from a preoperative x ray). A second layer of graft is placed perpendicular to the first. The layers of graft are secured by oversewing the still posteriorly attached reflected head of the rectus femoris. Postoperative care includes maintaining the femoral head in the acetabulum while the shelf consolidates (6 to 8 weeks). Theoretic advantages of this procedure over the Chiari are technical simplicity, lack of postoperative stiffness, and flexibility in placement of the augmentation.[54] Only one small series with relatively short follow-up is reported in the literature, however.

FEMORAL HEAD RESECTION

Proximal femoral resection interposition arthroplasty is an appropriate salvage procedure for patients with a painful dislocated hip with degenerative changes on x ray or seen at surgery, and who are nonambulatory. This procedure is also an appropriate alternative to hip fusion for patients with scoliosis and hip dislocation (see next section). Success of the procedure appears to depend on resection to the level of the gluteus maximus insertion, closing the capsule over the acetabulum and the rectus femoris and vastus lateralis over the proximal femur, and releasing adductors and hamstrings if they limit motion.[56] In our experience, applying skeletal traction with a threaded pin inserted through the distal femur and incorporated into a spica cast for 4 to 6 weeks is also important. It minimizes heterotopic bone formation, maintains better length of the leg, and avoids the development of abduction contracture. Splinting the leg in 30 degrees of abduction, extension, and neutral rotation at night for 6 months or until the end of growth helps maintain flexibility. The problem of possible impingement from appositional bone growth of the femur can be reduced by delaying the procedure until the patient is close to skeletal maturity.[57]

HIP FUSION

Arthrodesis of the hip is appropriate for nonambulating patients with spasticity and unilateral painful hip degeneration. It also may be advisable in young ambulatory patients with unilateral involvement. Significant abnormality of the lumbosacral spine and pelvic obliquity with scoliosis are contraindications. The presence of scoliosis that has been fused, or for which fusion is anticipated, is a relative contraindication to hip fusion. The combination of a spine fusion that includes the pelvis with a hip fusion will make comfortable positioning difficult and increase the risk of femoral fracture by creating a long lever arm.[58] The optimal position for a fusion depends on ambulatory status. For nonambulators, 50 degrees of flexion, 10 degrees of abduction, and neutral rotation are preferred. In ambulatory patients, the hips should be arthrodesed in less flexion, neutral abduction, and rotation.[59] Soft tissue releases may be required to correct flexion and adduction contractures. Proximal femoral osteotomy with internal fixation should be done to correct anteversion and reduce stress on the fusion site. Combined intra-articular and extra-articular fusion, internal fixation, and a muscle pedicle graft from the ilium will minimize the chance of nonunion. Spica cast immobilization is used postoperatively until evidence of arthrodesis is seen radiographically, usually in 3 to 4 months.

TOTAL HIP REPLACEMENT

Early results of total hip arthroplasty in a small series of patients with spasticity have been encouraging.[59] Consideration of this option should be restricted to older patients and those with bilateral hip degeneration or significant lumbosacral abnormality. The increased potential for dislocation and loosening should be anticipated by the surgeon and understood by the patient or family. Soft tissue releases may be required to correct flexion and adduction contractures. The acetabular components should be positioned in the true acetabulum. An extra small component may be necessary, and bone graft may be required to correct lateral deficiency. In nonambulators, the acetabulum should be positioned in more flexion and anteversion for better sitting stability. The need for a small, straight-stem femoral component or customized stem should be anticipated from the preoperative radiographs. A walking spica cast is used for 4 weeks postoperatively to avoid dislocation, secondary to hip flexor or adductor spasm.[59]

PROCEDURES FOR THE SPINE

SCOLIOSIS

Scoliosis is the most frequent and surgically significant spinal deformity seen in patients with spasticity. Incidence has been variously reported from 6 to 67% in children with CP or mental retardation, with the highest prevalence in nonambulatory, severely involved patients.[60] The cause of this deformity remains controversial. An association with hip dislocation and pelvic obliquity has been proposed, as discussed above.[39] Asymmetric persistence of the infantile incurvatum reflex has also been suggested.[61] Two major curve patterns have been identified: double curves which include both the thoracic and lumbar component, and C-shaped lumbar or thoracolumbar curves with pelvic obliquity.[60] Untreated progressive scoliosis leads to loss of erect posture and balance in the ambulatory patient, loss of sitting balance and

endurance in the nonambulatory, and compromise of cardiopulmonary function in both groups.[62] The use of a spinal orthosis in young patients with smaller curves improves sitting balance and may retard progression, but frequently has a high failure rate in severely involved patients.[60] Indications for spine fusion include curve progression beyond 50 degrees, pain or behavioral changes which can be related to the scoliosis, pressure sores from rib collapse into the ilium, and loss of sitting balance.[60,63,64] Fusion to the sacrum should be done if significant pelvic obliquity is present[60] and considered if there is no sitting balance. This will achieve the goal of a vertical torso positioned over a level pelvis. A complication rate as high as 80% has been reported in an early series for spine fusions in spastic patients.[60] Complications have included wound infection, pseudarthrosis, pressure sores, instrumentation problems, and pneumonia. The use of segmental spinal instrumentation has decreased this rate, as has the evolution of better preoperative assessment. The importance of the patient's nutritional status and gastro-intestinal function in avoiding complications postoperatively has recently been documented.[65] Although the height/weight charts for children frequently cannot be used to assess adequacy of nutrition in severely involved patients, serum proteins and total lymphocyte counts are helpful. Because of the frequency of disorders of the swallowing mechanism, the upper gastrointestinal tract should be studied radiographically before spine fusion. If evidence of gastroesophageal reflux and tracheal aspiration is found, gastrostomy and fundoplication are indicated. If the patient has a poor caloric intake and decreased serum proteins and/or lymphocyte count, preoperative placement of a gastrostomy should be strongly considered. Cardiopulmonary evaluation should also be done preoperatively, including blood gases, and if right heart enlargement is suspected, an echocardiogram should be obtained.

Several new surgical techniques have revolutionized the approach to neuromuscular scoliosis. The advent of segmental

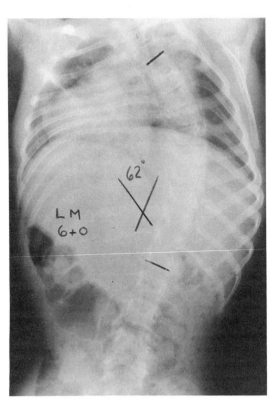

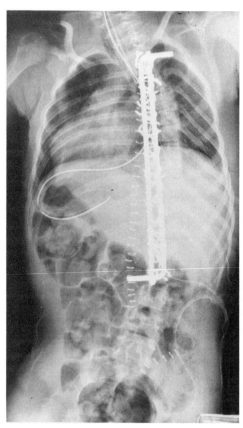

A   B

FIG. 13–12. A and B, Correction of scoliosis with segmental spinal instrumentation. See text.

spinal instrumentation (SSI), with the concept of sublaminar wire fixation to 2 prebent L-rods, has allowed early patient mobilization with significant reduction in the need for external support.[66] Figure 13–12A is a radiograph of a patient with quadriplegia and progressive scoliosis. In Figure 13–12B, the postoperative correction, obtained with Luque rod fixation and sublaminar wiring, is shown. The Galveston pelvic fixation technique of implanting prebent L-rods between the cortices of the ilium has extended the use of SSI to fusions to the sacrum. The development of bone bank technology has allowed use of cadaveric bone for a stronger fusion mass. Cell-saving techniques allow intraoperative blood recycling, thus decreasing the number of blood transfusions required. Spinal cord monitoring has provided a more sensitive and intraoperative indicator of potential neurologic injury.

Results with SSI technique have been such that posterior fusion alone is used, except for curves that cannot be reduced to 70 degrees on a traction anteroposterior radiograph. For these rigid curves, an anterior release is performed, with a partial discectomy and excision of 5 mm of subchondral bone at each disc space. The ribs excised during the approach are used for bone graft, and halo or halo-femoral traction is used for 10 to 14 days postoperatively. This is followed by posterior fusion with double L-rods, sublaminar wire fixation, decortication, and grafting.[62] Interspinous process wiring using an L-rod on the convex side of the curve and a Harrington rod on the concave side has also been reported as an alternative to passage of sublaminar wires.[63]

Postoperatively, we have used either solid or removable fiberglass jackets for 6 months, extending from the axilla to the pubis to allow sitting. Although many centers have reported early unencumbered mobilization, we have been concerned about stress on the fixation during transfers and when the patient is sitting fully upright.[62,63]

KYPHOSIS, LORDOSIS

Kyphosis and lordosis, encountered much less frequently than scoliosis, are usually secondary deformities. Kyphosis can be seen as a compensation for poor trunk control, tight hamstrings, or lumbar lordosis. The primary cause should be identified and treated appropriately. If the kyphosis is primary, bracing, if initiated early enough in the growth period, is usually sufficient. Lordosis is frequently an adaptation to hip flexion contracture. Iliopsoas recession will correct this deformity if performed before the lordosis becomes structural. X rays of the spine should always be taken, however, to avoid missing a spondylolisthesis.[61]

Scoliosis, kyphosis, and lordosis can all be seen following spinal cord injury at or above the T12 level in children. The younger the child at the time of the injury, the more certain the chance of developing a significant deformity. All patients with such injuries at birth will develop deformity. Sixty percent of those injured before the age of 13 develop scoliosis or kyphosis, severe enough to require spine fusion. The ligaments of the spine are not capable of maintaining normal alignment against gravity without muscle support. Hyperlordosis is seen in 20% of these patients, related to severe hip flexion contractures.[67] Prophylactic bracing is therefore recommended for all juvenile spinal cord injury patients, unless the lesion is low-level or the patient is near skeletal maturity. Bracing, however, frequently only delays the progress of spinal deformity.[68] If progression occurs and the child is too young to consider fusion, Harrington rod fixation can be placed without fusion, protected by

bracing.[67] When fusion is performed, the sacrum should be included, and SSI technique without double L-rod and sublaminar wiring at each level is recommended.[67] The L-rod should be prebent to maintain the normal sagittal curves of the spine.

PROCEDURES FOR THE UPPER EXTREMITY

Thumb in palm, wrist and finger flexion, elbow flexion and pronation, and shoulder adduction and internal rotation are the most common deformities seen in the spastic upper extremity. Successful surgical intervention requires more precise evaluation and goal definition than in the lower extremity, because of the role played by sensibility and intellectual function in the skilled use of the upper extremity. Because there are no surgical procedures to restore sensation, expectations from surgery must be limited in cases of sensory impairment. Realistic goals include improving grasp, release, and pinch, facilitating the use of the hand for gross assistance and improving appearance. In cerebral palsy patients, surgery should not be done before the central nervous system has matured sufficiently to permit accurate evaluation, and cooperation with post-operative therapy. Similarly, in patients with acquired spasticity, surgery should be considered only after maximal recovery has occurred. An exception to this would be severe pronator spasticity that threatens to produce posterior radial head dislocation.[11]

Several hand patterns can be defined that are useful in determining appropriate surgery. The hand that has adequate grasp, release, and pinch but lacks dexterity and speed will not be helped by operative intervention. If the wrist must be flexed to extend the fingers, surgery may improve function. If the fingers cannot actively be extended, even with the wrist flexed, cosmetic improvement only is the most realistic goal.[11]

In addition to observation of deformity patterns, specific functions should be evaluated, including stereognosis, hand placement, strength, general intelligence, and motivation. Within limits, motivation may be as important as intelligence.[69] Hand placement from the opposite knee to the head and back to the knee should be accomplished within 5 seconds to demonstrate adequate speed and proprioception.[70] Stereognosis can be tested with textures (from age 2 to 3), objects (from age 4 to 5), and graphesthesia or 2-point discrimination (from age 6 to adulthood), and appears to correlate best with surgical results[71,72] Adequate stereognosis is demonstrated by identifying 3 out of 5 objects or numbers, or 2-point discrimination of 10 millimeters.[71] Muscle strength may need to be evaluated with the assistance of Marcaine nerve blocks (e.g., a median nerve block at the elbow to assess wrist and finger extension and thumb adduction). Dynamic electromyography can be helpful in determining whether muscles are phasic or fire continuously. The ideal muscle for transfer rates "good" in strength, is under voluntary control, and is phasic with the activity for which it is transferred.[73]

THUMB IN PALM

Surgery should not be considered before age 4. Passive stretching of the thumb metacarpal into abduction and the entire thumb into extension should be carried out as soon as the deformity is detected, and an opponens splint used part-time during the day as soon as the hand is large enough.[74] If adductor contracture persists at age 4, Z-plasty of the web space and limited myotomy of the adductor pollicis and first dorsal interosseous are carried out until the thumb metacarpal can be easily brought into extension.[75] More established contractures in older patients may require release of the adductor origin from the second and third metacarpals. If the metacarpal-phalangeal joint is unstable in extension, it can be stabilized by volar plate capsulodesis (proximal advancement on the metacarpal) or by fusion.[11] Augmentation of thumb extension and abduction can be achieved by rerouting the extensor pollicis longus and transferring either the branchioradialis, flexor carpi radialis, or flexor digitorum superficialis.[11] It should not be done, however, if there is a fixed contracture or weak pinch.[70] Postoperatively, a well molded cast is applied, holding the thumb in maximal abduction, the metacarpophalangeal joint in neutral extension, and the interphalangeal joint in 10 degrees of flexion. Three weeks postoperatively, the cast is removed and an opponens splint is applied. Active and active-assisted exercises are initiated. An active therapy program and night splinting should be maintained until skeletal maturity, or for 6 months to avoid recurrent deformity.

WRIST FLEXION

Spasticity of the flexor carpi ulnaris is the most common cause of wrist flexion deformity in cerebral palsy.[11] Weakness of active wrist extension caused by this muscle imbalance may at first only compromise grasp by placing the finger flexors at a mechanical disadvantage. If it remains untreated, however, fixed contractures of the wrist and fingers may develop. Transfer of the flexor carpi ulnaris to the central wrist extensor can be used reliably, not only to prevent contracture but also to improve function.[76] Brachioradialis, pronator teres, and extensor carpi ulnaris have also been reported as successful donor tendons.[70] These procedures alone should usually not be considered if there is less than full passive wrist and finger extension, inability to actively extend the fingers with the wrist extended 45 degrees, or poor hand placement and astereognosis.[74] If contractures are present at the elbow, wrist, or fingers, an attempt should be made to correct them with serial solid casting and subsequent stretching and splinting. Fractional lengthening of the wrist and finger flexors at the musculotendinous junction can be performed if this fails. Inability to actively extend the fingers with the wrist held in extension, even in the absence of fixed finger flexion contractures, suggests the presence of increased finger flexor tone. This can be confirmed by an electromyogram showing constant firing of the finger flexors during both grasp and release.[70] Serial casting and therapy should be tried initially to decrease this tone, with fractional lengthening only if they are unsuccessful.

In the Banks-Green procedure, the flexor carpi ulnaris tendon is mobilized as far proximally as its nerve supply will allow. If additional supination is desired, it is transferred subcutaneously around the ulna. A large window is made in the interosseous membrane if a direct line of action is desired. The ulnaris tendon is usually sutured to itself through a buttonhole in the extensor carpi radialis brevis. Enough tension is obtained that the wrist will rest in 45 degrees of extension, but will allow 15 degrees of passive flexion. A long arm cast is applied postoperatively with the wrist extended 60 degrees, the thumb in abduction, metacarpophalangeal joints flexed 30 degrees, the interphalangeal joints neutral, and the elbow flexed 90 degrees, and in full supination. The cast is bivalved for active exercises only at 3 weeks. At 6 weeks, a splint is used for day support, holding the wrist extended 45 degrees with the thumb abducted and opposed. Night splinting is continued often until skeletal maturity with a long-arm bivalved cast. Support is maintained during the day until wrist extension is fair. An active exercise program is crucial to gaining maximal function.[74] In patients with weak release and fully flexible wrist and fingers, transfer of the flexor carpi ulnaris or brachioradialis into the finger extensors can be considered. An electromyogram, confirming phasic activity during release only, is helpful in selecting the appropriate donor tendon.[70]

In patients with severe fixed wrist and finger flexion contractures for which correction is being done for cosmetic and hygienic reasons, superficialis to profundus release, proximal row carpectomy (removal of the scaphoid, lunate, and triquetrum), or wrist fusion are possible options. In the superficialis to profundus release, the profundus tendons are cut at the level of the musculotendinous junction and attached to the superficial finger flexors, which are cut just proximal to the wrist. Fractional lengthenings of the thumb and wrist flexors are also done, or the flexor carpi ulnaris is transferred to act as a wrist extensor. It is difficult to determine the correct degree of tendon tension for the finger flexors. Swan-neck deformities may develop in the fingers requiring further surgery, and severe fixed contractures may not be correctable with this technique.[77] Proximal row carpectomy combined with tendon lengthenings allows more correction and maintains some wrist motion.[78] Wrist fusion permits maximum decompression of flexion deformity when combined with tendon lengthenings, but should be reserved for situations where contracture of the neurovascular structures precludes consideration of other alternatives.

ELBOW FLEXION

Flexion contactures at the elbow are primarily cosmetic or hygienic problems, although reaching activities or crutch walking may be adversely affected. In general, contractures less than 40 degrees can be accepted in hemiplegics, somewhat more in totally involved patients.[11] Serial casting techniques and exercises should be tried before consideration of surgery except in the most severe deformities. Musculocutaneous neurectomy has been reported effective for contractures of less than 30 degrees, in which increased tone is the major problem.[70] A Marcaine block of the musculocutaneous nerve can be tried preoperatively to determine if the brachioradialis will provide sufficient elbow flexion. For more significant contractures, the lacertus fibrosis is resected, the biceps Z-lengthened, and the brachialis fascia incised.[76] Brachialis myotomy, release of wrist flexor origin, transfer of the ulnar nerve, and anterior capsulotomy can be added as needed.[79] The neurovascular structures may limit ultimate correction in severe long standing contractures. The elbow is splinted in extension full-time for three weeks, followed by graduated exercises and long-term night splinting.

SHOULDER

Spasticity of the deltoid may rarely produce an abduction contracture at the shoulder. If this results in a cosmetic problem, the anterior ⅔ of the deltoid can be released from its insertion on the humerus.[74] The more common internal rotation and adduction deformity can usually be managed by an appropriate exercise program. Some patients with acquired spasticity develop restricted abduction (less than 45 degrees), external rotation (less than 15 degrees), and a persistent or increasing pain pattern. These patients are candidates for subscapularis and pectoralis major release.[80] An anterior deltopectoral groove approach is used. The subscapularis tendon is resected from its humeral insertion to the musculotendinous junction at the glenoid. The tendon is carefully dissected from the capsule, which is spared to avoid instability. After the pectoralis major tendon is released from the humerus, the shoulder is gently manipulated through a range of motion. Postoperatively, passive pulley exercises and active assisted range of motion are started within 24 hours and continued for a minimum of 3 months.[80]

HETEROTOPIC OSSIFICATION

Although not directly related to spasticity alone, ectopic ossification is frequently seen in patients with head injuries (15%),[81] and spinal cord injuries (2 to 25%).[67] The mechanism of bone formation is unknown, but may be related to the absence of a neurotropic factor, which results in undifferentiated connective tissue cells differentiating into osteoblasts.[67] The hip joint is most frequently involved, and the onset may mimic deep vein thrombosis because of the intense local inflammatory response. Loss of joint motion and local inflammation may occur as soon as 2 months post-injury, and precede radiographic changes. Early treatment includes gentle range of motion and splinting. Timing of operative intervention to restore motion is controversial. Most authors advise delay until radiographs suggest maturation of the bone to avoid recurrence. This may require deferring surgery for up to 2 years.[82,83] A recent report suggests that excision can be done as soon as motion restriction interferes with function if salicylates are used postoperatively to prevent recurrent bone formation.[81] A definitive answer will require a larger multicenter series.

SUMMARY

Surgery can be an effective way to maximize function and simplify care in patients with spasticity. Accurate preoperative assessment and a well supervised postoperative program are critical in achieving these goals. To optimize surgical results, the assessment must be in the context of the patient's overall functional goals. The likelihood of further growth, recovery, or deterioration will shape plans for surgical intervention, as will the patient's prognosis for achieving important functional goals, both with and without surgery. In addition, the patient's history of prior conservative treatment will affect the level of surgical aggressiveness chosen.

ACKNOWLEDGMENT

The authors wish to express their appreciation to Henry Banks, M.D., for stimulating and guiding their interest in the treatment of patients with spasticity.

REFERENCES

1. Rang, M.: Anthology of Orthopedics. Edinburgh, Livingstone, 1966.
2. Green, W.T.: Historical notes—The past generation. *In* Orthopaedic Aspects of Cerebral Palsy. Ed. R.L. Samilson. Philadelphia, J.B. Lippincott, 1975.

3. Green, W.T., and McDermott, L.J.: Operative treatment of cerebral palsy of spastic type. JAMA *118*:434, 1942.

4. Phelps, W.M.: Long-term results of orthopedic surgery in cerebral palsy. J. Bone Joint Surg. *39A*:53, 1957.

5. Banks, H.H.: Cerebral palsy. *In* Pediatric Orthopaedics. Ed. W.W. Lovell and R.B. Winter. Philadelphia, J.B. Lippincott, 1978.

6. Hoffer, M.M., Brink, J., Marsh, J., and Florin, R.: Head injuries. *In* Pediatric Orthopedics. 2nd Ed. Ed. W.W. Lovell and R.B. Winter. Philadelphia, J.B. Lippincott, 1986.

7. White, J.W.: Torsion of the Achilles tendon. Arch. Surg. *46*:784–787, 1943.

8. Banks, H.H., and Green, W.T.: The correction of equinus deformity in cerebral palsy. J. Bone Joint Surg. *40A*:1359–1379, 1958.

9. Vulpius, O., and Stoffel, A.: Orthopaedische Operationslebre. 2nd Ed. Stuttgart, Ferdinand Enke, 1920.

10. Tachdjian, M.O.: The Child's Foot. Philadelphia, W.B. Saunders, 1985.

11. Bleck, E.E.: Orthopaedic Management in Cerebral Palsy. Philadelphia, J.B. Lippincott, 1987.

12. Zimbler, S., and Craig, C.: Subtalar arthrodesis for stabilization of the valgus foot in neuromuscular disease. J. Pediatr. Orthop. *7*:490, 1987.

13. Duckworth, T.: The surgical management of cerebral palsy. Prosthet. Orthot. Int. *1*:96, 1977.

14. Banks, H.H. and Panagakos, P.: Orthopaedic evaluation in the lower extremity in cerebral palsy. Clin. Orthop. *47*:117, 1966.

15. Rang, M., Silver, R., and de la Garza, J.: Cerebral palsy. *In* Pediatric Orthopedics. Ed. W.W. Lovell and Winter, R.B. Philadelphia, J.B. Lippincott, 1986.

16. Turner, J.W., and Cooper, R.R.: Anterior transfer of the tibialis posterior through the interosseous membrane. Clin. Orthop. *83*:241, 1972.

17. Sneider, M., and Balon, K.: Deformity of the foot following anterior transfer of the posterior tibial tendon and lengthening of the Achilles tendon for spastic equinovarus. Clin. Orthop. *125*:113, 1977.

18. Banks, H.H.: The foot and ankle in cerebral palsy. *In* Orthopaedic Aspects of Cerebral Palsy. Ed. R.L. Samilson. Philadelphia, J.B. Lippincott, 1976.

19. Hoffer, M.M., Barakat, G., and Koffman, M.: 10-year follow-up of split anterior tibial tendon transfer in cerebral palsied patients with spastic equinovarus deformity. J. Pediatr. Orthop. *5*:432, 1985.

20. Barenfed, P.A., Weseley, M.S., and Shea, J.M.: The congenital cavus foot. Clin. Orthop. *79*:119, 1971.

21. McBride, E.D.: A conservative operation for bunions. J. Bone Joint Surg. *10*:735, 1928.

22. Banks, H.H.: The foot and ankle in cerebral palsy. Clin. Dev. Med. *52/53*:195, 1975.

23. Perry, J., Antonelli, D., and Ford, W.: Analysis of knee joint forces during stance phase. J. Bone Joint Surg. *57A*:961, 1975.

24. Banks, H.H., and Green, W.T.: Correction of hamstring contracture in cerebral palsy. J. Bone Joint Surg. *40A*:1205, 1958.

25. Sharps, C.H., Clancy, M., and Steel, H.H.: A long-term retrospective study of proximal hamstring release for hamstring contracture in cerebral palsy. J. Pediatr. Orthop. *4*:443, 1984.

26. Hoffer, M.M.: Management of the hip in cerebral palsy. J. Bone Joint Surg. *68A*:629, 1986.

27. Hollinshead, W.H.: Functional Anatomy of the Limbs and Back. Philadelphia, W.B. Saunders, 1951.

28. Bleck, E.E.: Surgical management of spastic flexion deformities of the hip with special reference to iliopsoas recession. J. Bone Joint Surg. *53A*:1468, 1971.

29. Steel, H.H.: Gluteus medius and minimus insertion advancement for correction of internal rotation gait in spastic cerebral palsy. J. Bone Joint Surg. *62A*:919, 1980.

30. Samilson, R.L.: Dislocation and subluxation of the hip in cerebral palsy. J. Bone Joint Surg. *54A*:863, 1972.

31. Magilligan, D.J.: Calculations of the angle of anteversion by means of horizontal lateral roentgenography. J. Bone Joint Surg. *38A*:1231, 1956.

32. Ryder, C.T., and Crane, L.: Measuring femoral anteversion: the problem and a method. J. Bone Joint Surg. *35A*:321, 1953.

33. Szalay, E.A., et al.: Extension-abduction contracture of the spastic hip. J. Pediatr. Orthop. *6*:1, 1986.

34. Hoffer, M.M., Stein, G.A., Koffman, J., and Prietto, M.: Femoral varus-derotation osteotomy in spastic cerebral palsy. J. Bone Joint Surg. *67A*:1229, 1985.

35. Lonstein, J., and Beck, K.: Hip dislocation and subluxation in cerebral palsy. J. Pediatr. Orthop. *6*:521, 1986.

36. Baker, L.D., Dodelin, N.D., and Bassett, F.H.: Pathological changes in the hip in cerebral palsy: Incidence, pathogenesis, and treatment. J. Bone Joint Surg. *44A*:1131, 1962.

37. Sharrard, W.J.W.: The hip in cerebral palsy.

In Orthopaedic Aspects of Cerebral Palsy. Ed. R.L. Samilson, Philadelphia, J.B. Lippincott, 1975.

38. Drummond, D.S., Rogala, E.J., Cruess, R., and Moreau, M.: The paralytic hip and pelvic obliquity in cerebral palsy and myelomenigocele. AAOS Intr. Course Lect. *28:*7, 1979.

39. Letts, M., Shapiro, L., Mulder, K., and Klassen, O.: The windblown hip syndrome in total body cerebral palsy. J. Pediatr. Orthop. *4:*55, 1984.

40. Pritchett, J.W.: The untreated unstable hip in severe cerebral palsy. Clin. Orthop. *173:*169, 1983.

41. Moreau, M., Drummond, D.S., Rogala, E.J., and Ashworth, A.: Natural history of dislocated hip in spastic cerebral palsy. Dev. Med. Child Neurol. *21:*749, 1979.

42. Sherk, H.H., Pasquariello, P.D., and Doherty, J.: Hip dislocation in cerebral palsy: selection for treatment. Dev. Med. Child Neurol. *25:*738, 1983.

43. Cooperman, D.R., Bartucci, E., Dietrick, E., and Millar, E.A.: Hip dislocation in spastic cerebral palsy: long-term consequences. J. Pediatr. Orthop. *7:*268, 1987.

44. Reimers, J.: The stability of the hip in children. A radiological study of the results of muscle surgery in cerebral palsy. Acta Orthop. Scan. Suppl. *184:*1, 1980.

45. Honkom, J.A., et al.: Treatment of acquired hip subluxation in cerebral palsy. J. Pediatr. Orthop., *4:*48, 1984.

46. Wheeler, M.E., Weinstein S.L.: Adductor tenotomy-obturator neurectomy. J. Pediatr. Orthop. *4:*48, 1984.

47. Reimers, J., and Poulsen, S.: Adductor transfer versus tenotomy for stability of the hip in spastic cerebral palsy. J. Pediatr. Orthop., *4:*52, 1984.

48. Schultz, R.S., Chamberlain, S.E., and Stevens, P.M.: Radiographic comparison of adductor procedures in cerebral palsied hips. J. Pediatr. Orthop. *4:*741, 1984.

49. Silver, R.L., Rang, M., Chan, J., and de la Garza, J.: Adductor release in nonambulant children with cerebral palsy. J. Pediatr. Orthop., *5:*672, 1985.

50. Shapiro, D., Craig, C., and Zimbler, S.: Management of the unstable hip of patients with cerebral palsy. J. Pediatr. Orthop., *7:*493, 1987.

51. Craig, C.L., Sosnoff, F., Murray, S., and Zimbler, S.: Fixed hip abduction contracture in the cerebral palsy patient—Treatable and preventable deformity. J. Pediatr. Orthop. *7:*492, 1987.

52. Carr, C., and Gage, J.R.: The fate of the non-operated hip in cerebral palsy. J. Pediatr. Orthop. *7:*262, 1987.

53. Chiari, K.: Medial displacement osteotomy of the pelvis. Clin. Orthop. *98:*55, 1974.

54. Zuckerman, J., Staheli, L.T., and McLaughlin, J.F.: Acetabular augmentation for progressive hip subluxation in cerebral palsy. J. Pediatr. Orthop. *4:*436, 1984.

55. Staheli, L.T.: Slotted acetabular augmentation. J. Pediatr. Orthop. *1:*321, 1981.

56. Castle, M.E., and Schneider, C.: Proximal femoral resection-interpostion arthroplasty. J. Bone Joint Surg. *60:*1051, 1978.

57. Kalen, V., and Gamble, J.G.: Resection arthroplasty of the hip in paralytic dislocations. Dev. Med. Child Neurol. *26:*341, 1984.

58. Baxter, M.P., and D'Astons, J.L.: Proximal femoral resection-interposition arthroplasty: Salvage hip surgery for the severely disabled child with cerebral palsy. J. Pediatr. Orthop. *6:*681, 1986.

59. Root, L., Goss, J.R., and Mendes, J.: The treatment of the painful hip in cerebral palsy by total hip replacement of hip arthrodesis. J. Bone Joint Surg. *68A:*590, 1986.

60. Lonstein, J.E., and Akbarnia, B.A.: Operative treatment of spinal deformities in patients with cerebral palsy or mental retardation. J. Bone Joint Surg. *65A:*43, 1983.

61. Bleck, E.E.: Deformities of the spine and pelvis in cerebral palsy. *In* Orthopaedic Aspects of Cerebral Palsy. Ed. R.L. Samilson. Philadelphia, J.B. Lippincott, 1975.

62. Allen, B.L., and Ferguson, R.L.: L-Rod instrumentation for scoliosis in cerebral palsy. J. Pediatr. Orthop. *2:*87, 1982.

63. Sponseller, P.D., Whiffen, J.R., and Drummond, D.S.: Interspinous process segmental spinal instrumentation for scoliosis in cerebral palsy. J. Pediatr. Orthop. *6:*559, 1986.

64. Winter, R.B.: Spinal problems in pediatric orthopaedics. *In* Pediatric Orthopedics. 2nd Ed. Ed. W.W. Lovell and R.B. Winter. Philadelphia, J.B. Lippincott, 1986.

65. Drvaric, D.M., et al.: Gastroesophageal evaluation in totally involved cerebral palsy patients. J. Pediatr. Orthop. *7:*187, 1987.

66. Luque, E.R., Ed.: Segmental Spinal Instrumentation. Thorofare, N.J., C.B. Slack, 1984.

67. Denis, F., and Krach, L.: Spinal injuries in the growing person. *In* Pediatric Orthopaedics. 2nd Ed. Ed. W.W. Lovell and R.B. Winter. Philadelphia, J.B. Lippincott, 1986.

68. Brown, J.C., Swank, S.M., Matta, J., and Barras, D.M.: Late spinal deformity in quadriplegic children and adolescents. J. Pediatr. Orthop. *4:*456, 1984.

69. Mowery, C.A., Gelberman, R.H., and

Rhoades, C.E.: Upper extremity tendon transfers in cerebral palsy: Electromyographic and functional analysis. J. Pediatr. Orthop., *5*:69, 1985.

70. Hoffer, M.M.: Cerebral palsy. *In* Operative Hand Surgery. Ed. D.P. Green. New York, Churchill Livingstone, 1982.

71. Hoffer, M.M., Waters, R.L., and Garland, D.E.: Spastic dysfunction of the elbow. *In* The Elbow and Its Disorders. Ed. B.F. Morrey. Philadelphia, W.B. Saunders, 1985.

72. Green, W.T., and Banks, H.H.: Flexor carpi ulnaris transplant and its use in cerebral palsy. J. Bone Joint Surg. *44A*:1343, 1962.

73. Boyes, J.H.: Selection of a donor muscle for tendon transfers. Bull. Hosp. Jt. Dis. Orthop. Inst. *23*:1, 1962.

74. Tachdjian, M.O.: Pediatric Orthopedics. Philadelphia, W.B. Saunders, 1972.

75. Gelberman, R.: Cerebral palsy. *In* The Pediatric Upper Extremity. Ed. F.W. Bora, Jr. Philadelphia, W.B. Saunders, 1986.

76. Mital, M.A.: Lengthening of the elbow flexors in cerebral palsy. J. Bone Joint Surg. *61A*:515, 1979.

77. Braun, R.M.: Stroke rehabilitation. *In* Operative Hand Surgery. Ed. D.P. Green. New York, Churchill Livingstone, 1982.

78. Omer, G.E., and Capen, D.A.: Proximal row carpectomy with muscle transfers for spastic paralysis. J. Hand Surg. *1*:197, 1976.

79. Goldner, J.L.: The upper extremity in cerebral palsy. *In* Orthopaedic Aspects of Cerebral Palsy. Ed. R.L. Samilson. Philadelphia, J.B. Lippincott, 1975.

80. Braun, R.M.: Surgical treatment of the painful shoulder contracture in the stroke patient. J. Bone Joint Surg. *53A*:1307, 1971.

81. Mital, M.A., Garber, J.E., and Stinson, J.T.: Ectopic bone formation in children and adolescents with head injuries: its management. J. Pediatr. Orthop. *7*:83, 1987.

82. Hoffer, M.M., et al.: The orthopedic management of brain injured children. J. Bone Joint Surg. *53A*:567, 1971.

83. Roberts, J.B., and Pankratz, D.G.: The surgical treatment of heterotopic ossification of the elbow following long-term coma. J. Bone Joint Surg. *61A*:760, 1979.

14

CASE EXAMPLE: THE MANAGEMENT OF SPASTICITY AFTER TRAUMATIC BRAIN INJURY

MEL B. GLENN

Spasticity can be among the most disabling sequelae of traumatic brain injury (TBI). Effective treatment of spasticity can help maximize mobility and communication skills, improve ability to perform activities of daily living, aid prevention and remediation of contractures, promote hygiene and improved nursing care, and facilitate positioning and comfort.

Clinicians working with patients with TBI should be familiar with the fundamental principles of spasticity evaluation and management, and with the considerations that are specific to this population in particular.

GENERAL CONSIDERATIONS

As in other populations with disabilities related to central nervous system dysfunction, the clinician's first consideration before embarking on a course of treatment for spasticity should be whether or not the problem being evaluated is actually related to spasticity. This is particularly important when working with the patient with TBI because so many areas can potentially be injured with severe trauma. The differential diagnosis of spasticity was discussed in Chapter 1, and will not be treated in detail in this chapter. Rigidity, however, including cogwheel rigidity, dystonia, and primitive motor behaviors, are commonly seen in conjunction with spasticity, as well as in

isolation. Spontaneous "spasms," or nociceptive reflexes, are occasionally seen, although not with the frequency with which they occur after spinal cord injury. Gegenhalten, or motor negativism, another cause of increased resistance to passive stretch of muscle, can result from bilateral frontal lobe lesions,[1] and can be mistaken for spasticity. Deep tendon reflexes may be normal, however, and resistance does not depend on initial positioning. It increases markedly, however, if the velocity of movement is increased or if the patient is pressured to relax the extremity. Perhaps most notable is the quality of active opposition, which may cause the clinician to feel that the patient is resisting treatment. Each of these motor disorders may, at times, respond to some of the approaches used to manage spasticity. In addition, particular treatment approaches may be indicated for each of these disorders. The overlap in treatment approaches to these distinct but related motor problems has not been well explored, and specific guidelines are difficult to formulate.

When the clinician has confirmed that spasticity is contributing to motor dysfunction, contracture, or other disability, an initial concern should be whether a medical or physical condition is exacerbating the spasticity. Respiratory, urinary tract, and other infectious processes, fractures, heterotopic ossification, and decubitus ulcers are just a few of the common medical problems that occur in association with TBI. Painful conditions such as ingrown toenails can increase spasticity. The development of post-traumatic hydrocephalus or cerebral abscess can result in an increase in muscle tone by worsening the CNS lesion. Among the initial interventions, then, should be the treatment of medical illness or the removal of inciting physical factors, such as tight shoes or orthoses that are digging into the skin. Further treatment, however, does not necessarily have to be withheld while waiting for a medical condition to resolve. If spasticity is contributing to contracture formation, for instance, aggressive treatment can be initiated while a large decubitus ulcer heals over a period of many months. In fact, effective management of spasticity may aid in the healing of the ulcer when it results in pressure relief from the affected area.

Anxiety can also increase spasticity. This is particularly important in individual therapy sessions, where anxiety can be addressed by education, by active involvement of the patient in therapeutic exercise and other treatments, and by the use of relaxation techniques, such as counting or the use of imagery. Education of the patient, including instruction or explanation of the procedures being used in therapy, must take into account the patient's cognitve strengths and weaknesses. An explanation that is misunderstood can be worse than no explanation at all. On the other hand, some patients are comforted by the nonverbal communication that takes place, even if they are unable to understand the verbal content. Modalites that emphasize relaxation, such as gentle rocking and superficial heat, play a more prominent role with the anxious patient. A busy environment can increase anxiety in the distractible patient, and individual or small treatment rooms should be used, if available, in these instances.

Before considering a more specific treatment approach to spasticty in a patient with TBI, the clinicians working with the patient must do a functional evaluation of the problem at hand to determine the goals of treatment. Spasticity can cause difficulties with active motion, resulting in loss of function; or with passive motion, leading to functional loss, discomfort, or interference

with care provided by others (e.g., maintenance range of motion, hygiene, or skin care). Spasticity can contribute to the development of contractures, which, in turn, exacerbate these problems. Spasticty can also cause scoliosis and hip subluxation or dislocation, particularly in children.

THE COMATOSE OR EARLY UNRESPONSIVE PATIENT

The framing of the goals, as well as the choice of treatment, depends on the time since injury, the history of the motor problem to date, and the patient's prognosis for functional improvement. If the patient has only recently been injured, a good prognosis should usually be assumed even if the patient is comatose or in a vegetative state.[2,3] The treating team will want to do everything possible to prevent contractures that might later limit function or affect positioning. Passive range-of-motion exercises, physical modalites, and the application of orthotic devices are the focus of treatment at this time (Table 14–1).

Some controversy remains over the use of passive range-of-motion exercises in the patient at high risk for heterotopic ossification. Although the cause of heterotopic bone formation has not yet been determined, aggressive passive range of motion in the face of severe spasticity in an unresponsive patient may indeed be a contributing factor.[4,5] On the other hand, whether heterotopic ossification is developing or not, if the patient is not ranged, contracture will almost certainly result. The therapist, then, has the difficult task of finding a balance at which range of motion will be maintained as well as possible without

TABLE 14–1. TREATMENT OF THE EARLY UNRESPONSIVE PATIENT

Goals	Goals are unlimited
Conservative treatments	PROM, orthotics, modalities are focus of treatment
Medications	Avoid sedating medications
Nerve blocks	Use cautiously when contractures are developing
Surgical procedures	Avoid permanent destructive procedures

being overly aggressive in pursuit of that goal. This dilemma underscores the need for optimal management of spasticity, so that ranging does not traumatize the joint.

Destructive procedures are infrequently used in the early weeks and months after a severe TBI, but can be considered with caution when more conservative measures fail. Although nerve blocks with phenol are unlikely to adversely affect the recovery of strong, isolated contraction of muscle, they can cause functional deficits in patients who rely upon spasticity or primitve motor behaviors for function, and the practitioner will not be able to predict in advance who these patients will be. Nerve blocks with phenol are generally not permanent (see Chapter 11), however, and can be used cautiously if contracture is developing despite the use of more conservative approaches.[6] A more cautious way to proceed with nerve blocks is to do intermittent local anesthetic blocks to allow for full range of motion exercises or casting. Another conservative approach is the use of intramuscular alcohol wash, which has been reported to last for only 1 to 6 weeks, thus minimizing the danger of loss of function at a later date. The effects of alcohol on the injured central nervous system must be considered if the injury was recent,[7] for the alcohol may be absorbed to a substantial degree.

Concerns about the use of destructive procedures also apply to the patient whose pattern of spasticity is fluctuating. If an agonist is effectively treated with a nerve block, for instance, and the antagonist later becomes more spastic, contracture or functional loss may ensue in the direction opposite that over which there was initial concern. One might be able to predict such fluctuations based on a recent history of changing patterns, but early on, this may not be possible. If such a "reverse contracture" does occur, nerve blocks to the responsible muscle or muscle group usually result in an adequate balance about the affected joint.

Medications can also be problematic early after injury, when sedating side effects can mask recovery. This is particularly true of diazepam, although baclofen can be neurotoxic as well. Dantrolene is probably the least sedating of the three commonly used medications[8] (see Chapter 10). Clonidine can also be considered, although it also carries a risk of sedation. Concern about sedation can be minimized by the willingness of the physician to titrate drug effect carefully so that the lowest possible dose is used, and to withdraw medications periodically to determine whether recovery proceeds more rapidly without the drug.

As the time of injury becomes more remote, the clinician will become progressively better able to assess the prognosis of the patient, and should then formulate goals that are consistent with that prognosis. It is probably best to err on the side of optimism so that if the patient should be among those to improve toward the better end of the spectrum of possibilities, he or she will have been given the maximal opportunity to benefit from rehabilitation. Many clinicians still underestimate the potential of a severely head-injured patient. Many individuals continue to make gains for years after their injury if rehabilitation continues. It is a mistake to rely too heavily on statistical studies of recovery based on large groups of patients. A given individual may vary considerably from the average, and most studies look at broad measures of recovery that do not reflect gains in a limited but significant area of function. The best way to assess the potential for improvement in a given head-injured person is to look back on the course of recovery to date in the context of an aggressive rehabilitation program, allowing the possibility that a stepwise pattern of recovery may take place, with periodic plateaus. If a patient has never been given the opportunity to participate in such a program, it may be difficult to judge the potential. If behavioral dysfunction has limited a patient's ability to participate and benefit from rehabilitation, a well coordinated behavioral rehabilitation program must be pursued along with the physical and cognitive efforts.

THE PATIENT WITH LIMITED RECOVERY

If a patient's prognosis is felt to be for limited or no recovery, one should not, of course, abandon all treatment, but rather

TABLE 14–2. TREATMENT OF THE PATIENT
WITH LIMITED RECOVERY

Goals	Goals are limited (e.g., comfort, positioning, hygiene)
Conservative treatments	Use as needed, but supplement with more intensive treatments
Medications	Use more aggressively
Nerve blocks	Use more aggressively
Surgical procedures	Use more aggressively

modify one's goals accordingly (Table 14–2). The treating team is likely to have a few modest but significant goals, even for a patient who remains in PVS.[2] Despite the uncertainty as to what such an individual may or may not be experiencing, those who care for the patient should assume that he or she may be capable of feeling pain or discomfort. Although it is entirely possible that grimacing, groaning, and other expressions of discomfort, in a patient in PVS, are reflexive responses that do not reflect the internal experience of the person, there is truly no way of knowing, and a primitive experience of pain is certainly possible in such patients.[9] Therefore, proper positioning, skin care, and hygiene should be maintained whenever possible. Passive range-of-motion exercises are necessary regardless of whether spasticity is present or not, but treating the spasticity makes ranging easier, less painful to the patient, and less time-consuming. Physical modalities applied before ranging can be useful, but if long-term management of spasticity is needed, modalities are not a cost-effective way to proceed. Proper bed and wheelchair positioning are fundamental to the management of spasticity in the severely involved individual (see Chapter 6). Sidelying often reduces the postural influences on muscle tone, and the use of custom-made sidelyers can aid in positioning the extremities, trunk, head, and neck in a manner that will further break up primitive motor patterns that may be associated with increased tone. Patients who are difficult to position comfortably in a wheelchair because, for instance, they have a tendency toward extensor synergy in the lower extremities that causes them to slide out of the chair will benefit from a firm seat and back,

a well-applied seat belt, and a tilted seat and back that take advantage of gravity to hold them in flexion at the hips and knees. Custom-made head and neck positioners are valuable when spasticity forces the head and neck into flexion or rotation. Bivalved casts or other orthotic devices that immobilize a joint or hold it in a tone-inhibiting posture may decrease spasticity and maintain proper positioning (see Chapters 8 and 9).

If conservative measures fail to address the problem adequately, more aggressive approaches are indicated. For the patient in PVS or with limited function, the most important of these to consider are medications, nerve blocks, and radiofrequency rhizotomy. Each of these treatments has advantages and disadvantages that lend themselves to use in particular situations.

Medications, when they are effective, are likely to be so over long periods, and may allow one to avoid invasive procedures. Although the potential for sedation or impairment of other aspects of cognition that may mask recovery is particularly worrisome in this population, if a patient has been in PVS for an extensive period, the problem is not as significant, and only occasional withdrawal of the medication is necessary. No convincing clinical evidence has yet been published that one agent is more effective than another in treating spasticity in patients with TBI. In fact, few studies have even investigated the effects of these medications on spasticity after TBI (see Chapter 10). Because the loss of inihibitory influences in this population results from supraspinal lesions, pharmacologic inhibition could conceivably be useful at any level of the nervous system, or in the muscle itself, in the case of dantrolene sodium. Indeed, the subjective experience of most clinicians is that dantrolene, baclofen, and diazepam may all be effective in some patients with TBI, and that it is difficult to predict which patients are more likely to respond to one medication or the other. More than one medication can be used simultaneously if the effect is greater than with either alone.[10] Because of the concern for inducing sedation or other cognitive side effects, dantrolene is generally preferable to either baclofen or diazepam, even in patients with little potential for recovery. Diazepam and other benzodiazepines are usually reserved for situations in which other medications have not been effective, and frequently, in fact, should be withheld until more invasive procedures have been exhausted as well, particularly if follow-up is uncertain. Clonidine might be considered even before diazepam, although its use in spasticity has been limited.

Medications are often not effective enough to ameliorate problems caused by severe spasticity. Nerve blocks are often a good alternative, and offer the advantage of selectively treating the muscle or muscle group that is causing a specific problem (see Chapter 11). When motor branches are lysed, complications other than local pain or swelling for a short time after the procedure are unlikely. When comfort, positioning, and proper nursing care are addressed in a patient who has been unresponsive for a long period of time, potential loss of function is not a major concern. If mixed motor and sensory nerves are lysed, the possibility of causing dysesthesias in the distribution of the sensory nerve must be considered and weighed against the other alternatives. This is usually a temporary condition, and in situations where spasticity is unusually severe or in which motor branch blocks have been unsuccessful or short-lived, mixed nerve blocks can be beneficial, and do not frequently result in a significant problem. The duration of effect of nerve blocks varies, however, and repeat blocks may need to be performed periodically. This can be a limiting factor, particularly if the patient is in a locality where no physicians perform nerve blocks.

Although recurrent spasticity can also be a problem with radiofrequency rhizotomy (see Chapter 12), it is more likely to have a long-lasting effect, and is, therefore, a good procedure for patients with recurrent, long-standing lower extremity spasticity, with little potential for significant functional use. Uncertainty about the effect of this procedure on sensation limits its usefulness for those with good motor recovery, but this is not a major concern in the patient who will be relying on others for turning and positioning. Radiofrequency rhizotomy, a relatively selective procedure, carries little risk of causing undesired bowel, bladder, or sexual dysfunction. It does, however, require general anesthesia for the patient with intact sensation, and therefore respiratory compromise can be a relative contraindication. In addition, it is not generally performed in the cervical area, so that upper extremity spasticity cannot usually be addressed in this manner.

THE RECOVERING PATIENT

When the patient has been recovering function to the point where he or she is achieving some degree of independence in one or more areas, or might be expected to do so in the context of an active therapy program, the treatment approach will, of course, reflect the goals that the treatment team has set with the patient. The team must carefully delineate the patient's physical and cognitive skills, and choose therapeutic measures that are consistent with these skills and that are not likely to result in further impairment (Table 14–3).

Functionally oriented therapeutic exercise is the mainstay of treatment for most patients, and the effects of other interventions are therefore judged in this context. Physical modalities often play a crucial role as daily or intermittent adjuncts to this program (see Chapter 7). Although their effect on spasticity may be short-lived, this temporary benefit may provide a stepping stone for improved motor control that results in a more permanent diminution in spasticity. For instance, any modality that reduces spasticity and thereby gives the patient greater active control of a muscle group will, in turn, lead to greater inhibi-

TABLE 14–3. TREATMENT OF THE RECOVERING PATIENT

Goals	Establish goals appropriate to predicted level of recovery
Conservative treatments	Therapeutic exercise, etc. are focus of treatment
Medications	Cognition should be monitored when medications are used
Nerve blocks	Use selectively
Surgical procedures	Use selectively

tion of the spastic antagonist by that group. Electrical stimulation promotes motor control by both strengthening the agonist and inhibiting the antagonist simultaneously. Ultrasound can cause a significant reduction in spasticity in the patient with contracture, both by directly diminishing the sensitivity of the muscle spindle and by allowing for greater extensibility of the muscle-tendon unit before the spindle is excited. Electromyographic biofeedback can also promote greater motor control. Impairment of memory is not necessarily a contraindication to the use of biofeedback. If attentional function is good enough that the patient can consistently attend to the task, he or she can learn procedurally even if unable to recall the task from day to day.[11] Learning may, however, proceed more slowly. Likewise, Bailliet et al.[12] have demonstrated that patients with severe language problems can benefit from biofeedback through repeated nonverbal presentation. For the patient with TBI, who is likely to have some compromise of attentional and organizational skills, simple and colorful feedback displays are most likely to be successful.

The physician prescribing medications for the treatment of spasticity in the patient with TBI who has made significant recovery must be particularly alert to the potential for these medications to cause cognitive side effects. Diazepam usually causes significant sedation in these patients. In addition, even when obvious sedation is not present, various components of attentional function may be affected and memory impaired.[13,14] Some patients appear to accommodate to these adverse effects over time, although some studies suggest that attention may continue to be affected even with chronic administration.[14] Longer-acting benzodiazepines such as clorazepate may not affect attention and memory[15] and are therefore preferable to diazepam in the brain-injured patient. Nonetheless, they can still be quite sedating. Baclofen is not as consistently sedating, but one limited study documented a reduction in the ability to learn and remember new information in brain-injured patients taking baclofen.[16] Attentional capacity (the ability to hold onto information for brief periods) can also be af-

fected.[8] The functional consequences of these changes can be dramatic or can be minor enough to go unnoticed by most observers, yet still have an impact on performance in therapies and daily activities, or on the ability to interpret the environment and to communicate effectively. Cognitive dysfunction that is insignificant at one point may become more important as the patient improves in other areas.

The potential for such side effects diminishes the relative value of medications in the armamentarium of therapeutic interventions available to the treatment team. When medications are used, cognitive skills must be monitored. If available, specific neuropsychologic assessment of the functions most likely to be affected can be performed on and off the medication, in addition to evaluation of performance in therapy tasks and activities of daily living. As mentioned previously, dantrolene is probably less likely to cause cognitive dysfunction than are diazepam or baclofen, although it can be sedating to some individuals and has not been studied as extensively in this regard. Liver functions must be tested periodically when a patient is taking dantrolene. This is generally not a problem as long as the patient is an inpatient, but once he or she is discharged to the community, his or her reliability for follow-up must be considered. Clonidine can also be problematic in the patient who might refuse or forget medications because of the potential for rebound hypertension.

Because medications are often limited in their effect on spasticity and frequently cause untoward side effects in this population, nerve blocks play a particularly important role in the treatment of spasticity in the patient who is continuing to recover after TBI. Nerve blocks can be used as an adjunct to range-of-motion exercises, traction, positioning techniques, physical modalities, and serial casting for correction of contractures. Serial casting of knee flexion contractures can cause posterior subluxation of the tibia on the femur. Blocking the branches of the sciatic nerve that innervate spastic hamstring muscles can decrease the dorsally directed moment of force and reduce the risk of subluxation.

Nerve blocks can be useful for improving

function in a muscle or muscle group that is being opposed by a spastic antagonist or an atagonist that is co-contracting. For example, when spastic ankle plantarflexors prevent adequate dorsiflexion during ambulation, nerve blocks can result in improved clearance of the foot and a heel-toe gait. Blocking spastic finger flexors can allow functioning extensors to open the hand so that objects can be grasped and held. Voluntary use of the finger flexors themselves is generally not lost. At times, isolated voluntary use of a muscle actually improves after it is blocked. Function based entirely on spasticity or synergistic movements, particularly weak synergies, however, can be reduced or lost after nerve blocks (see Chapter 11).

Radiofrequency rhizotomies can be effective in patients who have active use of the lower extremites, but the possiblity of sensory loss is more worrisome in the more functional individual. Selective dorsal rhizotomy minimizes this risk, and is a promising procedure, although it has not been used extensively in patients with TBI. In addition, it is a major surgical endeavor requiring laminectomy. It is, however, likely to be more consistently long-lasting than nerve blocks with phenol, and entails less risk than cordotomy, which is rarely indicated given the available alternatives. Pumps for the intrathecal administration of morphine or baclofen have not been used extensively in brain-injured patients, and their potential for treating severe spasticity in this population is unknown (see Chapter 12).

Musculotendinous releases or lengthenings are indicated when contractures do not respond to more conservative approaches, and when spasticity is a significant contributing factor, the use of nerve blocks or medications can help to maintain the gains made surgically. Hamstring lengthening should be considered as an alternative to serial casting or traction when severe knee flexion contractures are present, particularly in patients with potential for weight bearing on the affected extremity, for whom subluxation of the tibia on the femur can limit that potential. Musculotendinous transfers can be useful in some instances to correct a muscular imbalance about a joint caused by spasticity or primitive motor behaviors (see Chapter 13). For example, the split lateral anterior tibialis tendon transfer (SPLATT) can correct forefoot inversion during ambulation.[17] Extreme care must be taken to carefully evaluate all the components of such a problem, as well as the patient's ability to successfully participate in a postoperative rehabilitation program, before proceeding with surgery. Nerve blocks or polyelectromyographic evaluation can be useful in determining which muscles are most actively contributing to the imbalance. A nerve block, however, does not precisely predict the results of a surgical procedure. More conservative approaches, such as nerve blocks with phenol or the use of orthotic devices, should be considered first. Tone-inhibiting orthoses can be particularly useful in controlling spasticity in a weight-bearing extremity, and, when working effectively, are not necessarily cumbersome to the patient (see Chapter 9).

CASE HISTORY

PART 1

An 18-year old woman has a severe TBI. At 1 month postinjury, she opens her eyes but does not communicate in any meaningful way. Both arms are held adducted and internally rotated at the shoulders, flexed at the elbows, the forearms pronated, and the wrists and fingers flexed. Resistance to passive stretch of muscle is moderately increased in the right upper extremity, but is severely increased in the left upper extremity, particularly when ranging in the direction opposite to the posturing. The "clasp-knife" phenomenon is present when most joints are stretched in either direction, and deep tendon reflexes are hyperactive throughout. Passive range of motion is close to normal at most joints, but despite daily ranging, significant contractures are developing at the left shoulder and elbow. Both lower extremities are held in an extensor pattern with intermittent posturing in flexion, and range of motion is within normal limits, though ranging is easier on the right. Incontinence of urine is managed with a Foley catheter, and feeding is accomplished by means of a gastrostomy tube. A tracheostomy tube has been removed, and the stoma is healing.

Clinical Approach. Although the patient's prognosis is completely uncertain at this time, considering the relative recency of the injury and the patient's youth, we must assume that this young woman could make an excellent recovery. Therefore our ultimate goals include the possibility of independence in mobility and activities of daily living at some time in the future, and, for the moment, we strive to maintain range of motion as close to normal as possible.

Any possible contributing medical factors must be evaluated. Her Foley catheter could be removed, and attempts made to sterilize her urine. If repeated urinary tract infections ensue, a urologic workup is indicated. Attempts should be made to regularize her bowel movements to prevent constipation. A follow-up CT scan of the head should be done at some point during the first few months after injury. X rays of the left elbow and shoulder, or a bone scan, as well as a serum alkaline phosphatase level, should be considered to determine if heterotopic ossification might be contributing to the contractures at these joints. In any event, this patient, having been unresponsive for one month, and having significant spasticity, is at high risk for the development of heterotopic ossification, and she should be given disodium etidronate for prophylaxis.

Daily or twice-daily ranging should, of course, continue, and the left upper extremity splinted and positioned appropriately. This might include an axillary wedge while the patient is in bed to hold the left shoulder in abduction and a bivalved cast, air splint, or other elbow extension orthosis. The cast could extend to the wrist and incorporate a cone for the fingers, or a separate wrist-finger control orthosis could be used. If a long-arm cast is used, it can be fabricated with the forearm in supination. Ultrasound could be used before ranging to try to increase the extensibility of the elbow flexors while decreasing spasticity. Ultrasound could be applied at the shoulder as well. If x ray or bone scan indicates that heterotopic ossification might be forming, ultrasound should probably be withheld because the deep heating might contribute to the inflammatory process.

If contractures continue to develop or cannot be substantially reduced, more aggressive approaches are indicated. Serial casting at the left elbow should be attempted first to maximize range of motion at this joint. If spasticity remains severe, it may be necessary to reduce the spasticity before attempting serial casting to prevent skin problems. Dantrolene sodium can be tried while liver function tests are monitored, and baclofen added if the effect is only partial. If dantrolene has no effect, it should be replaced with baclofen if the physician chooses to continue with pharmacologic intervention. If medications are successful, they should be withdrawn periodically to determine whether they are still needed and whether or not they are interfering with recovery.

Nerve blocks can be attempted if medications fail to control spasticity, or tried before medications to avoid cognitive side effects, particularly if the patient is beginning to show behavioral evidence of cerebral cortical function. If contractures are developing rapidly, the treating team may not be able to afford to wait to see whether a medication will be helpful. Because of the possibility of good recovery of upper extremity function that might include the use of spasticity or primitive motor behaviors for functional purposes, the treating physician might want to proceed first with alcohol washes. Careful assessment must be undertaken by the physician and the treating therapists to determine which muscles are responsible for the contracture formation. If alcohol washes are not successful, or as an alternative, nerve blocks with phenol can be used in these circumstances because the risk of loss of function resulting from the nerve block is quite small, and must be weighed against that resulting from contracture. One could also attempt intermittent local anesthetic nerve blocks before or instead of serial casting.

PART 2

Two months later, the patient has made substantial gains and is actively participating in therapies, although her performance tends to deteriorate after 15 to 20 minutes. She has moderately increased resistance to stretch of the left upper extremity muscle groups described above, and mildly increased tone in their antagonists. Tone is only mildly increased in the right upper extremity. Range of motion is within normal limits except for mild but stable left shoulder adduction, elbow flexion, and forearm pronation contractures. Although she has a tendency to flex her elbows, wrist, and fingers when stimulated, anxious, or excited, she can break the tendency with encouragement, and is using a communication board slowly but effectively with her right arm. Attentional, organizational, and memory problems are prominent.

When she is sitting in a reclining wheelchair, her hips tend to adduct and extend, while her knees extend, her ankles plantarflex, and her feet invert. In turn, her trunk extends, and she begins to slide out of the chair. When the patient is sat upright, she leans to the left with a right convex, flexible thoracolumbar scoliosis. Tone is increased in the left thoracic and lumbar paraspinal muscles and in the left quadratus lumborum, and is greater on the left in general.

Her Foley catheter has been removed, and her urine has been sterile. She has regular bowel movements every other day with the aid of a suppository, and her tracheostomy has healed. She is still fed by gastrostomy, but has begun a feeding program, and can do some limited self-feeding with her right arm.

Clinical Approach. The patient's course of recovery has been relatively rapid over the past two months, and therefore significant gains are likely in the coming months. Contractures are mild and stable, and spasticity management should now emphasize active function and positioning. Therapeutic exercise and positioning will be the major interventions in the coming months. She should be given a wheelchair with a good pelvic belt, a solid seat, and a back reclined just enough to hold her in the chair with her hips and knees at 90 degrees, and lateral supports and hip pads arranged to create a 3-point pressure system that will hold her scoliosis in check. Among the modalities, electromyographic biofeedback might be particularly useful, if she can participate, for teaching her to relax the antagonists that are interfering with upper extremity function. One must be particularly cautious with medications during this time of rapid recovery, particularly when there is already significant impairment of attentional function, with a limted ability to sustain attention over time. Medications, in particular dantrolene sodium, can be used, however, if the progress being made with motor control diminishes or if positioning problems continue despite optimal conservative intervention. Baclofen, too, can be tried if dantrolene is not successful or if hepatotoxicity occurs, although there is a greater likelihood of attentional problems. Rather than risk lost time from a temporary setback caused by a medication, the physician might want to consider whether nerve blocks could successfully address one or more focal problems caused by

spasticity. For instance, if active elbow extension were present, but limted by flexor tone, nerve blocks to the biceps and/or brachioradialis muscles would be likely to facilitate extension.

Before either medications or nerve blocks are tried, however, specific functional goals should be identified that would be likely to improve if spasticity were to diminish. Because the patient is substantially more functional with the right than with the more spastic left arm, it is not clear that reducing spasticity would lead to significant gains in, for example, self-feeding or use of the communication board. With minimal spasticity on the right side, the slowness that is seen is probably secondary to negative symptoms of the upper motor neuron syndrome, such as weakness, and perhaps to cognitve impairment, rather than to spasticity. On the other hand, should she improve to the point where a reduction in left arm spasticity could give her the ability to assist the right arm with feeding or washing, for example, it would be worthwhile to pursue these interventions.

Were the treatment team to conclude that right elbow flexor hypertonicity is indeed slowing her abilty to reach for objects or for the plate during feeding, nerve blocks could be considered. If, however, elbow flexion is part of a synergy pattern being used to bring utensils to the mouth during feeding, or if the strength here is tenuous, the physician might want to do marcaine blocks before using phenol.

Positioning problems could also be addressed with nerve blocks if more conservative approaches fail. If the patient continues to slide out of her wheelchair due to an extensor thrust, the left inferior gluteal nerve or its branches could be blocked to reduce gluteus maximus muscle tone. If the scoliosis were to develop a structural component, the nerve to the left quadratus lumborum could be blocked.

PART 3

At one year postinjury, the patient has made great strides and is left largely with a left hemiparesis. She is independent in all activities of daily living (ADLs) and is walking independently with a cane. Her major gait deviation is inversion at the left forefoot during swing phase, causing her to land on the lateral border of her foot.

Clinical Approach. Strengthening and electrical stimulation of the evertors of the foot might be the first approach to this problem. If inversion continued to be significant, a plastic inhibitory orthosis might be tried. If she could benefit from an orthosis that did not prevent dorsiflexion at the ankle, this would be ideal. If this were not entirely successful, nerve blocks could be considered. It would be important, however, to determine which muscles were responsible for causing the inversion. If a strong tibialis anterior were fighting a spastic gastrocnemius and soleus that were cocontracting during dorsiflexion, forceful inversion would result. Blocking the plantarflexors would then allow easier dorsiflexion, and inversion would be reduced. If a plantarflexion contracture were present, attempts should be made to reduce it before proceeding with nerve blocks. Blocking the tibialis anterior itself would be riskier, even it if were spastic, because dorsiflexion related to a synergy pattern might be weakened or endurance diminished. If it could be determined that the tibialis posterior was the major contributor to inversion, the branch of the tibial nerve to this muscle could be blocked. The tibialis posterior, however, helps to support the arch of the foot, and pes planus could result, requiring the use of an arch support or other orthotic device. Evaluation to determine the contributing muscles should be done by physical examination and observation, but also with polyelectromyography and/or local anesthetic block before using phenol, if the situation is not straightforward. Both nerve block and orthosis might be necessary to maximize the result.

Medications could be tried as well, but would be unlikely to resolve the problem without other interventions, and might cause some cognitive regression. If all else fails, and inversion continues to be a major problem during the next year, a surgical procedure such as SPLATT, with release of other contributing muscles, could be considered after careful evaluation.

REFERENCES

1. Plum, F., and Posner, J.B.: The Diagnosis of Stupor and Coma. 2nd Ed. Philadelphia, F.A. Davis, 1972.
2. Whyte, J., and Glenn, M.B.: The care and rehabilitation of the patient in a persistent vegetative state. J. Head Trauma Rehabil. 1(1):39, 1986.
3. Berrol, S.: Evolution and the persistent vegetative state. J. Head Trauma Rehabil. 1(1):7, 1986.
4. Spielman, G., Gennarelli, T.A., and Rogers, C.R.: Disodium etidronate: Its role in preventing heterotopic ossification in severe head injury. Arch. Phys. Med. Rehabil. 64:539, 1983.
5. Izumi, K.: Study of ectopic bone formation in experimental spinal cord injured rabbits. Paraplegia 21:351, 1983.
6. Garland, D.E., Lilling, M., and Keenan, M.A.: Percutaneous phenol blocks to motor points of spastic forearm muscles in head-injured adults. Arch. Phys. Med. Rehabil. 65:243, 1984.
7. Sparadeo, F.R., and Gill, D.: Effects of prior alcohol use on head injury recovery. J. Head Trauma Rehabil. 4(1):75, 1989.
8. Glenn, M.B., and Wroblewski, B.: Update on pharmacology: Antispasticity medications in the patient with traumatic brain injury. J. Head Trauma Rehabil. 1(2):71, 1986.
9. Doherty, D.L.: Can vegetative patients feel pain? (Abstract) Arch. Phys. Med. Rehabil. 69:721, 1988.
10. Griffith, E.R.: Spasticity. In Rehabilitation of the Head Injured Adult. Ed. M. Rosenthal, E.R. Griffith, M.R. Bond, and J.D. Miller. Philadelphia, F.A. Davis, 1983.
11. Nissen, M.J.: Neuropsychology of attention and memory. J. Head Trauma Rehabil. 1(3):13, 1986.
12. Balliet, R., Levy, B., and Blood, K.M.T.: Upper extremity sensory feedback therapy in chronic cerebrovascular accident patients with impaired expressive aphasia and auditory comprehension. Arch. Phys. Med. Rehabil. 67:304, 1986.
13. Romney, D.M., and Angus, W.R.: A brief review of the effects of diazepam on memory. Psychopharmacol. Bull. 20:313, 1984.
14. McLeod, D.R., Hoehn-Saric, R., Labib, A.S., and Greenblatt, D.J.: Six weeks of diazepam treatment in normal women: Effects on psychomotor performance and psychophysiology. J. Clin. Psychopharm. 8:83, 1988.
15. Scharf, M.B., Hirschowitz, J., Woods, M., and Scharf, S.: Lack of amnestic effects of clorazepate on geriatric recall. J. Clin. Psychiatry 46:518, 1985.
16. Sandy, K.R., and Gillman, M.H.: Baclofen-induced memory impairment. Clin. Neuropharmacol. 8:294, 1985.
17. Smith, C.W., and Leventhal, L.: Surgical treatment of lower extremity deformities in adult head-injured patients. J. Head Trauma Rehabil. 2(2):53, 1987.

15

CASE EXAMPLE: THE MANAGEMENT OF SPASTICITY IN MULTIPLE SCLEROSIS

DENNIS S. GORDAN

EVALUATION OF SPASTICITY IN MULTIPLE SCLEROSIS

Unlike the specific disease entities covered in other chapters, multiple sclerosis (MS) is a progressive degenerative disease. For that reason, the spasticity associated with MS and its management become worsening problems over time. Patient tolerance for intervention varies, not only with the psychologic changes brought on by the disease, but with the realization that treatments become increasingly complicated and improvement diminishes as the disease progresses. In spite of general progression of the disease, the importance of intervening with any particular symptom may wax and wane. Timing of treatment, therefore, is most important, both in initiating or increasing interventions and in decreasing or discontinuing them. A large therapeutic armamentarium is of little avail if the right weapon is not used at the appropriate time in the course of the disease. That course is comprised of the physical, cognitive, and emotional manifestations of the disease, all of which must be considered.

Only aspects of the disease germane to spasticity need be discussed here. Standard texts and references offer more complete coverage of pathology.[1,2]

NEUROPHYSIOLOGIC CONSIDERATIONS

The most important neurophysiologic aspect of MS is the distribution of its lesions throughout the central nervous system (CNS) (Fig. 15–1 and Table 15–1). Spasticity in MS may thus stem from involvement of multiple sites. In most patients it is futile to try to sort out which lesion is responsible for what element of the spasticity. There are, however, a few patterns of distribution in which an educated guess could be made:

1. Devic's syndrome. The plaques of MS are located in the optic nerve and spinal cord exclusively. These represent about 13% of American cases according to one autopsy study.[3]
2. Optic nerve, cerebral, and spinal cord distribution. This is the most common (66%) situation in the study cited above.
3. Cerebellar involvement. Extensive plaques are found in the cerebellum in only 39% of autopsied patients who also had extensive involvement of cerebrum.[1]

What these figures mean in terms of treatment has not been worked out, but they may help explain the occasional patient who is not showing the expected cognitive and emotional effects despite visual, spas-

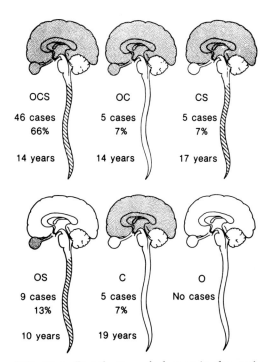

FIG. 15-1. Distribution of plaques in the optic nerves and tracts (O), cerebrum (C), and spinal cord (S) of 70 autopsied patients with multiple sclerosis in the U.S. (with permission from Ikuta, F., and Zimmerman, H.M.: Distribution of plaques in seventy autopsy cases of multiple sclerosis in the United States. Neurology (Minneapolis) 26 (6 Part 2):26–28, 1976).

tic, and autonomic effects of a Devic type involvement. Also, they lend support to the notion that what is frequently described as ataxia, in patients with evidence of other CNS involvement, is not truly cerebellar in origin.

Lesions can also be classed as active and inactive.[4] While finer classifications can be made, it can be expected that an active lesion, being inflammatory, will cause symptoms of two kinds: fixed, from the anatomic loss of myelin and secondary axonal effects, and variable, related to the physiologic effects of inflammation. Plaques are known to be edematous,[1] and this may cause some pressure effects on surrounding tissue. Inactive lesions are scars and cause only fixed symptoms by means of anatomic alterations. Thus, during an exacerbation, symptoms referable to an active lesion can wax as the lesion involves a greater volume of tissue directly in inflammation and indirectly through associated edema, and wane as the edema subsides and the lesion contracts.

EXACERBATING FACTORS

At any particular examination, a number of transient factors may influence the level of spasticity in a particular patient. One must distinguish between an increase resulting from a true exacerbation and one from an exacerbating factor. In the former the disease activity itself is increased and

TABLE 15-1. A COMPARISON OF THE OCCURRENCE OF EXTENSIVE MULTIPLE SCLEROSIS PLAQUES IN THE OPTIC NERVE, CEREBRUM, CEREBELLUM, OR SPINAL CORD, WITH SIMULTANEOUS OCCURRENCE OF PLAQUES IN SIX OTHER REGIONS OF THE CENTRAL NERVOUS SYSTEM*

Extensive Plaques	Optic Nerve	Cerebrum	Cerebellum	Midbrain	Pons	Medulla	Spinal Cord
Optic nerve		17 cases	9	10	15	12	22
32 cases		(53%)	(28%)	(31%)	(47%)	(38%)	(69%)
Cerebrum	19 cases		13	14	24	14	19
36 cases	(53%)		(36%)	(39%)	(67%)	(39%)	(53%)
Cerebellum	9 cases	13		8	12	7	8
13 cases	(69%)	(100%)		(62%)	(92%)	(54%)	(62%)
Spinal cord	22 cases	19	18	12	17	14	
37 cases	(59%)	(51%)	(22%)	(32%)	(46%)	(38%)	

*With permission from Ikuta, F., and Zimmerman, H.M.: Distribution of plaques in seventy autopsy cases of multiple sclerosis in the United States. Neurology (Minneapolis) 26 (6 Part 2):26–28, 1976.

evidence of new lesions may appear along with a worsening of previous symptoms; in the latter, something extrinsic (to the CNS, at least) causes a worsening of symptoms. In both cases, the worsened spasticity is best addressed indirectly when possible, through treatment of the exacerbation or exacerbating factor.

Exacerbations may be aborted with a course of ACTH or prednisone.[2]

Well-known exacerbating factors include heat, which is easily identified and removed (by avoidance, air conditioning, or antipyretics), stress, infections, and other illnesses, which may also be treatable. The relatively short term worsening under all these circumstances usually does not justify a permanent change in chronic antispasticity treatment. The patient, nevertheless, is likely to suffer a permanent worsening after an exacerbation, and possibly some worsening after an exacerbating factor is removed. It is on the basis of these chronic changes that long-term alterations in spasticity management should be made.

TEMPORAL FACTORS

Beside the above temporary variations in level of spasticity, MS patients show long-term changes related to the progressive nature of the disease. Stepwise with each exacerbation, or gradually in the case of progressive disease, any body part usually becomes more spastic. Additionally, with time, more body parts show evidence of spasticity. These lasting and worsening symptoms and signs are valid indications for alteration in antispasticity treatment. In the rare acute form, a patient's general condition may deteriorate so rapidly that medical control of spasticity becomes fraught with difficulty because the rapidly changing clinical picture may make assessment of therapeutic and side effects impossible.

In these patients, positioning and range of motion are important in preventing contractures. They may, however, not be enough. Under that circumstance, direct intervention with nerve or motor point blocks may be the only actions that are effective, uncomplicated by side effects, and nonsurgical. Even if contractures do supervene

(and this is true whatever the clinical course has been), there may still be a contribution to the worsening of those contractures by spasticity; for this reason antispasticity medications or blocks can help reduce the contractures. While no active functional goal may be realized, nursing care can be facilitated.

FUNCTIONAL CONSIDERATION

Spasticity is the great fooler of the uninitiated. On one hand, its mere presence may spark a desire to treat even though no benefit may be obtained. On the other, an examiner can easily be tricked into thinking that voluntary muscle strength is good to normal grade if the examination provokes a powerful spasm that does not really represent what the patient can muster at will.

It is necessary, therefore, to see the patient more than once, at different times of the day and during different stages of fatigue, to get a true picture of what spasticity means. Treatment aimed at reducing tone that is high during a single examination, but not functionally limiting, may itself become functionally limiting when the patient finds that he or she can no longer rely on it, e.g., knee extensor spasticity to hold himself or herself up.

Most frequently, spasticity is manifest in the lower extremities and causes problems with mobility. Tripping, an early symptom, may result from toe dragging, often the result of gastrocsoleus spasticity and/or weakness of the ankle dorsiflexors. Frequently, the ambulatory patient next experiences adductor spasticity with a "scissoring" gait resulting. Hip and knee flexor spasticity is often seen concurrently, so that the patient stands and walks in a minimally squatted position with knees together with some internal rotation of the hips, and, during weight bearing, the ankles may be passively dorsiflexed and everted. The forefoot is frequently pronated. Depending on the relative weakness and spasticity of the ankle motors, during the abortive "swing" phase, the ankle may be dorsiflexed or in spastic or passive plantarflexion. Despite the flexion at the hip and knee, the patient usually relies on some degree of knee extensor spasm to keep the leg from collapsing. Patients generally give up walking by the time they experience spontaneous hip and knee flexor spasms of major degree.

Other problems resulting from adductor spasticity are difficulty using the toilet, hygiene, and dressing.

In the upper extremities, spasticity, although evident during tone and reflex examination, shows up symptomatically first as clumsiness and progressive loss of control. While there may be true ataxia mixed with the spasticity, the flexed posturing and eventual contracture generally indicate the underlying tone alteration rather than cerebellar influences. These upper extremity effects impede writing, feeding, dressing, grooming, and other skills.

TREATMENT CONSIDERATION SPECIFIC TO MULTIPLE SCLEROSIS

The patient, physician, or therapist whose goal of treatment is improvement of function has only temporary success with MS. Improvement may simply reflect a remission rather than the effects of treatment, and can be washed away in the wave of the next exacerbation. Treatment goals should therefore be reasonable compromises between what is possible and what is tolerable.

Because the course is so protracted, most patients adapt gradually to each symptom or worsening of symptoms, to the point that such inconveniences are incorporated into their homeostatic patterns. A treatment that results in notable improvement in the clinicians' eyes may be rejected by the patient because it upsets an overall adaptive pattern. The upset may be as specific as an intolerable sensation of heaviness caused by a new brace, even though it produces a vast improvement in gait, or as general as an unacceptable decrease in dependency brought about by provision of training and equipment for self-care. Some adverse reactions certainly arise from simple changes in habits. In the cognitive and emotional effects of the disease, however, reasons for the patient's poor tolerance of change range from subtle to blatant.

Progression in the physical manifestations of the disease is accompanied by progression in the emotional and cognitive aspects. While the organic problems worsen, one may find increasingly oppositional behavior, or, on the other hand, patient cooperation with treatment may improve. The latter actually represents worsening because of decreased volition; the patient is now passive as a result of frontal lesions. Exactly what is seen, of course, depends on the locations of lesions.

SPECIFIC TREATMENT

Although many articles have been written about particular treatment for spasticity, few of lasting worth are specific to the spasticity of MS. Indeed, two recent compendia of treatment for MS[5,6] have relatively little to say on the subject.

Aside from the cautions regarding the use of dantrolene sodium, which have been discussed earlier in this text (Chapter 10), the only significant problem specific to MS patients relates to the potential for cognitive impairment. Because of the effects of MS on the brain, diazepam, which carries a greater propensity for sedation than baclofen[7] in any patient, is even more likely to produce that effect in these patients. Baclofen, however, when taken concurrently with antidepressants, has been reported to affect cognition in a more subtle manner than diazepam,[8] so those who know the patient well should observe closely for changes. In practice, the patient will probably determine which of these medications will be tolerated and therefore used.

Physicians and therapists, who see the results of medication treatment during only short periods of observation, are not usually able to cite enough good objective evidence of beneficial change to modify the patient's opinion when it conflicts with their own.

Leaving the area of systemic drug therapy, one may offer local nerve or muscle blocks either in place of, or in addition to, such medications. Because of the focality of MS lesions and the spasticity they produce, these focal treatments are often the best means available, and there are no problems with central effects.

For the advanced patient in whom other interventions have been unsuccessful, intrathecal phenol has been advocated to change a spastic paraplegia to a flaccid one. This treatment causes bowel, bladder, and sexual dysfunction, however,[9] and should rarely, if ever, be used. While radiofrequency rhizotomy may circumvent these problems, no studies of this procedure on MS patients could be found.

In the experience of the Boston Veterans Administration (VA) Outpatient Clinic, which follows a group of about 200 MS patients, long-term physical therapy, mainly range-of-motion exercises, provided on a regular basis, can keep spasticity and its complications under sufficient control that more aggressive approaches are often not necessary. The physicians involved have experience with similar patients in various settings, including academic and private practices. Only in the VA, however, is such maintenance therapy covered. VA patients suffer few of the deforming problems seen in MS patients in other situations. The key to success here is probably the enforced performance provided by regular sessions with a therapist.

The value of some physical therapy maneuvers aimed at tone reduction is open to question. These have often been advocated for cerebral palsy and stroke patients, and seem to have been extrapolated to MS patients. As indicated earlier, MS produces much of its spasticity by means of spinal cord lesions. The rationale for inhibiting primitive reflexes and putting the patient through the developmental sequence,[6] which is advocated for brain-damaged patients, makes almost no more sense, however, for the MS patient than it does for the spinal cord-injured patient. On the practical level, the variability of spasticity in MS through each day and over the course of the disease makes any objective assessment of the effects of these maneuvers nearly impossible. Most likely, any benefit seen relates to the general effects of exercise, stretching, and attention.

Air conditioning is a reasonable therapeutic modality for all the symptoms of MS, including spasticity, and may be covered by insurance on prescription from the physician. In this connection, it should be re-membered that although local heat may reduce spasticity, local cold is more effective, and in MS, if the core temperature is raised, all symptoms, including spasticity, worsen. If thermoregulation is impaired, it is particularly likely that general cooling will decrease symptoms.

Bracing or splinting can help prevent contractures and improve gait in MS, but they are not a permanent or stable solution as in nonprogressive diseases.

CASE HISTORY

PART 1

A 15-year-old right-handed boy has problems with coordination, which partially resolve without treatment. At age 18, he has an episode of blurry vison and diplopia, and 1 year later, a worsening of his clumsiness. At age 27, he develops weakness and spasticity in his left leg, as well as an intention tremor. The following year he begins to experience falls related to the onset of diplopia. At age 30, he develops visual field deficits and frequency of urination, and after a neurologic evaluation is undertaken, a diagnosis of multiple sclerosis is made. Several weeks later, he is admitted to the hospital for the treatment of severe debilitating anxiety and for evaluation and treatment of multiple sclerosis. At this time, he is independent in activities of daily living (ADLs), but is experiencing difficulty ambulating. He has a toe-heel gait on the left with intermittent recurvatum. There is moderate resistance to passive stretch of the left plantarflexors, and ankle clonus is present. Sensation is intact. Knee extensor tone is moderately increased as well. Voluntary strength is decreased throughout in the left leg, and he is unable to dorsiflex the ankle actively more than a few degrees. Left knee extensor strength is 4-/5. In the left arm, there are mild increases in tone in the wrist and finger flexors, and in the pronators. Deep tendon reflexes are increased throughout on the left. He has bilateral upper extremity intention tremors, worse on the right than on the left. Range of motion is slightly decreased in dorsiflexion at the left ankle, but can be brought to neutral.

Clinical Approach. At this point, the patient has problems with spasticity on the left, particularly in the leg, where it is causing him the most difficulty with function. Before this time, he has never received any rehabilitation. Therefore, it makes sense to begin with basics. He should be seen by physical and occupational therapists for range-of-motion exercises, including the teaching of self-ranging, which he can do on a daily basis, for strengthening exercises, which should be monitored closely to be sure that he does not begin to develop further weakness, and for ambulation training. Although he claims that he does not have any major limitations of upper extremity use, this should be evaluated carefully. He should be advised regarding the possible effects of overwork and heat on his disease process. A urologic evaluation should be undertaken because an untreated neurogenic bladder or a urinary tract infection might be an exacerbating factor. Skin integrity and bowel regulation should be investigated as well.

He probably can benefit from an ankle-foot orthosis (AFO) at this time. A metal AFO with double metal uprights and double-action ankle joint would be best from the point of view of knee control through control of the ankle once range of motion was increased into dorsiflexion, and would provide maximum flexibility in an ever-changing neurologic situation. The heel, however, might tend to pop out of the shoe unless a high-top were used. This problem might be better managed with a plastic AFO that captured the heel, and cosmesis would be improved.

If his hypertonicity cannot be adequately controlled with the above interventions, or if there appears to be a possibility of eventually eliminating the AFO, functional electrical stimulation to the dorsiflexors during gait or biofeedback might assist him in gaining further control of his ankle dorsiflexion. A medication could be added as well, and baclofen would probably be the first-line drug to use in a patient with MS. In patients with MS, in whom cognitive impairment is common, changes in mental status should be watched for. If baclofen does not prove beneficial, dantrolene sodium might be tried next, but increased weakness might be problematic, and liver function tests would have to be monitored. Diazepam could also be tried, but problems with memory and attention might be expected to worsen with this drug. On the other hand, diazepam might also help the patient to control his anxiety, and if it is psychiatrically felt to be indicated, could have a beneficial effect on spasticity as well. If it is found that left upper extremity hypertonia is interfering with function in some way, these interventions might be beneficial here as well.

One must be cautious about using nerve blocks in a patient with multiple sclerosis, although they should not automatically be eliminated as a possible alternative in a patient such as this, should other approaches fail to adequately control the spasticity that is causing the patient problems. This patient appears to have a progressive form of multiple sclerosis rather than a disease process characterized by exacerbations and remissions. This significantly diminishes the possibility that a nerve block with phenol, for instance to the plantarflexors of the ankle, would provide some benefit while the patient is more impaired, only to cause him problems when his spasticity diminishes because of neurologic improvement. He has never received any medical treatment for multiple sclerosis, however, and if such treatment is undertaken at this time, some response might be seen. More worrisome in this situation is the chance that he might suffer a further neurologic insult that would, for example, result in further weakening of his left quadriceps. In this case, his knee extension might be aided by some spasticity of the plantarflexors by increasing the extension moment at the knee. One would have to wait for the nerve block to lose its effect, which could take months or years. An AFO, on the other hand, could simply be adjusted to provide slightly more plantarflexion, and a medication could be discontinued.

PART 2

At age 33, the patient is admitted to the hospital confused and disoriented following a fall in the bathtub, where he was found unconscious. A workup yields a diagnosis of toxic encephalopathy secondary to administration of diazepam, baclofen, and whiskey. After detoxification, he is unable to walk or transfer, but has relatively good use of his arms. He has greater weakness and spasticity on the left than he had 3 years previously, and cannot actively dorsiflex his left ankle to greater than 30 degrees from neutral. When he attempts to walk, weight bearing on the left produces a painful extensor hypertonus of the entire leg, with ankle plantarflexion and inversion and knee and hip extension that cannot be broken voluntarily.

When the hip and knee are flexed, however, he is able, with difficulty, to extend them actively. There is some mild weakness and spasticity in the right leg as well. Sensation is decreased on the left also.

Clinical Approach. Medications no longer appear to be a viable alternative in this patient. Diazepam and baclofen have combined with alcohol to result in a toxic encephalopathy, and the likelihood of ongoing alcohol abuse precludes the use of dantrolene sodium as well because of the possibility of hepatotoxicity and unreliable follow-up. He has just had a fall and intercurrent illness, however, and with an intensive inpatient program including the interventions discussed in Part 1, he might once again be able to walk and transfer independently, perhaps with the use of Lofstrand crutches. Nerve blocks still might be considered, but the relative contraindications discussed in Part 1 must still be taken seriously.

PART 3

Six years later, at age 39, he is able to walk a few steps using Lofstrand crutches and a metal AFO with a double action ankle joint and a lateral T-strap on the left, but otherwise relies on a power wheelchair for most community ambulation, and takes a manual wheelchair with him if he is going somewhere by car. Physical examination is similar to that seen on the previous admission, but now there are significant left arm weakness and spasticity as well, and right arm ataxia has worsened. His ankle tends to plantarflex and invert within the AFO when he is walking.

Clinical Approach. At this time, nerve blocks in the left leg probably offer the greatest likelihood of improvement in the patient's gait, and there appears to be less likelihood that they would eventually cause a problem because any further neurologic deterioration will probably leave him unable to walk in any event. Because there is an increase in both flexor and extensor tone, however, and because he is probably relying to a large extent on extensor tone to support his left leg, any nerve blocks done with phenol should be preceded by a local anesthetic block followed by observation of his ambulation and transfer skills while the block is still in effect. The nerve blocks with phenol should probably be done at the level of the motor nerves and titrated carefully. Branches of the tibial nerve to the plantarflexors should certainly be blocked first if a block with a local anesthetic shows no loss of his ability to maintain his knee in extension during weight bearing. If knee flexor tone begins to predominate while the local anesthetic block of the tibial nerve is still in effect, further blocking of the branches of the sciatic nerve to the hamstring muscles could be performed to see if this could offset the imbalance created. Nerve blocks with phenol could then be cautiously undertaken, perhaps over several sessions so that careful titration can be done.

REFERENCES

1. Vinken, P.J., and Bruyn, G.W. (eds.): Handbook of Clinical Neurology. Vol. 9. Multiple Sclerosis and Other Demyelinating Diseases. New York, American Elsevier, 1970.
2. McFarlin, D.E., and McFarland, H.F.: Multiple sclerosis. N. Engl. J. Med. 307:1183–1188 and 1246–1251, 1982.
3. Ikuta, F., and Zimmerman, H.M.: Distribution of plaques in seventy autopsy cases of multiple sclerosis in the United States. Neurology (Minneapolis) 26(6 PT 2):26–28, 1976.
4. Adams, C.W.M.: The progression of the lesion in multiple sclerosis. Neurology (Minneapolis) 26(6 PT 2):33–34, 1976.
5. De Loya, A., Arndt, J., and Schapiro, R.T.: Spasticity. *In* Symptom Management in Multiple Sclerosis. Ed. R.T. Schapiro. New York, Demos, 1987.
6. Maloney, F.P., Burkes, J.S., and Ringel, S.P. (eds.): Interdisciplinary Rehabilitation of Multiple Sclerosis and Neuromuscular disorders. Philadelphia, J.B. Lippincott, 1985.
7. Young, RR., and Delwaide, P.F.: Drug therapy—Spasticity. N. Engl. J. Med. 304:28–33, 96–99, 1981.
8. Sandyk, R., and Gillman, M.A.: Baclofen-induced memory impairment. Clin. Neuropharmacol. 8(3):294–295, 1985.
9. Browne, R.A., and Catton, D.V.: The use of intrathecal phenol for muscle spasms in multiple sclerosis. Can. Anaesth. Soc. J. 22:208–218, 1975.

INDEX

Page numbers in *italics* indicate figures; those followed by t indicate tables.

313